Interventional Cardiology

FUNDAMENTAL AND CLINICAL CARDIOLOGY

Editor-in-Chief
Samuel Z. Goldhaber, M.D.
*Harvard Medical School
and Brigham and Women's Hospital
Boston, Massachusetts*

Associate Editor, Europe
Henri Bounameaux, M.D.
*University Hospital of Geneva
Geneva, Switzerland*

ADDITIONAL VOLUMES IN PREPARATION

Interventional Cardiology

New Techniques and Strategies for Diagnosis and Treatment

edited by

Christopher J. White
Health Care International Medical Center
Glasgow, Scotland

Stephen R. Ramee
Ochsner Medical Institutions
New Orleans, Louisiana

Marcel Dekker, Inc.   New York • Basel • Hong Kong

Library of Congress Cataloging-in-Publication Data

Interventional cardiology : new techniques and strategies for diagnosis and treatment /
edited by Christopher J. White, Stephen R. Ramee.
    p. cm. — (Fundamental and clinical cardiology ; 25)
    Includes bibliographical references and index.
    ISBN 0-8247-9415-X (alk. paper)
    1. Coronary heart disease—Surgery. 2. Coronary heart disease—Diagnosis.   3.
Thrombolytic therapy. I. White, Christopher J. II. Ramee, Stephen R. III. Series:
Fundamental and clinical cardiology ; v. 25.
    [DNLM: 1. Coronary Disease—therapy. 2. Angioplasty—method. 3.
Technology, Medical.   4. Heart Catheterization—methods.   5. Cardiovascular
Diseases—diagnosis.   W1 FU538TD v. 25 1995 / WG 30 I6444 1995]
    RD598.I546   1995
    617.4'12—dc20
    DNLM/DLC
    for Library of Congress   94-44825
                                                         CIP

The publisher offers discounts on this book when ordered in bulk quantities. For
more information, write to Special Sales/Professional Marketing at the address below.

This book is printed on acid-free paper.

Marcel Dekker, Inc.
270 Madison Avenue, New York, New York   10016

Current printing (last digit):
10 9 8 7 6 5 4 3 2 1

PRINTED IN THE UNITED STATES OF AMERICA

Series Introduction

Marcel Dekker, Inc., has focused on the development of various series of beautifully produced books in different branches of medicine. These series have facilitated the integration of rapidly advancing information for both the clinical specialist and the researcher.

My goal as editor of the Fundamental and Clinical Cardiology series is to assemble the talents of world-renowned authorities to discuss virtually every area of cardiovascular medicine. In the current monograph, *Interventional Cardiology: New Techniques and Strategies for Diagnosis and Treatment*, Drs. White and Ramee have edited a much needed and timely book. Future contributions to this series will include books on molecular biology, other aspects of interventional cardiology, and clinical management of such problems as coronary artery disease and ventricular arrhythmias.

Samuel Z. Goldhaber

Preface

The clinical practice of interventional cardiology does not advance in a predictable linear fashion; rather, progress is made by trial and error with major changes in the approach to some lesion subsets occurring relatively "overnight" while others continue to be managed much the same way that they were more than 10 years ago. Changes in our practice may be characterized as "device-dependent," relating to new technologies, or "strategy-dependent," implying that conventional equipment or drugs are employed in a novel algorithm to solve difficult clinical problems.

The difficulty in summarizing the state of the art in interventional cardiology is that the technology and treatment strategies are constantly evolving and changing to optimize the percutaneous treatment of coronary artery disease. It is our intention to provide the reader with clinically relevant information regarding new devices and the most current percutaneous treatment strategies being employed in this rapidly changing and challenging field of medicine.

To this end, we have invited experienced clinical investigators to contribute their expertise and insights regarding the clinical application of new devices and treatment strategies used to approach difficult clinical problems in interventional cardiology. The book has three main divisions. Part I is devoted to advanced diagnostic methods, including intravascular ultrasound, coronary angioscopy, intracoronary Doppler flow measurements, quantitative coronary angiography, and assessment of myocardial viability. These chapters will familiarize the reader with these new techniques and highlight their potential clinical application in everyday practice.

Part II focuses on new therapeutic technologies, and includes chapters on laser angioplasty, intracoronary stents, and the application of atherectomy techniques. These new devices are being employed to expand the current indications for angioplasty, to improve the primary success rates of angioplasty (particularly in unfavorable lesion subsets), and, finally, in an attempt to improve the long-term outcomes of patients treated percutaneously.

Part III illustrates advanced therapeutic strategies for handling difficult clinical problems such as treatment of occluded saphenous vein grafts, adjunctive use of thrombolysis with angioplasty, percutaneous treatment of vein graft stenoses, techniques for supported angioplasty, strategies for reducing restenosis, and, finally, an overview of techniques used for salvaging a failed angioplasty. These chapters give the reader insight into some of the innovative techniques and strategies employed by experienced clinical investigators to solve some of the most challenging problems facing the interventional cardiologist.

We are grateful to the many authors who have contributed to this work. Without their willing sacrifice this book would not have been possible. We also would like to thank Mr. James O'Meara for his talented assistance with medical illustrations. Finally, we are deeply grateful for the thoughtful assistance and expertise of our medical editor, Ms. Angela Lorio, whose sharp eye and critical reading of the manuscript improved the clarity of our writing.

Christopher J. White
Stephen R. Ramee

Contents

Contributors

Alaa E. Abdelmeguid, M.D., Ph.D. Assistant Professor, Division of Cardiology, Brooklyn Veterans Affairs Medical Center, Brooklyn, New York

Jorge Cheirif, M.D. Director of Echocardiography, Department of Cardiology, Ochsner Medical Institutions, New Orleans, Louisiana

Tyrone J. Collins, M.D. Director, Interventional Cardiology, Section of Cardiology, Ochsner Medical Institutions, New Orleans, Louisiana

Lawrence Deckelbaum, M.D. Director, Cardiac Catheterization Laboratory, West Haven Veterans Affairs Medical Center, and Associate Professor, Department of Internal Medicine (Cardiology), Yale University School of Medicine, New Haven, Connecticut

Peter J. Fitzgerald, M.D., Ph.D. Assistant Professor, Department of Cardiovascular Medicine, Stanford University Medical School, Stanford, California

Michael S. Flynn, M.D. St. Louis University Health Sciences Center, St. Louis, Missouri

Guy F. Friedrich, M.D.   Staff Cardiologist, Department of Invasive Cardiology, Innsbruck Medical School, Innsbruck, Austria

Joseph R. Hartmann, M.D.   Director, Department of Cardiology, Good Samaritan Hospital, Downer's Grove, Illinois

Dirk Hausmann, M.D.   Department of Cardiology, Hannover Medical School, Hannover, Germany

David R. Holmes, Jr., M.D.   Mayo Clinic and Mayo Foundation, Rochester, Minnesota

Morton J. Kern, M.D.   Professor of Medicine, Director, J.G. Mudd Cardiac Catheterization Laboratory, Department of Internal Medicine/Cardiology, St. Louis University Health Sciences Center, St. Louis, Missouri

Richard E. Kuntz, M.D., M.Sc.   Assistant Professor of Medicine, Harvard Medical School, and Interventional Cardiology Section, Beth Israel Hospital, Boston, Massachusetts

John R. Laird, M.D.   Director, Cardiac Catheterization Laboratories, Director, Interventional Cardiology, Division of Cardiology, Walter Reed Army Medical Center, Washington, DC

E. Magnus Ohman, M.D.   Associate Professor, Department of Medicine, Division of Cardiology, Duke University Medical Center, Durham, North Carolina

Jeffrey J. Popma, M.D.   Director, Angiographic Core Laboratory, Washington Hospital Center, Washington, DC

Stephen R. Ramee, M.D.   Director, Cardiac Catheterization Laboratory, Section of Cardiology, Ochsner Medical Institutions, New Orleans, Louisiana

Robert S. Schwartz, M.D.   Associate Professor, Division of Cardiovascular Diseases, Mayo Clinic and Mayo Foundation, Rochester, Minnesota

Christopher J. White, M.D.   Director, Invasive Cardiology, Health Care International Medical Center, Glasgow, Scotland

Patrick L. Whitlow, M.D.   Director, Interventional Cardiology, Department of Cardiology, The Cleveland Clinic Foundation, Cleveland, Ohio

John S. Wilson, M.D.   Cardiology Fellow, Duke University Medical Center, Durham, North Carolina

Dale C. Wortham, M.D.   Chief, Division of Cardiology, Walter Reed Army Medical Center, Washington, DC

Paul G. Yock, M.D.   Associate Professor, Division of Cardiovascular Medicine, Stanford University Medical School, Stanford, California

1

Intravascular Ultrasound Imaging

Peter J. Fitzgerald and Paul G. Yock
Stanford University Medical School, Stanford, California

Dirk Hausmann
Hannover Medical School, Hannover, Germany

Guy F. Friedrich
Innsbruck Medical School, Innsbruck, Austria

I. INTRODUCTION

In the past 5 years there have been considerable technical advances in intravascular ultrasound and a building experience among interventionalists in the clinical use of imaging. Because of its ability to visualize beneath the luminal surface, ultrasound is generating new insights into the effect of plaque morphology and composition on the various catheter-based therapies. With preprocedural ultrasound imaging, it is becoming possible to predict the results of a particular intervention, offering the potential for developing strategies of lesion-targeted therapy based on certain plaque characteristics. This chapter will describe the design of ultrasound catheters, discuss image interpretation, outline the results of clinical trials using imaging during interventions, and explore the potential use of tissue characterization to predict plaque types.

II. CATHETER DESIGN

There are two basic designs of stand-alone imaging catheters—mechanical and solid state. Mechanical systems develop images either by rotating a mirror that directs the ultrasound beam orthogonal to the axial direction of the catheter or by directly rotating the transducer (1). The delivery systems allowing mechanical imaging catheters to be introduced over standard coronary guidewires are eccentric, with the imaging core offset from the guidewire. Thus the guidewire appears in the image as a raylike artifact. In the mirror construction, the effective path length is increased, so near-field distortion is consumed within the cathether. Thus the beam exiting the catheter is well behaved and can be focused. The major advantage of the mechanical catheter is enhanced image quality due to larger dynamic range and improved resolution. Transducer frequencies for coronary applications are in the range of 20–30 MHz. The current size of mechanical coronary ultrasound catheters ranges from 2.9–4.3 French.

The solid-state catheter is equipped with 64 transducer elements located circumferentially around the catheter, and is the only truly coaxial over-the-wire configuration (2). Images are obtained by the recruitment of signals to produce an electronically reconstructed cross section. Solid-state catheters are advantageous in that no guidewire artifact is present in the image, there are no moving parts, and the possibility of manipulating the beam electronically allows focusing at different depths. Current clinical solid-state catheters operate between 20 and 25 MHz and are sized between 3.5 and 5.5 French.

Each of these catheter designs come prepared in sterile packaging and is connected to a central processing unit. This "ultrasound cart" is slightly smaller than a commercially available echocardiographic scanner. Both mechanical and solid-state designs integrate easily into diagnostic and/or interventional procedures, typically adding approximately an extra 10–15 min to the overall case time. At this point in time, all catheter-based imaging devices are constructed for single use only. In this country a single catheter is being used for each human study; careful flushing and handling at the end of the procedure allows for multiple uses in animal or in vitro studies.

The current size of ultrasound imaging catheters allows preprocedural imaging to be accomplished in a significant number of cases — perhaps 70–80%. Since the ultrasound beam is directed orthogonal to the catheter, intralesional imaging is accomplished only by crossing the lesion. Distal lesions or lesions located in severely tortuous vessels are often difficult to negotiate with the current size imaging catheters. Passage of the imaging device into critically stenotic lesions may mechanically "dotter" the lesion but, in general, few clinical sequelae have resulted. The most common side effect has been vessel and target lesion spasm — estimated to occur in approximately 1–3% of the cases. This spasm typically responds favorably to nitroglycerin (3). A recent case report illustrated a "snow-plow" effect of an imaging device in a right coronary artery. Following ultrasound catheter instrumentation alone, the severity of the lesion was reduced by nearly 50% (4). In our experience, nearly all lesions selected for directional atherectomy are "pre-imaged" successfully, whereas in small, diffusely diseased lesions targeted for angioplasty or rotational atherectomy, imaging requires initial dilation.

III. IMAGE INTERPRETATION

A. Acoustic Properties

In muscular vessels such as the coronary arteries the different layers of the vessel wall can be defined due to their unique acoustic properties. The medial layer consists primarily of smooth muscle cells with little elastin and collagen. With high-frequency ultrasound, imaging of this layer results in the appearance of an "echo lucent" band. On the other hand, the intima and adventitia contain large amounts of collagen and elastin which produce a brighter ultrasound signal. Thus, the typical coronary artery imaged in the catheterization laboratory has a three-layered appearance (Fig. 1) (5,6). In advanced disease, the medial layer is invaded by plaque, resulting in a loss of clear medial layer identification (7). To overcome this, it is useful to move the catheter back and forth to adjacent vessel areas in order to identify the adventitial layer which often has a different appearance than advanced plaque. This also helps to obtain a relative measure of the vessel size.

B. Plaque Composition

One of the major advantages of intravascular ultrasound is the ability to assess plaque composition. The discrimination among calcification, dense

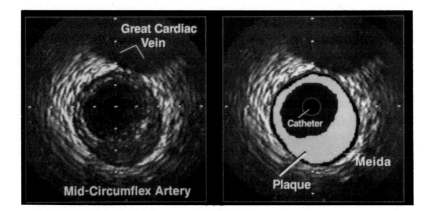

Figure 1   Two views of the ultrasound image from mid-circumflex artery using a 2.9 French catheter-imaging device. The catheter is the dark circle central to the vessel lumen and plaque is observed in the 3–7 o'clock region, as labeled on the right panel image.

fibrous tissue, and soft plaque is possible. Calcified plaques are represented by highly reflective echoes with intense shadowing, and acoustic reverberations. Reverberations are generated because the ultrasound signal completely reflects off the calcium, returns back to the catheter, reflects back off the catheter, and so forth. This oscillation of the signal produces equally spaced "ghost" signals in the far field behind the calcium. Because of shadowing and reverberation, it is often difficult to estimate the vessel boundary beyond the calcium. Dense fibrous tissue is also bright but without intense shadowing. In fact, signal drop-out is usually observed in the far field because of attenuation by the plaque, but reverberations are usually absent. Soft plaque is defined as a relatively homogeneous appearing plaque without significant attenuation or shadowing (Fig. 2). At present, imaging alone cannot reliably distinguish lipid pools within plaque or uniformly discriminate soft plaque from other entities such as thrombus.

C. Plaque Encroachment

Angiography provides a contrast silhouette reflecting the encroachment by plaque into the lumen. Pathological studies and in vivo intravascular ultrasound studies have shown that plaque encroachment into the lumen represents a relatively late stage of atherogenesis. Glagov (8) demonstrated that vessel remodeling occurs early in the process of plaque development. As plaque accumulates, the overall size of the vessel stretches to accommodate this growth and thus minimize lumen encroachment (Fig. 3). Thus

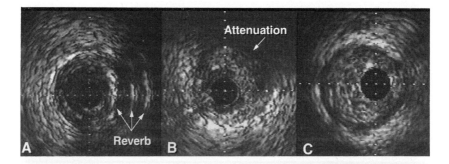

Figure 2 Common plaque types observed during routine intracoronary ultrasound imaging. In panel A, calcium is seen to generate a bright signal with shadowing and signal reverberations (arrows). Although fibrous tissue (panel B) can result in a bright signal return, it generally does not produce reverberations, but rather a progressive signal attenuation (arrow). Panel C shows soft plaque in which the signal passes with enough power to reflect adventitial signals.

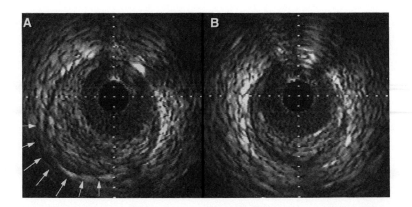

Figure 3 These two coronary images were obtained in a circumflex vessel between the first and second marginal branches. They are separated by approximately 5 mm with no branching vessels between. The relatively increased accumulation of plaque (arrows, panel A) is associated with vessel stretch so as to keep the lumen approximately the same as the vessel segment with less plaque (panel B).

it is not surprising that ultrasound imaging within the coronary arteries detects disease before it becomes visible on the angiogram.

D. Morphological Data in Transplant Patients

Experience with intracoronary ultrasound in heart transplant patients has demonstrated the utility of this imaging modality in the early detection of atherosclerosis (9). The most common cause of death among transplant patients beyond 2 years is coronary disease. Detecting disease in angiographically "silent" vessels may be important to the medical management of these patients. Figure 4 shows the presence of eccentric plaque accumulation in the proximal LAD by ultrasound in this angiographically normal vessel. Sequential studies with ultrasound may provide information regarding the risk factors associated with plaque acceleration and potential strategies to arrest or regress plaque in this patient population.

Intravascular ultrasound in heart transplant recipients has shown that coronary vasodilation after nitroglycerin is reduced in the presence of angiographically silent coronary vasculopathy (10); this implies that morphological changes detected only by ultrasound imaging are already associated with functional impairment. In our laboratory we have shown that coronary segments with plaque involvement of the entire vessel circumference (concentric disease) show more impairment than those with only partial involvement of the circumference (eccentric disease) (Fig. 5) (11). Thus endothelium-

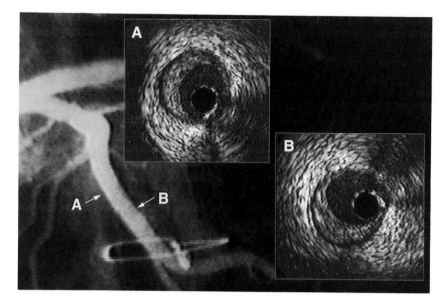

Figure 4 Images from an angiographically normal proximal coronary vessel. At points A and B, a moderate amount of eccentric plaque is noted by ultrasound in corresponding insets.

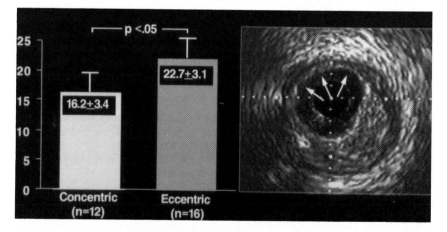

Figure 5 The bar graph on the left illustrates the difference in vasodilatory response to nitroglycerin for mild lesions that are primarily distributed as concentric or eccentric. Ultrasound image on the right shows the normal vessel arc (arrows) in an eccentric lesion probably responsible for vasoreactivity.

independent vasoreactivity in transplant recipients is related to the extent of disease-free wall.

IV. ULTRASOUND VERSUS ANGIOGRAPHY

In order to systematically determine the differences between intravascular ultrasound and angiography in the assessment of lesion morphology, a multi-center prospective trial was organized among centers with experience in catheter ultrasound. Phase I of the GUIDE trial (Guidance by Ultrasound Imaging for Decision Endpoints) has recently closed enrollment and some of the initial findings have been presented in preliminary form. Phase I of the trial concentrated on the assessment of PTCA and directional coronary atherectomy (DCA) with respect to (1) comparison of ultrasound and angiography (12); and (2) change in approach of therapy based on information from the ultrasound images (13). A total of 152 patients from 12 centers were enrolled in this phase of the study resulting in the analysis of 158 lesions (112 angioplasty, 46 atherectomy).

In the GUIDE study, the morphological findings by angiography and ultrasound were found to be significantly discrepant: (1) lesions were classified

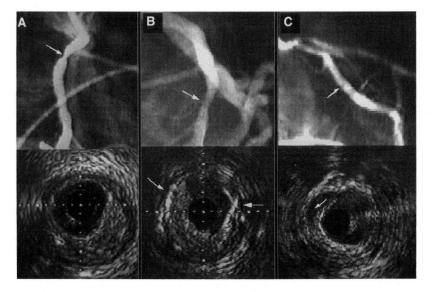

Figure 6 Comparison between angiographic lesion characteristics (top) and ultrasound lesion characteristics (bottom). The presence of (A) calcium, (B) dissection, and (C) lesion shape is often underestimated by angiography.

as eccentric in 77% with ultrasound whereas the lesions were judged eccentric in 33% by angiogram; (2) target lesion calcification was observed in 62% of cases by ultrasound but in only 35% of cases by angiogram; (3) following angioplasty, ultrasound evidence for plaque fracture/dissection was seen in 49% of lesions compared to 22% of lesions by conventional angiography. Figure 6 illustrates morphological differences between angiography and ultrasound in two sample coronary target lesions. This discrepancy between ultrasound and angiography highlights the need for outcome studies to determine if the ultrasound information regarding plaque and vessel wall morphology is important for the choice and guidance of interventional strategies.

V. INTRAVASCULAR ULTRASOUND AND INTERVENTIONS

A. Angioplasty

Up to this point the greatest experience with intravascular ultrasound imaging has been in the context of coronary angioplasty (14–16). Many interventional laboratories now routinely use intravascular ultrasound imaging to guide balloon size and inflation pressures, and to assess final neolumen dimensions following angiographically successful angioplasty. The two most important ultrasound characteristics in the target segment during angioplasty are the presence of preprocedural lesion calcium and residual plaque burden.

Lesion response to balloon angioplasty is strongly influenced by the presence of calcium deposits within plaque and vessel wall. When calcium is present within plaque, high shear forces during balloon inflation occur at the junction between the stiff calcium and soft plaque increasing the likelihood for fracture at that point (17). Figure 7 shows sequential ultrasound images from a coronary artery in which an elongated dissection tracks a rim of calcium following angioplasty. The exact relationship between clinical outcome and ultrasound evidence of dissection is still controversial. Tenaglia and coworker (18) found that an increase in clinical events occurred in patients with resultant dissection seen by ultrasound after angioplasty. On the other hand, data from the GUIDE trial suggest that a greater acute lumen gain is observed with less recoil in lesions that fracture in association with calcium deposits (19). In addition, the depth of dissection may be controlled in lesions with deep calcium as the rigidity of this substance blocks the direction of fracture from penetrating deep into the medial or adventitial layers. Multicenter trials are now underway to determine if the presence of these dissections influences patient outcome at 6 months follow-up (20,21).

Besides the ability to detect fractures, ultrasound provides a more accurate measurement of true lumen dimensions following angioplasty than angio-

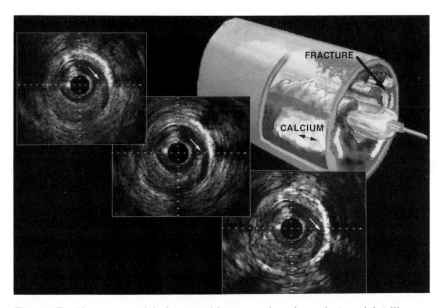

Figure 7 Three sequential ultrasound images and a schematic (top right) illustrating the association of dissection and calcium following balloon dilation.

graphy alone. Ultrasound has shown that filling defects seen with angiography following PTCA cover a wide spectrum of actual morphological features including thrombus, ulceration, and the presence of one or many dissected "tissue arms" extending into the neolumen. When these irregular lumens are quantitated by ultrasound, it is not surprising that they do not match measurements made by quantitative angiography—i.e., lesions that appear well dilated by angiography often appear to have small cross-sectional area by ultrasound. In addition to neolumen irregularities, overestimation by angiography may also be related to vessel remodeling in the target lesion (22) as well as a significant plaque accumulation in the angiographically "normal" reference segment (23).

Successful long-term outcome following angioplasty is the net result of increase in lumen size immediately after the procedure less the amount of intimal response over the ensuing months (late lumen loss). Acute lumen gain is both device-dependent and lesion-dependent (24). However, late lumen loss may be less dependent upon the device and more a function of the response of a particular lesion to the magnitude of vessel trauma (25–27). In both human and animal studies, the magnitude and depth of vessel wall injury directly correlates to the amount of reactive smooth muscle cell migration and proliferation (28,29). In the GUIDE trial, acute lumen gain by PTCA was measured by computing the ratio of the post-procedure neoluminal area to the nominal balloon cross-sectional area (neolumen:balloon ratio, NLBR). The higher the NLBR the larger the acute lumen expansion in response to balloon dilation; the lower the index, the greater the degree of recoil. In 112 lesions following successful angioplasty, the single most important ultrasound feature predicting high NLBR was the presence of plaque dissection. In dissected lesions, the NLBR was 0.90 ± 0.08 which was significantly higher ($p < 0.001$) than lesions in which dissection did not occur following balloon dilation (0.74 ± 0.11).

Lesion shape (eccentricity) also played a role in acute lumen gain following angioplasty. Results from the GUIDE study demonstrate that concentric lesions that dissect during balloon dilation achieve a higher NLBR (0.82 ± 0.07) compared to concentric lesions that do not dissect during angioplasty (0.69 ± 0.06). In addition, there was a trend (which did not achieve statistical significance) for eccentric lesions that dissected following angioplasty to have a higher acute lumen expansion (NLBR = 0.73) compared with eccentric lesions that did not tear (NLBR = 0.68).

One of the critical issues for the future of intravascular ultrasound during intervention is the demonstration of clear clinical benefit derived from the imaging information. Several ongoing studies are addressing this issue at an initial level by analyzing the impact that ultrasound imaging has on operator decision making during the course of an intervention. In phase I of the GUIDE trial, a time-based data form recorded operator's therapeutic decisions before ultrasound imaging (based on angiography alone) and then after analysis of the ultrasound images. Significant changes in therapeutic approach occurred in 43% of cases overall. For PTCA these changes included additional inflations with the same balloon, change to a larger balloon, and change in primary approach to directional atherectomy.

B. Directional Atherectomy

Intravascular ultrasound imaging provides a tomographic "slice" of the lesion and vessel wall. This is a particularly attractive format in the context of DCA. The ability to identify areas of greatest plaque accumulation by ultrasound provides useful information for the longitudinal positioning and rotational orientation of the atherectomy cuts.

Scanning the target segment with ultrasound prior to DCA can establish a cutting sequence for optimizing the tissue retrieval. Figure 8 demonstrates ultrasound images pre- and post-DCA in a mid-LAD artery. Directing the cutting sequence toward maximal plaque buildup can be accomplished by identifying a reference branch close to or within the lesion (30). The branch can then be used to spatially relate the ultrasound and angiographic information. In the rotational coronary atherectomy (RCA), for example, the

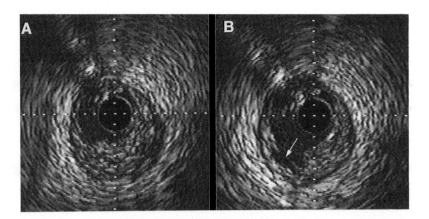

Figure 8 Ultrasound images showing plaque configuration (A) prior to and (B) following DCA. Following two cuts by the device (B), the ultrasound image shows evidence of tissue excision directly into the largest accumulation of plaque (4–7 o'clock). The arrow denotes plaque excision.

emergence of the right ventricular (RV) marginal branch close to the target lesion is selected. The ultrasound catheter is placed at the ostium of the branch vessel and the position of the ostium on the image (referenced to quadrants) is noted. The catheter is then advanced into the lesion and the orientation of the maximal plaque buildup is noted. By this method the rotational orientation of the deepest area of plaque accumulation relative to the ostium of the marginal branch can be determined (Fig. 9). The imaging catheter is then withdrawn, and the atherectomy device is inserted and rotated into the position known to have the major accumulation of plaque with respect to the emergence of the marginal branch. If the plaque is truly eccentric, with normal vessels on the other side of the wall, the cuts are made only in this area. Repeat imaging can be performed while the housing of the cutting device is being emptied. The images of the remaining plaque in the target segment help indicate where to perform further cuts, and whether to perform them at a higher pressure or with a larger device.

Despite excellent primary success rates with directional coronary atherectomy, tissue excision appears to account for only 30–50% of the contribution to acute lumen gain (31). Several intravascular ultrasound studies have shown that significant amounts of plaque remain within the target lesion following angiographically successful atherectomy (32–34). With intravascular ultrasound, residual stenosis within the lesion can be computed directly from the vessel and lumen areas. This is in contrast to the indirect measurement of stenosis by angiography in which the diameter of proximal reference

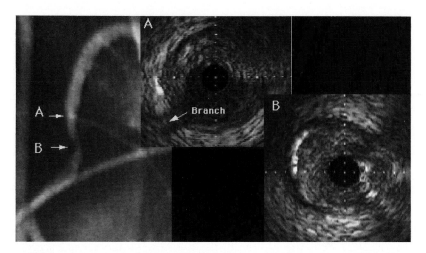

Figure 9 Angiogram (left) and corresponding ultrasound images (A,B) showing the spatial relationship to the emergence of the RV marginal branch and maximal plaque accumulation. Although the angiogram may be interpreted to show plaque on the opposite side of the branch vessel, ultrasound demonstrates plaque to be on the same side as the branching vessel.

segments is compared to the lesion diameter. From the atherectomy arm of the GUIDE trial, the average residual area stenosis was 48% by ultrasound following angiographically successful atherectomy.

Effective tissue debulking with directional atherectomy also depends upon the exact nature of plaque composition within the target lesion. Calcification within a target segment is a known negative risk factor for directional atherectomy (35,36). Recent experience with intravascular ultrasound imaging suggests that fluoroscopy is a relatively insensitive technique for identifying calcium within plaque. Localized calcium deposits are detected by ultrasound in 50–70% of lesions approached with therapeutic catheters, compared to 20–30% by fluoroscopy (37,38). Intravascular ultrasound has also demonstrated that the pattern of calcium within lesions is highly variable. Calcium may be principally deposited at the luminal surface of a plaque in a superficial rim, or can occur deeper within the plaque substance.

Our early experience with directional atherectomy and intravascular ultrasound suggested that the distribution of calcium had a significant impact on the mechanical response of the plaque to the device (39). Recently, a more detailed study was conducted at three centers with experience in directional atherectomy as well as intravascular imaging (40). The objective of this study was to investigate the relationship between the pattern of lesion calcification seen by ultrasound and excised tissue. A total of 51 patients (54 lesions) with successful atherectomy procedures and good quality images were included in the study. Target lesions were classified into three groups with respect to the pattern of calcification detected by ultrasound: (1) soft plaque with no calcium detected (NC); (2) superficial calcium (SC) located at the intimal border; and (3) deep calcium (DP) deposited within the intimal layer near the medial border (Fig. 10). The presence of calcium was identified within the lesion by intravascular ultrasound in 31/54 cases (57%), but detected in only 12/54 cases (22%) by fluoroscopy. Analysis of tissue weights as a function of lesion composition revealed that significantly less ($p < 0.001$) tissue was extracted from SC lesions (10.3 ± 6.8 mg) versus DC (19.7 ± 6.9 mg) or NC (22.5 ± 7.2 mg) lesions. From this and other similar studies (41) it is becoming increasingly apparent that certain lesions have a variable response to directional atherectomy and identification of these lesion subgroups may be important for optimal debulking. Intravascular ultrasound imaging offers critical information about the plaque and vessel wall characteristics that may provide rationale for specific lesion therapy.

C. Rotational Atherectomy

Rotational atherectomy is a relatively new second generation device that ablates plaque by a high-speed rotational burr. Experience is rapidly growing with this device in complex lesions that are difficult to approach by conventional balloon or directional atherectomy (42). These lesions include long, diffusely diseased vessel segments with large amounts of plaque containing dense fibrous tissue and/or calcification. Since this debulking device pulverizes plaque in a coaxial manner, intravascular ultrasound may be a useful format to determine true vessel cross-sectional dimensions and assess

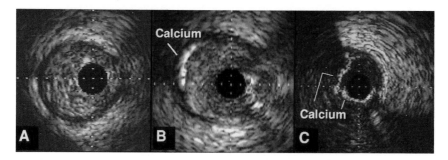

Figure 10 Panel A shows mildly eccentric soft plaque. Panel B shows calcium deep to the plaque (10–11 o'clock), and panel C shows calcium to be at the intimal border with resultant far-field shadowing (superficial calcium).

the extent and distribution of calcium. Superficial calcium may inhibit efficient debulking with directional atherectomy whereas this type of lesion may be optimal for rotational atherectomy, since it preferentially ablates inelastic tissue components.

In addition to the utility of ultrasound to identify fibrocalcific deposits, its ability to penetrate beyond plaque may be useful in choosing burr sizes. In our early experience in collaboration with Stertzer and colleagues (Seton Medical Center), decisions about burr sizes have been influenced by imaging in over 50% of the cases. Figure 11 demonstrates coronary imaging during rotational atherectomy. Mintz et al. (43) have proposed the strategy of initial debulking of a lesion by rotational ablation to change the biomechanics of the plaque, followed by balloon dilation. In their experience, pulverizing superficial plaque with rotational atherectomy achieves the largest luminal diameter following adjunctive angioplasty.

As previously discussed, balloon angioplasty in the presence of calcification can predispose to target lesion dissection. In our small series of 27 coronary

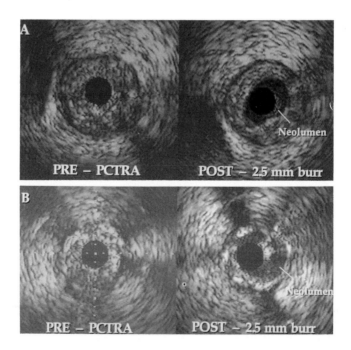

Figure 11 Ultrasound morphology before (left) and after (right) rotational atherectomy for soft plaque (panel A) and calcific plaque (panel B). Note that the soft plaque lesion appears elliptical whereas the calcified lesion is smooth and circular (images obtained in conjunction with Simon Stertzer, MD, at Seton Medical Center).

lesions using rotational atherectomy with adjunct angioplasty, we encountered 5 of 27 with evidence of dissection by ultrasound. Additionally, plaque composition may be related to vessel spasm following rotational ablation. We have observed that intralesional spasm occurs less frequently (9%) in calcified lesions compared to lesions primarily composed of soft plaque (42%). However, a higher rate of distal vessel spasm (29%) was observed in lesions with calcium compared to lesions with soft plaque (16%) (Fig. 12). Immediately following Rotablator® with a 2.5-mm burr, the overall vessel size is reduced by 26%. One possible explanation for this observation may be that intralesional calcium acts as a rigid scaffolding in the lesions and prevents local spasm. However, ablation in calcified lesions may lead to increased embolic debris that could initiate spasm in noncalcified distal vessel segments. As experience with this device increases, intravascular ultrasound will provide an ideal imaging strategy to determine the primary mechanism of this ablation therapy and study vessel response of a particular lesion type to this device.

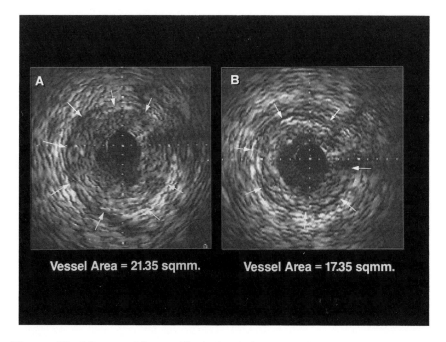

Figure 12 Ultrasound images illustrating lesion spasm in soft plaque following rotational atherectomy. The image on the right (panel B) was acquired 15 min following successful debulking with a 2.5-mm burr shown on the left (panel A) (images obtained in conjunction with Simon Stertzer, MD, at Seton Medical Center).

D. Stents

Intracoronary stents have already shown promise in the setting of rescue angioplasty and favorable results are accumulating for coronary stent placement as primary treatment in certain lesions (44,45). Since metallic struts are highly visible with intravascular ultrasound, several institutions are proposing that ultrasound is a useful tool for initially sizing the target lesions and assessing proper stent deployment (46,47). The relationship between struts to the vessel wall can be tracked throughout the body of a deployed stent thus providing an accurate method to assess tissue opposition (Fig. 13). The situation of incomplete strut opposition is of particular concern due to the increased likelihood of stent thrombosis. Stents with incomplete deployment expose a larger amount of metallic surface to local flow disturbances, providing a nidus from thrombus formation. Identification of stents not fully expanded in the coronary artery may encourage operators to redilate the stent and establish complete strut apposition. The results of several ongoing studies using intravascular ultrasound as a guidance for stent deployment will soon become available.

VI. TISSUE CHARACTERIZATION

Acute ischemic syndromes are most commonly precipitated when mild-to-moderate coronary lesions become disruptively transferred into complete occlusions (48,49). Spontaneous plaque fracture usually involves fissuring of the fibrous cap with intraplaque hemorrhage and lumen thrombosis.

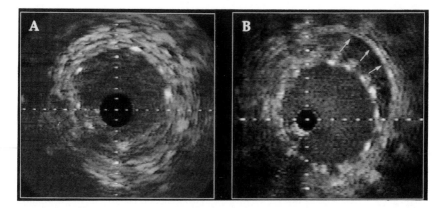

Figure 13 Ultrasound images following successful deployment of an intravascular stent. Panel A shows good strut-to-tissue apposition whereas Panel B illustrates incomplete strut-to-tissue apposition (arrows).

Plaque at high risk for such fissuring generally has a large core of lipid substance roofed by a structurally weak fibrous cap (50). Spontaneous rupture and thrombosis result in unstable angina or myocardial infarction. The majority of the lesions undergoing this process have an underlying stenosis of < 50% (46). Thus, angiographic detection of the "culprit" lesions may be difficult. Intravascular ultrasound imaging has already shown its value in detecting lesions that are angiographically silent (9). The next issue is whether ultrasound can discriminate lesions at high risk for rupture on the basis of different underlying histological composition and morphology. Figure 14 demonstrates two coronary lesions of approximately 40–50% stenosis from two different patients in which the eccentric lesions have different ultrasound characteristics. On the left, a band of highly reflective echoes seems to represent a "cap" over a hypoechoic area deep within the plaque body. This may represent plaque with a fibrous intimal layer roofing an underlying lipid collection. The image on the right shows a more homogeneous speckle pattern throughout the plaque which may represent primarily fibrous tissue.

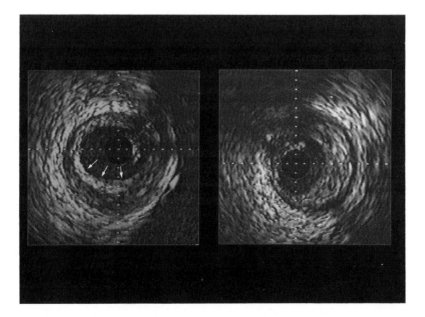

Figure 14   Ultrasound images from two individuals with mild plaque accumulation. The plaque speckle on the left panel is somewhat heterogeneous, possibly representing a fibrous cap with soft plaque below. The plaque speckle on the right panel is more uniform, possibly a result of less fatty tissue and more fibrous components.

A. Homogeneous Versus Inhomogeneous Tissue

With respect to high-frequency ultrasound, atherosclerotic plaque can be categorized into two broad groups. Plaque such as fibrous (de novo), intimal hyperplasia (restenosis), and thrombus can be modeled as homogeneous architecture, whereas fibrofatty plaque can be modeled as inhomogeneous. Each of these plaque types will theoretically scatter ultrasound uniquely. Wave mechanics applied to this model predict that the statistical fluctuation of the radio-frequency (RF) backscatter, as reflected in the morphology of the probability distribution function (PDF), will be different for homogeneous and inhomogeneous tissue samples (51). Thus, by computing the PDF from each isolated backscatter region representing plaque types or thrombus, a registry of signal morphologies can be accumulated for correlation with histological classification. For example, the cellular infrastructure of noncalcific plaque and thrombus is slightly different. Soft plaque is made up of an amorphous collection of lipid substances, fibrosis, cholesterol clefts, and a variable amount of collagen and elastin. A thrombus, on the other hand, consists of a fairly organized layering of fibrous strands packed with a dense collection of red blood cells. Although these subtleties cannot be appreciated by their gray-scale appearance on the ultrasound image, preliminary results from our laboratory, using a 30-MHz transducer, show significant differences in the shape of the PDF [as measured by mean to standard deviation ratio (MSR)] of the RF backscattered signal from these two tissue types (52).

B. Calcific Versus Fibrous Tissue

Perhaps an even more clinically useful application would be the ability to distinguish plaques composed of high lipid content from those composed mainly of fibrous tissue (i.e., plaques more susceptible for spontaneous rupture from less aggressive plaques). Preliminary work in this area has been attempted using higher frequencies than conventional imaging but still lower than those employed with intravascular ultrasound. Picano (53) showed that fibrous and fibrofatty plaque can be distinguished by evaluating the backscatter coefficient in vitro over the 7- to 11-MHz frequency range. Barzilai (54), using a 10-MHz transducer, was able to demonstrate delineation between calcific and fibrous disease in atherosclerotic sites. A major shortcoming of both studies with respect to intravascular ultrasound imaging is that, while possible in the aorta, these parameters will have insufficient resolution for small vessels such as coronary arteries. A recent study by Wickline and coworkers (55) demonstrated that higher frequency (50-MHz) tissue characterization techniques can discriminate between fibrous and fibrofatty disease in vitro based on integrated backscatter analysis. Ongoing studies in

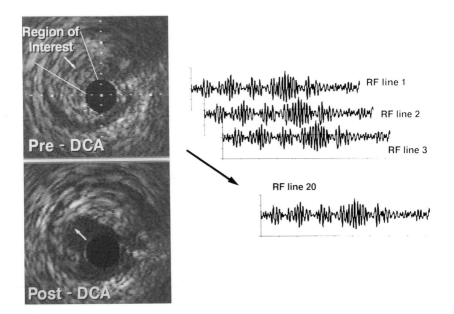

Figure 15 Ultrasound images from a human pre- and postatherectomy (left) and real-time acquisition of RF signals from the excised tissue (right).

our laboratory are investigating the spatial and temporal RF analysis in coronary plaques and comparing these signal characteristics to tissue specimens retrieved during directional atherectomy procedures (Fig. 15). This provides a convenient technique to compare signal characteristics with histology in order to test algorithms for plaque characterization.

VII. CONCLUSIONS

Rapid technological advances are occurring in the field of intravascular ultrasound imaging. The imaging catheters are now less than 1 mm in diameter and provide excellent image quality in lesions approached by conventional balloon angioplasty equipment. The clinical information provided by intravascular ultrasound has stimulated many new developments for imaging applications and generated enthusiasm for clinical decision making on a routine basis in the interventional laboratory. Single-center and multicenter trials using intravascular ultrasound for the choice of a particular interventional strategy and/or endpoint analysis of a given device are maturing and the results will begin to become available this year. In particular, optimizing the deployment of intracoronary stents with ultrasound and the effect it may have on anticoagulation protocols is an exciting evolving application for this imaging modality. Finally, advanced processing of the backscattered ultrasound signal may permit an in vivo bioassay of plaque and contribute to the understanding of plaque progression, regression, and response to various forms of therapy.

REFERENCES

1. Yock PG, Fitzgerald PJ, Linker DT, Angelsen BAJ. Two dimensional intravascular ultrasound: Technical development and initial clinical experience. J Am Soc Echo 1989;2:296–304.
2. Nissen SE, Grines CL, Gurley JC, et al. Application of a new-phased-array ultrasound imaging catheter in the assessment of vascular dimensions: In vivo comparison to cineangiography. Circulation 1990;81:660–666.
3. The SAFETY of ICUS Study Group. Safety of intracoronary ultrasound: A multicenter, multicatheter registry in 1837 patients (abstr.). Circulation 1993;88: I-2690.
4. Liebson PR, Klein LW. Intravascular ultrasound in coronary atherosclerosis: A new approach to clinical assessment. Am Heart J 1992;123:1643–1659.
5. Gussenhoven EJ, Essed CE, Lancee CT, et al. Arterial wall characteristics determined by intravascular ultrasound imaging: An in vitro study. J Am Coll Cardiol 1989;14:947–952.
6. Fitzgerald PJ, St. Goar FG, Connolly AJ, et al. Intravascular ultrasound imaging of coronary arteries: Is three layers the norm? Circulation 1992;86:154–158.
7. Isner JM, Donaldson RF, Fortin AH, Tischler A, Clarke RH. Attenuation of the media of coronary arteries in advanced atherosclerosis. Am J Cardiol 1986; 58:937–939.
8. Glagov S, Weisenberg E, Hiratzka LF, et al. Delineation of the extent of coronary atherosclerosis by high frequency epicardial echocardiography. N Engl J Med 1987;316:304–309.
9. St. Goar FG, Pinto FJ, Alderman EL, et al. Intracoronary ultrasound in cardiac transplant recipients: In vivo evidence of "angiographically silent" intimal thickening. Circulation 1992;85:979–987.
10. Yamagishi M, Nissen SE, Booth DC, Gurley JC, Fischer C, DeMaria AN. Impaired nitroglycerin induced vasodilation in coronary atherosclerosis: Evidence from intravascular ultrasound (abstr.). J Am Coll Cardiol 1992;19:95A.
11. Hausmann D, Mügge A, Fitzgerald PJ, Yock PG, Daniel WG. Nitroglycerininduced coronary vasodilation in heart transplant patients is impaired by intimal thickening (abstr.). J Am Coll Cardiol 1993;21:334A.
12. Fitzgerald PJ, Yock PG, and the GUIDE Trial Investigators. Discrepancies between angiographic and intravascular ultrasound appearance of coronary lesions undergoing intervention. A report of Phase I of the GUIDE trial (abstr.). J Am Coll Cardiol 1993;21:118A.
13. Mullen B, Fitzgerald PJ, Yock PG, and the GUIDE Trial Investigators. Impact of intravascular ultrasound on device selection and endpoint assessment of interventions (abstr.). J Am Coll Cardiol 1993;21:134A.

14. Werner GS, Sold G, Buchwald A, Kreuzer H, Wiegand V. Intravascular ultrasound imaging of human coronary arteries after percutaneous transluminal angioplasty. Morphologic and quantitative assessment. Am Heart J 1991;122: 212–220.
15. Honye JH, Mahon DJ, Jain A, et al. Morphological effects of coronary balloon angioplasty in vivo assessed by intravascular ultrasound imaging. Circulation 1992;85:1012–1025.
16. Gerber TC, Erbel R, Gorge G, Ge Jumbo, Rupprecht HJ, Meyer J. Classification of morphologic effects of percutaneous transluminal coronary angioplasty assessed by intravascular ultrasound. Am J Cardiol 1992;70:1546–1554.
17. Fitzgerald PJ, Ports TA, Yock PG. Contribution of localized calcium deposits to dissection after angioplasty. An observational study using intravascular ultrasound. Circulation 1992;86:64–70.
18. Tenaglia AN, Buller CE, Kissle KB, Phillips HR, Stack RS, Davidson CJ. Intracoronary ultrasound predictors of adverse outcomes after coronary artery interventions. J Am Coll Cardiol 1992;20:1385–1390.
19. The GUIDE Trial Investigators. Lumen enlargement following angioplasty is related to plaque characteristics. A report from the GUIDE trial (abstr.). Circulation 1992;86(suppl):I-531.
20. Stone GW, St. Goar F, Klette MA, Linnemeier TJ. Initial clinical experience with a novel low-profile integrated coronary ultrasound-angioplasty catheter: Implications for routine use (abstr.). J Am Coll Cardiol 1993;21:134A.
21. Pichard AD, Mintz GS, Satler LF, et al. The influence of pre-intervention intravascular ultrasound imaging on subsequent transcatheter treatment strategies (abstr.). J Am Coll Cardiol 1993:133A.
22. Stiel GM, Stiel LSG, Schofer J, Donath K, Mathey DG. Impact of compensatory enlargement of atherosclerotic coronary arteries on angiographic assessment of coronary artery disease. Circulation 1989;80:1603–1609.
23. Fitzgerald PJ, Yock PG. Mechanisms and outcomes of angioplasty and atherectomy assessed by intravascular ultrasound imaging. J Clin Ultrasound 1993; 21:579–588.
24. Kuntz RE, Safian RD, Levine MJ, Reis GJ, Diver DJ, Baim DS. Novel approach to the analysis of restenosis after the use of three new coronary devices. J Am Coll Cardiol 1992;19:1493–1499.
25. Haude M, Erbel R, Issa H, Meyer J. Quantitative analysis of elastic recoil after balloon angioplasty and after intracoronary implantation of balloon-expandable Palmaz-Schatz stents. J Am Coll Cardiol 1993;21:26–34.
26. Kuntz RE, Gibson CM, Nobuyoshi M, Baim DS. Generalized model of restenosis after conventional balloon angioplasty, stenting and directional atherectomy. J Am Coll Cardiol 1993;21:15–25.
27. Essed CE, van den Brand M, Becker AE. Transluminal coronary angioplasty and early restenosis: Fibrocellular occlusion after wall laceration. Br Heart J 1983;49:393–396.
28. Nobuyoshi M, Kimura T, Ohishi H, et al. Restenosis after percutaneous transluminal coronary angioplasty: Pathologic observations in 20 patients. J Am Coll Cardiol 1991;17:433–439.

29. Schartz RS, Huber KC, Murphy JG, et al. Restenosis and the proportional neo-intimal response to coronary artery injury: Results in a porcine model. J Am Coll Cardiol 1992;19:267–274.

30. Kimura BJ, Fitzgerald PJ, Sudhir K, Amidon TM, Strunk BL, Yock PG. Guidance of directed coronary atherectomy by intravascular imaging. Am Heart J 1992;124:1365–1369.

31. Safian RD, Gelbfish JS, Erny RE, Schnitt SJ, Schmidt DA, Baim DS. Coronary atherectomy. Clinical, angiographic, and histological findings and observations regarding potential mechanisms. Circulation 1990;82:69–79.

32. Smucker ML, Scherb DE, Howard PF. Intracoronary ultrasound: How much "angioplasty effect" in atherectomy (abstr.). Circulation 1990;82(suppl III):III-676.

33. De Lezo JS, Romero M, Medina A, et al. Intracoronary ultrasound assessment of directional coronary atherectomy: Immediate and follow-up findings. J Am Coll Cardiol 1993;21(suppl):298–307.

34. Matar FA, Mintz GS, Farb A. Tissue weight measurements underestimates "atherectomy effect" after directional atherectomy. An intravascular ultrasound study (abstr.). J Am Coll Cardiol 1993;21:193A.

35. Hinohara T, Rowe MH, Robertson GC, et al. Effect of lesion characteristics on outcome of directional coronary atherectomy. J Am Coll Cardiol 1991;17:1112-20.

36. Popma JJ, Decesare NB, Ellis SG. Clinical angiographic and procedural correlates of quantitative coronary dimensions after directional coronary atherectomy. J Am Coll Cardiol 1991;18:1183–1189.

37. Mintz GS, Douek P, Pichard AD, et al. Target lesion calcification in coronary artery disease: An intravascular ultrasound study. J Am Coll Cardiol 1992;20:1149–1155.

38. Davidson CJ, Sheikh K. Kisslo K. Intracoronary ultrasound evaluation of interventional technologies. Am J Cardiol 1991;68:1305–1309.

39. Yock PG, Fitzgerald PJ, Syles C. Morphologic features of successful coronary atherectomy determined by intravascular ultrasound imaging. Circulation 1990;82(suppl III):III-676.

40. Fitzgerald PJ, Mühlberger VA, Friedrich G, Yock PG. Calcium location within plaque as a prediction of atherectomy tissue retrieval. An intravascular ultrasound study. Circulation 1992;(suppl I):I-516.

41. De Lezo JS, Romero M, Medina A, et al. Intracoronary ultrasound assessment of directional coronary atherectomy: Immediate and follow-up findings. J Am Coll Cardiol 1993;21:298–307.

42. Stertzer SH, Rosenblum J, Shaw RE, et al. Coronary rotational ablation: Initial experience in 302 procedures. J Am Coll Cardiol 1993;21:287–295.

43. Mintz GS, Potkin BN, Keren G, et al. Intravascular ultrasound evaluation of the effect of rotational atherectomy in obstructive atherosclerotic coronary artery disease. Circulation 1992;86:1383–1393.

44. Roubin GS, Cannon AD, Agrawal SK, et al. Intracoronary stenting for acute and threatened closure complicating percutaneous transluminal coronary angioplasty. Circulation 1992;85:916–927.

45. Schatz RA, Golberg S, Leon M, et al. Clinical experience with Palmaz-Schatz coronary stent. J Am Coll Cardiol 1991;17:115B–159B.

46. Cavaye DM, Tabbara MR, Kopchock GE, Termin P, White RA. Intraluminal ultrasound assessment of vascular stent deployment. Ann Vasc Surg 1991;5: 241–246.
47. Diethrich EB, Santiago O, Gustafson G, Heuser RR. Preliminary observations on the use of the Palmaz stent in distal portion of the abdominal aorta. Am Heart J 1993; 125:490–501.
48. Davies MJ. A macro and micro view of coronary vascular insult in ischemic heart disease. Circulation 1990;82(suppl II):38–46.
49. Gertz SD, Roberts WC. Hemodynamic shear force in rupture of coronary arterial atherosclerotic plaques (editorial). Am J Cardiol 1990;66(19):1368–1372.
50. Lee RT, Grodzinsky AJ, Frank EH, Kamm RD, Schoen FJ. Structure-dependent dynamic mechanical behavior of fibrous caps from human atherosclerotic plaques. Circulation 1991;83:1764–1770.
51. Fitzgerald PJ, Popp RL. Computerized echocardiographic tissue characterization. Comput Cardiol 1981;276:395–398.
52. Fitzgerald PJ, Connolly AJ, Watkins RD, Yock PG. Distinction between soft plaque and thrombus by intravascular tissue characterization (abstr.). J Am Coll Cardiol 1991;17:11A.
53. Picano E, Landini I, Distante A, Benassi A, Sarnelli R, L'Abbate A. Fibrosis, lipids and calcium in human atherosclerotic plaque. Circ Res 1985;56:556–562.
54. Barzilai B, Saffitz JE, Miller JG, Sobel BE. Quantitative ultrasonic characterization of the nature of atherosclerotic plaques in human aorta. Circ Res 1987; 60:459–463.
55. Wickline SA, Barzilai B, Thomas LJ, Saffitz JE. Quantification of intimal and medial thickness of human coronary arteries by acoustic microscopy. Coronary Artery Dis 1990;1:333–340.

2

Percutaneous Coronary Angioscopy

Christopher J. White
Health Care International Medical Center, Glasgow, Scotland

I. INTRODUCTION

The general acceptance of percutaneous coronary revascularization, angioplasty, first performed in 1977 by Dr. Gruentzig (1), has dramatically changed our treatment strategies regarding coronary artery disease. New technologies are being developed in an attempt to maintain high procedural success rates and minimize complications as more complex and difficult lesions are accepted for percutaneous treatment. One such new technological advance, the angioscope, is a percutaneous catheter-based system designed to allow direct visual inspection of the endoluminal surface of the coronary arteries (2–31).

The promise of the angioscope is that direct visual examination of the surface morphology of a coronary artery will provide more accurate information than angiography, the current "gold standard." Theoretically, this enhanced ability to detect subtle details of plaque morphology will yield improved clinical outcomes for selected patients undergoing interventional procedures.

II. ANGIOSCOPY EQUIPMENT

The imaging system is made up of components including illumination fibers, imaging fibers, a video camera and monitor, and a videotape recorder. The illumination source provides a high-intensity "cold" light to avoid thermal damage to the vessel being imaged. The imaging bundle consists of at least 2000 optical fibers for adequate resolution. The video recorder provides an archival storage medium for review of the images.

The angioscope (Fig. 1) (Imagecath®, Baxter Healthcare Interventional Cardiology Division, Irvine, CA) is a catheter within a catheter. The inner catheter contains 3000 images fibers and is guided within the coronary artery over a 0.014-in. angioplasty guidewire. The outer catheter measures 4.5 French in diameter and has a lumen for inflating and deflating the occlusion balloon at its distal tip. Both the inner and outer catheters are guided by the same angioplasty guidewire in a "monorail" fashion. The occlusion balloon is a compliant balloon that achieves a variable final diameter depending on the volume of liquid introduced by hand injection up to a maximum diameter of 5.0 mm. In the space between the inner and outer catheters, there is room for a flush solution to be infused to clear the field of view during inflation of the occlusion balloon. The inner catheter may be advanced or withdrawn independently of the outer catheter a distance of 6 cm so that many segments of the vessel lumen can be examined.

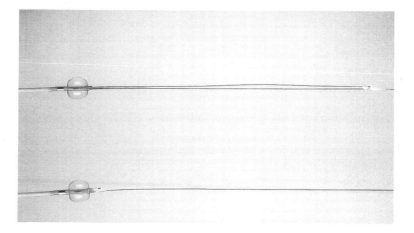

Figure 1 Photograph of the angioscope with the occlusion balloon inflated and inner image bundle extended (top) and retracted (bottom).

III. ANGIOSCOPY TECHNIQUE

To perform angioscopy, an 8-French conventional angioplasty guiding catheter is advanced to the coronary ostium of interest, and 10,000 units of heparin are administered. A 0.014-in. angioplasty guidewire is placed into the distal portion of the coronary artery. The angioscope, which is a monorail design, is advanced over a guidewire and into the coronary artery proximal to the segment of the vessel to be imaged. The flush lumen of the angioscope is connected to a power injector for infusion of warmed, lactated Ringer's at a rate of 0.5–1.0 cc/s. The occlusion balloon is hand inflated with a 1-cc syringe filled with a 50:50 mixture of saline and radiographic contrast. Special care is taken not to overinflate the balloon. The inner catheter, or the imaging bundle, is then advanced over the guidewire to view the intraluminal surface of the vessel. Each imaging sequence lasts approximately 30–45 s after which the balloon is deflated and the flush discontinued. These steps can be repeated several times until the region of interest has been adequately investigated.

When angioscopy is performed in conjunction with angioplasty, imaging may be performed before and/or after treatment. The target lesion is generally not crossed when performing preangioplasty imaging due to the size of the angioscope catheter. Complete imaging of the vessel can be performed after dilation to examine the distal segments of the vessel not accessible before angioplasty. The entire sequence from introducing the angioscope to obtaining images can usually be accomplished in less than 15 min.

IV. CLINICAL STUDIES

A. Coronary Artery Disease

Dramatic differences in plaque morphology have been observed between patients presenting with clinical symptoms of stable or unstable angina when undisturbed lesions were imaged with angioscopy before coronary angioplasty. Intracoronary angioscopy of undisturbed lesions (performed before coronary angioplasty) demonstrated a significantly higher incidence of complex plaque, including plaque ruptures (dissections) and associated intracoronary thrombi, in patients with unstable angina ($n = 11$) compared to those with stable angina (Fig. 2).

These results confirmed the intraoperative angioscopy study by Sherman et al. (12) in which they documented a surprisingly high incidence of intracoronary thrombi in patients with unstable angina as well as the insensitivity of angiography for detecting these thrombi. These in vivo findings are consistent with postmortem studies suggesting that the pathophysiology respon-

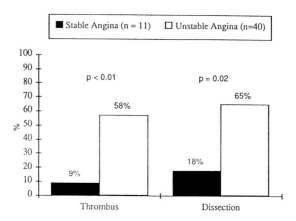

Figure 2 Angioscopic findings of undisturbed lesions (before angioplasty) in patients with stable and unstable angina.

sible for the occurrence of unstable angina is plaque rupture and thrombus formation.

We tested the hypothesis that the presence of intracoronary thrombus is related to procedural complications of angioplasty by performing percutaneous coronary angioscopy before and/or after angioplasty in 122 patients. Stable angina was present in 27 patients, and unstable angina was present in 95 patients. Patients were treated with routine angioplasty techniques and no thrombolytic therapy was administered.

In-hospital adverse outcomes, defined as either the occurrence of major complications (death, myocardial infarction, or emergency bypass) or the recurrence of ischemic events (abrupt occlusion, repeat angioplasty, or recurrent angina), were significantly associated with the presence of angioscopically identified intracoronary thrombus (Fig. 3). Angioscopy demonstrated that 70 of 95 patients (74%) with unstable angina had a much higher incidence of intracoronary thrombus than 4 of 27 patients (15%) with stable angina ($p < 0.001$). A major complication occurred in 10 of 95 patients (11%) with unstable angina and in none of the 27 stable angina patients ($p = 0.07$); recurrent ischemic events occurred in 22 of 95 unstable angina patients (23%) and in only 2 of 27 stable angina patients (7%) ($p = 0.05$). The presence of intracoronary thrombus appears to be associated with adverse outcomes after coronary angioplasty.

B. Abrupt Occlusion After Angioplasty

Abrupt occlusion of a coronary artery is the major cause of morbidity and mortality associated with percutaneous angioplasty. Therapy intended

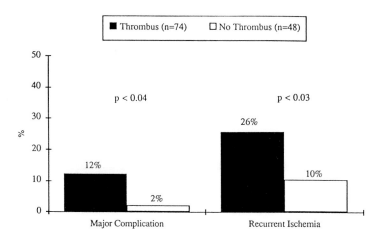

Figure 3 Incidence of major complications (death, myocardial infarction, and emergency coronary bypass) and recurrent ischemia (recurrent angina, repeat angioplasty, and abrupt occlusion) stratified by the presence or absence of angioscopically detected intracoronary thrombus.

to reopen occluded vessels is either empirical or guided by angiographic lesion morphology which has inherent limitations in specifically identifying the cause of the occlusion. We performed percutaneous coronary angioscopy in 17 patients with abrupt occlusion after coronary angioplasty to directly visualize the intravascular morphology of abruptly occluded vessels and compared the results of angioscopy with those of angiography.

Angioscopic lesion morphology was characterized by either mural or occlusive intracoronary thrombus and/or superficial or occlusive dissection (Fig. 4). Angioscopy demonstrated that the most common cause of the abrupt occlusion was dissection, with only a minority due to intracoronary thrombi (Fig. 5). When compared with angioscopy, angiography was significantly less accurate for identifying a specific cause of the occlusion and correctly identified only 4 of 14 occlusive dissections (29%) and 1 of 3 intraluminal thrombi (33%).

Diagnostic images were obtained in each case without complications attributable to the angioscopy procedure. Angioscopy was superior to angiography for detecting dissections and coronary thrombi. Dissections were visualized by angioscopy in all 17 vessels (100%) whereas angiography identified dissection in only 8 vessels (47%) ($p = 0.0005$). Dissection with bulky tissue fragments obstructing the lumen of the vessel was the primary cause of the occlusion in 14 of 17 vessels (82%), while an incidental superficial dissection was identified by angioscopy in the remaining three patients. None

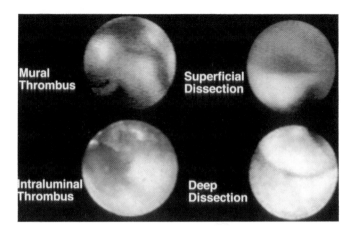

Figure 4   Angioscopy of intracoronary thrombus: Mural thrombus (top left) and occlusive thrombus (bottom left). Angioscopy of dissection: Superficial dissection (top right) and occlusive dissection (bottom right).

of the superficial dissections ($n = 3$) were detected by angiography, and only 8 of 14 occlusive dissections (57%) visualized with the angioscope were identified by angiography.

Intracoronary red thrombi were identified by angioscopy in 13 of 17 vessels (76%). Nonobstructive mural thrombi were present in 10 of 17 vessels (59%) and, in each case, were associated with occlusive dissections. In 3 of 17 vessels (18%), occlusive intraluminal thrombi were seen. In each of these

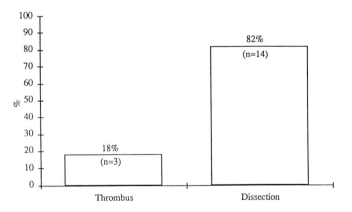

Figure 5   Causes of abrupt occlusion as determined by angioscopy.

thrombotic occlusions, superficial plaque disruptions, or shallow dissections, were also observed, but did not contribute to the luminal obstruction. All three patients with occlusive intraluminal thrombi had unstable angina, including two patients with postmyocardial infarction angina, and one patient with a crescendo pattern of angina.

We were able to use the angioscopic findings to guide our therapy. The three patients with occlusive thrombi were treated with a selective infusion of 250,000 units of intracoronary urokinase (Abbokinase, Abbott Laboratories, Abbott Park, IL) over 30 min (Fig. 6). Urokinase was used alone in one patient and as an adjunct to repeat balloon dilation in two patients. Two patients had their angioplasty procedures successfully salvaged without infarction; however, while the third patient's vessel was successfully recanalized, patency could not be sustained and the patient was sent for emergency bypass surgery with a perfusion balloon in place to maintain flow.

Among the procedures performed in the 14 patients with occlusive dissections, two occluded vessels were unable to be reopened with long balloon inflations and the patients were subsequently sent for emergency coronary bypass surgery. One of these patients suffered a non–Q-wave infarction. Of the remaining 12 patients with occlusive dissections, 8 were successfully treated with repeat balloon dilation, 3 were successfully reopened with repeat balloon dilation and directional coronary atherectomy, and 1 was salvaged with stent implantation. Two of the patients with successfully reopened arteries developed Q-wave infarctions.

There were no complications related to the angioscopy procedure. There were no deaths, strokes, sustained ventricular arrhythmias, or episodes of hemodynamic collapse in any of the patients. As described above, three

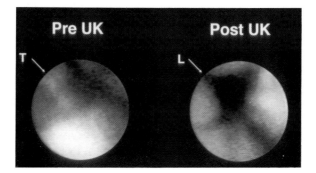

Figure 6 Angioscopy of intracoronary thrombus before intracoronary lytic therapy with urokinase (left) and after intracoronary lytic therapy with dissolution of the red thrombus (right).

patients required emergency coronary bypass surgery due to failure to maintain patency. Three patients (18%) suffered myocardial infarctions, including one non–Q-wave infarction and two Q-wave infarctions. Both Q-wave infarctions occurred when abrupt occlusion occurred outside of the catheterization laboratory, which unavoidably delayed attempts to reopen the vessel.

The lesion morphology we observed in these occluded arteries clearly demonstrated the primary cause of the obstruction. It is interesting to note that although the majority of the patients (88%) had unstable angina, a condition that has been associated with a high incidence of intracoronary thrombi, the majority of occlusions after angioplasty were due to dissection and not thrombus.

Angioscopy was superior to angiography for identifying specific lesion morphologies such as dissection and thrombus. Additionally, we were able to determine a "primary cause" of the abrupt occlusion with the angioscope when both thrombus and dissection were present. Angioscopic information was used in these patients to select specific treatment modalities directed at the underlying cause of the failed angioplasty attempt. For example, for intracoronary thrombus we used thrombolytic therapy, and for occlusive dissections we used repeat balloon dilation, directional atherectomy, or stent placement.

Specific information regarding the causes for the occlusion will allow the operator to select an appropriate treatment strategy more efficiently. This knowledge, if it can be gained rapidly and safely, should expedite the reestablishment of coronary flow and avoid inappropriate therapies, such as the use of thrombolysis for tissue obstruction, or unattractive treatments, such as the placement of stents in thrombus-filled arteries.

C. Saphenous Vein Grafts

The results of percutaneous angioscopy and angiography for detecting critical elements of surface lesion morphology were compared in 21 patients undergoing balloon angioplasty of saphenous vein coronary bypass grafts (30). Angioscopy and angiography were performed before and after angioplasty of "culprit lesions" in bypass grafts. All but one of the patients had unstable angina. The mean age of the saphenous vein coronary bypass grafts was 10.1 ± 2.4 years (range 5–15 years). Restenosis at a prior angioplasty site was present in seven patients. Intravascular thrombi were seen in 15 of 21 grafts (71%) by angioscopy and in 4 of 21 grafts (19%) by angiography ($p < 0.001$). Dissection was identified in 14 of 21 grafts (66%) by angioscopy and in 2 of 21 grafts (10%) by angiography ($p < 0.01$). The presence of friable plaque lining the luminal surface of the vein graft was detected in 11 of 21 grafts (52%) by angioscopy and in 5 of 21 grafts (24%) by angiography ($p < 0.05$). There was no correlation between age of the bypass graft and

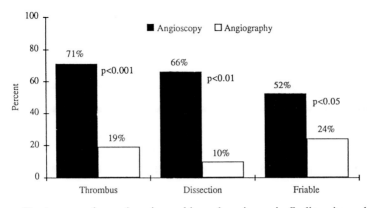

Figure 7 A comparison of angiographic and angioscopic findings in saphenous vein grafts ($n = 21$) before and/or after angioplasty.

presence of friable plaque. We concluded that angioscopy is superior to angiography for detecting complex lesion morphology in bypass grafts and for detecting the presence of friable plaque which does not preclude an uncomplicated angioplasty result (Fig. 7).

V. POTENTIAL CLINICAL UTILITY

The correlation of atherosclerotic lesion morphology with clinical outcomes has been the cornerstone of our understanding of this disease and has guided our treatment of these patients. The landmark study by DeWood et al. (32) made clear the role of intracoronary thrombosis in the pathogenesis of myocardial infarction and dramatically changed the standard therapy of this disease from supportive care to interventional therapy with thrombolytic agents. Angiographic morphology studies of coronary arteries in patients with stable and unstable angina have allowed us to stratify patients with high-risk lesions (33–35). These studies have been limited by the documented insensitivity of angiography for assessing residual stenosis after angioplasty, and for detecting subtle changes in coronary artery surface morphology, such as plaque fractures, dissections, and intracoronary thrombi (36–50).

When compared with angiography, angioscopy offers a superior sensitivity and specificity for identifying subtle changes in atherosclerotic plaque morphology. Like angiography, this is a percutaneous technique that can be used in conjunction with diagnostic angiography to examine more closely suspicious regions or lesions and, hopefully, to provide more precise data concerning the progression of coronary disease. Angioscopy allows the in vivo examination of the surface pathology present in the coronary artery. Our early studies suggest that angioscopy has the potential to improve our understanding of coronary artery lesion morphology in patients with acute ischemic syndromes, restenosis following angioplasty, atherosclerotic allograft coronary disease, and saphenous vein graft disease.

Percutaneous coronary angioscopy may play a role in guiding interventional coronary therapy. Angioscopy, when compared with angiography, is better able to detect small amounts of intracoronary thrombus which may have a negative impact on the outcome of angioplasty in patients with acute ischemic syndromes. Current studies are underway to determine if the angioscopic detection of intracoronary thrombus in patients undergoing balloon angioplasty can identify those at higher risk for complications from the procedure. Perhaps the administration of adjunctive thrombolytic therapy, either before or after balloon dilation, will be guided by angioscopic findings.

We have demonstrated the feasibility of performing diagnostic angioscopy in the setting of abrupt occlusion after coronary angioplasty. The angioscope allows the operator to specifically identify the causes of the obstruction reliably and quickly, and is superior to angiography. The primary cause of abrupt occlusion in our population of unstable angina patients was, surprisingly, dissection with obstruction secondary to tissue flaps. To determine whether the lesion-specific information provided by angioscopy will be both cost-effective and improve clinical outcomes will require a comparative trial. As alternative angioplasty techniques, such as atherectomy, laser angioplasty, and stent implantation, are more commonly used, perhaps the surface morphology of coronary lesions will become an important factor in device selection.

Our early experience in patients with stenotic saphenous vein coronary bypass grafts has demonstrated the ability to differentiate shaggy atheroma from smooth fibrotic-appearing lesions, which has not been possible with angiography alone. This suggests that the risk of distal embolism in older vein grafts following balloon dilation may be better assessed by angioscopy and that the choice of the revascularization procedure to be performed in patients with stenotic bypass grafts could be guided by angioscopic findings.

VI. CONCLUSIONS

Coronary angioscopy will not replace diagnostic angiography as the "gold standard" for imaging stenotic lesions in coronary arteries. However, there may well be a clinical niche for an imaging technology that gives accurate information regarding a specific lesion if that information can be used to improve the acute or chronic outcome of an interventional procedure.

Our initial experience with coronary angioscopy suggests that critical information regarding lesion morphology that is not available from angiographic images can be used to improve patient outcome and assess risk. With angioscopes, we now have access to information regarding arterial wall pathology that heretofore has only been available at necropsy. Whereas angiography provides a two-dimensional, gray-scale image of the coronary vessels, angioscopy offers a full-color, three-dimensional perspective of the intracoronary surface morphology.

REFERENCES

1. Gruntzig AR, Senning A, Siegenthaler WE. Nonoperative dilatation of coronary artery stenosis. Percutaneous transluminal coronary angioplasty. N Engl J Med 1979;301:61–68.
2. Mizuno K, Kurita A, Imazeki N. Pathological findings after percutaneous transluminal coronary angioplasty. Br Heart J 1984;52:588–590.
3. Cutler EC, Levine, Beck CS. The surgical treatment of mitral stenosis: Experimental and clinical studies. Arch Surg 1924;9:689–821.
4. Harken DE, Glidden EM. Experiments in intracardiac surgery. II. Intracardiac visualization. J Thorac Surg 1943;12:566–572.
5. Bolton HE, Bailey CP, Costas-Durieux J, Gemeinhardt W. Cardioscopy – simple and practical. J Thorac Surg 1954;27:323–329.
6. Sakakibara S, Ilkawa T, Hattori J, Inomata K. Direct visual operation for aortic stenosis: Cardioscopic studies. J Int Coll Surg 1958;29:548–562.
7. Litvack F, Grundfest WS, Lee ME, et al. Angioscopic visualization of blood vessel interior in animals and humans. Clin Cardiol 1985;8:65–70.
8. Grundfest WS, Litvack F, Sherman T, et al. Delineation of peripheral and coronary detail by intraoperative angioscopy. Ann Surg 1985;202:394–400.
9. Sanborn TA, Rygaard JA, Westbrook BM, Lazar HL, McCormick JR, Roberts AJ. Intraoperative angioscopy of saphenous vein and coronary arteries. J Thorac Cardiovasc Surg 1986;91:339–343.
10. Lee G, Garcia JM, Corso PJ, et al. Correlation of coronary angioscopic to angiographic findings in coronary artery disease. Am J Cardiol 1986;58:238–241.
11 Grundfest WS, Litvack F, Glick D, et al. Intraoperative decisions based on angioscopy in peripheral vascular surgery. Circulation 1988;78(suppl I):I-13-I-17.
12. Sherman CT, Litvack F, Grundfest W, et al. Coronary angioscopy in patients with unstable angina pectoris. N Engl J Med 1986;315:913–919.
13. Spears JR, Spokojny AM, Marais HJ. Coronary angioscopy during cardiac catheterization. J Am Coll Cardiol 1985;6:93–97.
14. Susawa T, Yui Y, Hattori R, et al. Direct observation of coronary thrombus using a newly developed ultrathin (1.2 mm) flexible angioscope (abstr). J Am Coll Cardiol 1987;9(suppl A):197A.
15. Takahashi M, Yui Y, Susawa T, et al. Evaluation of coronary thrombus by a newly developed ultra-thin (0.75 mm) flexible quartz microfiber angioscope [Abstract]. Circulation 1987;76(suppl IV):IV-282.

16. Uchida Y, Furuse A, Hasegawa K. Percutaneous coronary angioscopy using a novel balloon guiding catheter in patients with ischemic heart diseases (abstr). Circulation 1987;76(suppl IV):IV-185.
17. Uchida Y, Tomaru T, Nakamura F, Furuse A, Fujimori Y, Hasegawa K. Percutaneous coronary angioscopy in patients with ischemic heart disease. Am Heart J 1987;114:1216-1222.
18. Inoue K, Kuwaki K, Ueda K, Shirai T. Angioscopy guided coronary thrombolysis (abstr). J Am Coll Cardiol 1987;9(suppl A):62A.
19. Morice M-C, Marco J, Fajadet J, Castillo-Fenoy A. Percutaneous coronary angioscopy before and after angioplasty in acute myocardial infarction: Preliminary results (abstr). Circulation 1987;76(suppl IV):IV-282.
20. Inoue K, Kuwaki K, Ueda K, Takano E. Angioscopic macropathology of coronary atherosclerosis in unstable angina and acute myocardial infarction (abstr). J Am Coll Cardiol 1988;11(suppl A):65A.
21. Kuwaki K, Inoue K, Ueda K, Shirai T, Ochiai H. Percutaneous transluminal coronary angioscopy during cardiac catherization: The results of experiences in the first 30 patients (abstr). Circulation 1987;76(suppl IV):IV-186.
22. Uchida Y, Hasegawa K, Kawamura K, Shibuya I. Angioscopic observation of the coronary luminal changes induced by percutaneous transluminal angioplasty. Am Heart J 1989;117:769-776.
23. Uchida Y. Percutaneous coronary angioscopy by means of a fiberscope with a steerable guidewire. Am Heart J 1989;117:1153-1155.
24. Ramee SR, White CJ, Collins TJ, Mesa JE, Murgo JP. Percutaneous angioscopy during coronary angioplasty using a steerable microangioscope. J Am Coll Cardiol 1991;17:100-105.
25. White CJ, Ramee SR. Percutaneous coronary angioscopy: Methods, findings, and therapeutic implications. Echocardiography 1990;7:485-494.
26. Mizuno K, Arai T, Satomura K, et al. New percutaneous transluminal coronary angioscope. J Am Coll Cardiol 1989;13:363-368.
27. Ventura HO, White CJ, Ramee SR, et al. Percutaneous coronary angioscopy findings in patients with cardiac transplantation (abstr). J Am Coll Cardiol 1991; 17:273A.
28. Ventura HO, White CJ, Ramee SR, Colins TJ, Mesa JE, Jain A. Coronary angioscopy in the diagnosis of graft coronary artery disease in heart transplant recipients (lett). J Heart Lung Transplant 1991;10:488.
29. White CJ, Ramee SR, Mesa J, Collins TJ. Percutaneous coronary angioscopy in patients with restenosis after coronary angioplasty. J Am Coll Cardiol 1991; 17(suppl B):46B-49B.
30. White CJ, Ramee SR, Collins TJ, Mesa JE, Jain A. Percutaneous angioscopy of saphenous vein coronary bypass grafts. J Am Coll Cardiol 1993;21:1181-1185.
31. White CJ, Ramee SR, Collins RJ, Jain A, Mesa JE, Ventura HO. Percutaneous coronary angioscopy: Applications in interventional cardiology. J Interventional Cardiol 1993;6:61-67.
32. DeWood MA, Spores J, Notske R, et al. Prevalence of total coronary occlusion during the early hours of transmural myocardial infarction. N Engl J Med 1980;303:897-902.

33. Ambrose JA, Winters SL, Stern A. Angiographic morphology and the pathogenesis of unstable angina pectoris. J Am Coll Cardiol 1985;5:609–616.
34. Rehr R, Disciascio G, Vetrovec G, Cowley M. Angiographic morphology of coronary artery stenoses in prolonged rest angina: Evidence of intracoronary thrombosis. J Am Coll Cardiol 1989;14:1429–1437.
35. Levin DC, Fallon JT. Significance of the angiographic morphology of localized coronary stenoses: Histopathologic correlations. Circulation 1982;66:316–320.
36. Vlodaver Z, Frech R, Van Tassel RA, Edwards JE. Correlations of the antemortem coronary arteriogram and the postmortem specimen. Circulation 1973;47:162–169.
37. Grondin CM, Dyrda I, Pasternac A, Campeau L, Bourassa MG, Lesperance J. Discrepancies between cineangiographic and postmortem findings in patients with coronary artery disease and recent myocardial revascularization. Circulation 1974;49:703–708.
38. Pepine CJ, Feldman RL, Nichols WW, Conti CR. Coronary arteriography: Potentially serious sources of error in interpretation. Cardiovasc Med 1977;2:747–752.
39. Arnett EN, Isner JM, Redwood DR, et al. Coronary artery narrowing in coronary heart disease: Comparison of cineangiographic and necropsy findings. Ann Intern Med 1979;91:350–356.
40. Isner JM Kishel J, Kent KM, Ronan JA, Ross AM, Roberts WC. Accuracy of angiographic determination of left main coronary arterial narrowing: Angiographic-histologic correlative analysis in 28 patients. Circulation 1981;63:1056–1064.
41. Spears JR, Sandor T, Baim DS, Paulin S. The minimum error in estimating coronary luminal cross-sectional area from cineangiographic diameter measurements. Cathet Cardiovasc Diag 1983;9:119–128.
42. White CW, Wright CB, Doty DB, et al. Does visual interpretation of the coronary arteriogram predict the physiologic importance of a coronary stenosis? N Engl J Med 1984;310:819–824.
43. Isner JM, Donaldson RF. Coronary angiographic and morphologic correlation. Cardiol Clin 1984;2:571–592.
44. Gould KL. Quantification of coronary artery stenosis in vivo. Circ Res 1985;57:341–353.
45. Zijlstra F, van Ommeren J, Reiber HC, Surruys PW. Does the quantitative assessment of coronary artery dimensions predict the physiologic significance of a coronary stenosis? Circulation 1987;75:1154–1161.
46. Marcus ML, Skorton DJ, Johnson MR, Collins SM, Harrison DG, Kerber RE. Visual estimates of percent diameter coronary stenosis: "A battered gold standard" (edit). J Am Coll Cardiol 1988;11:882–885.
47. Katritsis D, Webb-Peploe M. Limitations of coronary angiography: An underestimated problem? Clin Cardiol 1991;14:20–24.
48. Block PC, Myler RK, Stertzer S, Fallon JT. Morphology after transluminal angioplasty in human beings. N Engl J Med 1981;305:382–385.

49. Duber C, Jungbluth A, Rumpelt HJ, Erbel R, Meyer J, Thoenes W. Morphology of the coronary arteries after combined thrombolysis and percutaneous transluminal coronary angioplasty for acute myocardial infarction. Am J Cardiol 1986;58:698–703.

50. Essed CE, Van Den Brand M, Becker AE. Transluminal coronary angioplasty and early restenosis: Fibrocellular occlusion after wall laceration. Br Heart J 1983;49:393–396.

3

Clinical Applications of Intracoronary Coronary Doppler Flow Velocity in Interventional Cardiology

Morton J. Kern and Michael S. Flynn
St. Louis University Health Sciences Center, St. Louis, Missouri

I. INTRODUCTION

Decisions for proceeding with coronary angioplasty and other newer interventional procedures are based on clinical presentation and findings from angiography and noninvasive stress testing. Unfortunately, ischemic stress testing is prone to occasional (10–30%) false positive or negative results and most clinicians employ nonquantitative angiographic assessment of lesion severity to determine the need for these procedures. A recent technological advance, a coronary Doppler-tipped angioplasty-style guidewire, allows physicians to measure blood flow velocity in individual coronary arteries beyond stenoses with relative ease and safety. Using the Doppler velocity guidewire, the interventionalist can determine the physiological significance of an individual coronary stenosis both before and following the procedure in a quantitative fashion. Distal arterial flow velocity information provides an objective measurement on which to base treatment decisions when angiographic findings are in question. This chapter will review intracoronary flow velocity measurements emphasizing the major clinical applications of translesional flow data (Table 1) (1,2).

Table 1 Clinical Applications of Intracoronary Doppler Guidewire Flow Velocity

Applications	Reference No.
Interventional Procedures	
Angioplasty	
End point	4, 5, 10, 11
Monitoring complications	12, 23, 29
Assessing additional lesions	11, 35
Collateral flow	13, 15, 16
Stent	12, 45, 46
Atherectomy	48, 49
Laser	49
Intermediate Coronary Lesion Assessment	35, 36, 65
Coronary Vasodilatory Reserve	1, 2, 51
Intermediate lesion assessment	35, 36, 65
Syndrome X	1
Transplant coronary arteriopathy	50
Coronary Physiology Research	
Pharmacological studies	64, 66
Intra-aortic balloon pumping	67, 68
Perfusion imaging correlation	36
Saphenous vein graft, internal mammary artery flow characteristics	69
Endothelial function	

II. CORONARY FLOW VELOCITY TECHNIQUES

A. Instrumentation

There are four commercially available Doppler catheters with two types of velocimeters for measuring blood flow velocity in the coronary arteries: (1) the nonselective Judkins Doppler catheter (Cordis Corp, Miami, FL); and (2) the 3-French subselective end-mounted catheter (Millar Instruments, Houston, TX); (3) the side-mounted ultrasonic crystal catheter (NuMed, Inc., Hopkinton, NY); and (4) the flowire/FloMap System (Cardiometrics, Inc., Mountain View, CA) (Fig. 1) (1). The two available velocimeters are the zero-crossing type (Millar Instruments, Houston, TX and Triton Medical, San Diego, CA) compatible with the three Doppler catheters, and the spectral velocity analyzer (Cardiometrics, Inc., Mountainview, CA) compatible only with the Doppler flowire. The 3-French subselective Doppler catheters have been proposed for assessing the hemodynamic significance of coronary lesions and interventions, but have not been incorporated into routine practice because of the large catheter size, measurements limited to only velocity

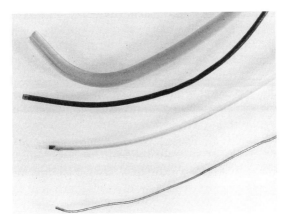

Figure 1 Intracoronary Doppler catheters. From top to bottom: Judkins Doppler (Cordis Corp., Miami, FL); Millar 3-French end-mounted crystal Doppler (Millar Instruments, Houston, TX); NuMed 3-French side-mounted catheter (NuMed, Hopkinton, NY); flowire 0.018-in. Doppler angioplasty tipped guidewire (Cardiometrics, Inc., Mountain View, CA). (Reprinted with permission from Ref. 4.)

proximal to a lesion, the necessity to exchange the catheter for the interventional device, and difficulty in ascertaining optimal signals with the zero cross technique. In addition, coronary vasodilatory reserve (i.e., the hyperemic/basal flow ratio) proved to be a poor indicator of procedural completion due to changing basal and hyperemic flow values. The Doppler flowire has features that overcome many of these limitations, making it suitable for routine clinical use (2). The flowire is small enough (0.014–0.018-in. diameter) to assess coronary flow velocity both proximal and distal to any coronary stenoses. It can also be used to determine whether normal blood flow velocity has been restored following angioplasty and to monitor flow changes during routine and complicated coronary angioplasty or other interventional procedures. During diagnostic angiography, the flowire can also identify whether there is flow velocity impairment caused by an intermediately severe coronary narrowing and which intermediate lesions might benefit from mechanical intervention. Coronary vasodilatory reserve before and after procedures can also be assessed.

B. Characteristics and Method of Use of the Doppler Flowire

The Doppler angioplasty guidewire (Flowire™, Cardiometrics, Inc., Mountain View, CA) is a 175-cm-long 0.014–0.018-in. diameter flexible steerable guidewire with a piezoelectric ultrasound transducer integrated into the tip. The 12-MHz crystal on the tip of the guidewire sends and receives ultrasound waves. The timing of the sending and receiving velocity allows the flowire to measure blood flow velocities up to 400 cm/s from moving red cells in a sample area 5 mm ($\times$ 2 mm) from the tip of the wire, a distance far enough away that the blood velocity is not affected by the wake of the wire. The returning signal is transmitted, in real time, to the display console. The gray-scale spectral scrolling display shows the velocities of all the red blood cells within the sample volume. When the sample area is constant, the peak velocity is accurately tracked in the center of the artery and the key parameters will remain relatively positionally insensitive and reliable. As described and validated by Doucette et al. (3), the forward-directed ultrasound beam diverges in a 27° arc from the long axis (measured to the -6 dB round-trip points of the ultrasound beam pattern) (Fig. 2). The pulse repetition frequency of >40 kHz, pulse duration of $+0.83$ ms, and sampling delay of 6.5 ms are standard for clinical usage. The system is coupled to a real-time spectrum analyzer, videocassette recorder, and video page printer. The quadrature/Doppler audio signals are processed by the spectrum analyzer using on-line fast Fourier transformation. The frequency response of the system calculates approximately 90 spectra/s. Simultaneous electrocardiographic and arterial pressure are also input to the video display.

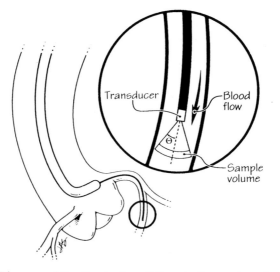

Figure 2 Diagram of the flowire in a 5-French diagnostic catheter. Transducer has a 27° beam spread from the mid axis. Sample volume is 5 mm from the tip. (Reprinted with permission from Ref. 4.)

Flow velocity spectra are printed on an integrated video page printer. Computerized parameters of intracoronary flow velocity, including peak and mean diastolic and systolic velocities, diastolic and systolic velocity integrals (obtained by planimetry of the total area under the peak instantaneous velocity profile), mean total velocities, and the total velocity integral are automatically analyzed (Fig. 3). These velocity parameters are validated using a custom software program and manual tracing of the spectral peak Doppler velocity signal on a digital computer bit pad (2–4).

C. Validation Studies

The Doppler guidewire has been validated during intravascular measurement of coronary arterial flow velocity by Doucette et al. (3). The velocity signals, processed on-line by fast Fourier transformation, have been found to correlate with absolute coronary flow measurements in in vitro and in vivo validation studies (3). The Doppler spectra were recorded in model tubes with pulsatile blood flow. In four straight tubes with internal diameters varying from 0.79–4.76 mm, the peak spectral flow velocity was linearly related to absolute flow velocity measured by in-line electromagnetic flow meters ($r > 0.98$ for each tube). Quantitative volumetric flow was calculated from vessel cross-sectional area and mean flow velocity. The average

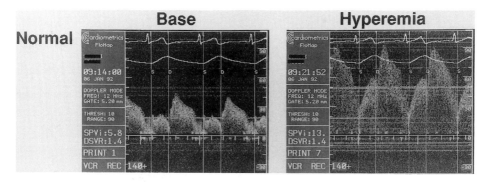

Figure 3 Normal basal (left) and hyperemic (right) coronary flow velocity spectra demonstrating small systolic and large diastolic velocity components. The diastolic velocity integral is the area under the velocity profile demarcated by the D-S (diastolic-systolic) lines; the systolic velocity integral (SPVi) by the S-D (systolic-diastolic) lines. Peak systolic and peak diastolic (PVd) velocities are obtained from the maximal signal during that phase of the flow cycle. The velocity scale is 0–140 cm/s on this example. DSVR = diastolic/systolic velocity ratio. Note the ECG and aortic pressure on top two tracings. The hyperemic response to intracoronary adenosine is shown on the right panel.

peak velocity was less accurate in larger tubes (>7.5-mm diameter) and a slightly reduced correlation with absolute flow was observed in some tortuous model segments. In four canine circumflex coronary arteries, the electromagnetic flow probe and Doppler flow velocities also demonstrated high correlations in both the proximal and distal segments ($r^2 = 0.93–0.99$ in the proximal vessel and $0.86–0.99$ in the distal vessel). Using quantitative angiography to determine arterial diameter, quantitative flow velocity correlations for the two techniques were $r = 0.95$ in the model cannula and $r = 0.85$ in the proximal coronary artery (Fig. 4). These data indicated that the Doppler guidewire accurately measures flow velocity and linearly tracks changes in flow rates in small (3–5 mm), predominantly straight coronary arteries.

The Doppler guidewire flow velocity signals were not importantly affected by increasing heart rates to 150 beats/min in the canine model. The motion artifact of rapidly changing heart rate might influence flow velocity, but this artifact was not identified in the initial validation studies. Changes of pulsatility intensity examined in the in vitro system also demonstrated satisfactory tracking and correlation with electromagnetic flow responses at rapid heart rates. In the in vivo pacing experiments, the relationship between the average peak velocity of the Doppler guidewire system and flow meter response at spontaneous heart rates and at paced rates of 150 beats/min demonstrated a high correlation. A small zero drift was observed in only one animal study, and it is known that differences of this magnitude represent a <21 ml/min change in flow and are likely to be of minimal clinical importance.

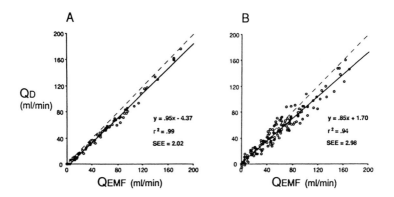

Figure 4 Linear regression of Doppler-derived flow (QD) vs blood flow by electromagnetic flow meter (QEMF) in canine circumflex arteries. (A) Flowire in coronary cannula. (B) Flowire in proximal circumflex. Dashed line is line of identity. Solid line is regression line. (Reprinted from Ref. 3.)

III. IMPORTANT FEATURES IN MEASURING DOPPLER FLOW VELOCITY

A. Normal Proximal and Distal Epicardial Coronary Flow Velocity Signal Interpretation

To assess normal flow velocity in patients, simultaneous flow velocity measurements in 55 angiographically normal, proximal, and distal coronary arteries (right coronary arteries = 12, left circumflex arteries = 19, and left anterior descending coronary arteries = 24) were measured (4,5) (Table 2). Coronary hyperemia was produced with intracoronary administration of 8–18 μg of adenosine (6).

Fundamental to using flow velocity as a marker of atherosclerotic lesion significance and flow obstruction is the difference between velocity and volumetric flow along the course of the epicardial vessel. Two anatomical features occur to preserve velocity while volume flow is normally reduced from the proximal to distal one-third portion of the major artery. First, coronary

Table 2 Baseline and Hyperemia Velocity Parameters in Individual Coronary Arteries

	Baseline			Hyperemia[a]		
	LAD (n = 24)	LCX (n = 19)	RCA (n = 12)	LAD	LCX	RCA
Proximal						
Peak D Vel	49 ± 20	40 ± 15	37 ± 12	104 ± 28[c]	79 ± 20	72 ± 13
Mean Vel	31 ± 15	25 ± 8	26 ± 7	66 ± 18[c]	50 ± 14	48 ± 13
D Vel Int	18 ± 11[b]	13 ± 5	11 ± 4	37 ± 55[c]	27 ± 7	22 ± 9
1/3 FF (%)	45 ± 4[b]	44 ± 5	40 ± 5	44 ± 5	43 ± 6	41 ± 4
D/S	2.0 ± 0.5[b]	1.8 ± 0.7	1.5 ± 0.5	2.0 ± 0.5	1.9 ± 0.6	1.9 ± 0.8
Distal						
Peak D Vel	35 ± 16	35 ± 8	28 ± 8	70 ± 17	71 ± 22	67 ± 16
Mean Vel	23 ± 11	21 ± 6	21 ± 9	45 ± 12	45 ± 12	42 ± 9
D Vel Int	13 ± 9	10 ± 3	8 ± 5	9 ± 6	11 ± 8	9 ± 2
1/3 FF (%)	46 ± 2	45 ± 9	39 ± 6	45 ± 3	42 ± 7	40 ± 9
D/S	2.4 ± 0.8[b]	2.1 ± 0.8	1.4 ± 0.3	2.2 ± 1.0	1.9 ± 0.8	1.6 ± 0.3

ANOVA: Scheffe F test $p < 0.05$.
[a]All three coronary arteries had significantly higher absolute velocity parameters during hyperemia ($p < 0.001$).
[b]LAD vs RCA.
[c]LAD vs LCX and RCA.
D = diastolic; D/S = peak diastolic/systolic velocity; D Vel Int = diastolic flow velocity integral (units); Vel = velocity (cm/s); 1/3 FF = one-third flow fraction.
Source: Modified with permission from Ref. 5.

arteries gradually taper from proximal to distal, on average about 0.5–1 mm in diameter. Second, branching vessels distribute blood volume across the myocardium with absolute volume flow lower in the distal region compared to proximal vessel region. Since volume flow is calculated as the product of vessel cross-sectional area and velocity (mean velocity or velocity integral), flow velocity, not volume, is maintained along the epicardial conduit from the proximal to distal part of the artery (Fig. 5). The ratio of proximal to distal flow velocity is approximately 1:1 while the ratio of proximal to distal flow volume is often > 2:1.

In normal human coronary arteries, distal coronary flow velocity is similar to proximal flow velocity in all three vessels. Proximal and distal mean velocity in each artery was not different at baseline or hyperemia (Fig. 6). There were differences among the three major coronary arteries, with the diastolic velocity integral at baseline significantly higher for the proximal left anterior descending artery compared to the proximal right coronary artery. Furthermore, hyperemia mean velocity, peak diastolic velocity, and diastolic velocity integral were significantly higher in the proximal left anterior descending coronary artery compared to proximal left circumflex and right coronary arteries (5).

For most subjects with angiographically normal vessels, the average proximal left anterior descending and circumflex flow velocity values are approximately 30 cm/s (mean diastolic velocity). Peak diastolic velocity ranges

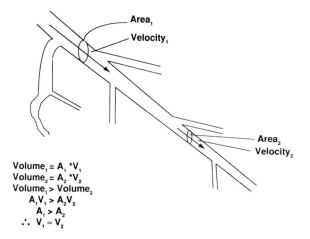

Figure 5 Diagram of branching coronary artery. Volumetric flow and cross-sectional vessel area gradually diminish from proximal to distal regions resulting in normalization of flow velocity. V = velocity; A = area.

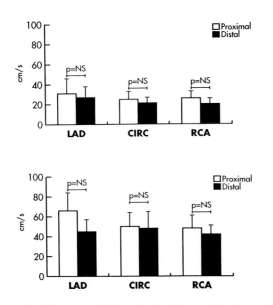

Figure 6 Normal and hyperemic flows in the left anterior descending, right coronary and circumflex arteries. LAD = left anterior descending coronary artery; CIRC = left circumflex coronary artery; RCA = right coronary artery. (Reprinted from Ref. 5.)

from 40–80 cm/s and peak systolic velocity from 10–20 cm/s. Right coronary artery and distal locations may be slightly reduced by ≤15% (4,5).

B. Diastolic–Systolic Phase Velocity Patterns

All three coronary arteries show a diastolic predominant pattern in both proximal and distal arterial segments. The normal diastolic/systolic flow velocity ratio (DSVR) >1.5 is maintained in both the proximal and distal segments in patients with normal left ventricles. This pattern is less marked in the right coronary artery, which had significantly lower peak diastolic to systolic flow velocity ratio than in the left anterior descending coronary artery (Fig. 7). However, right coronary branches extending over the inferior and lateral left ventricle (such as the posterior descending artery and posterolateral branches) will have distal DSVR resembling the left coronary artery (7). The reduced diastolic predominant pattern of the right coronary artery, described in canine coronary circulations, may be due to a relatively unimpeded right coronary systolic flow as a result of the lower right ventricular contractile force, compared to that of the left ventricle.

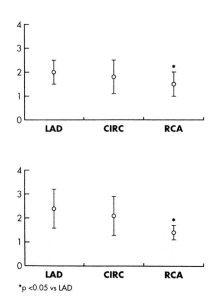

Figure 7 Diastolic/systolic velocity ratio in normal left anterior descending, right coronary and circumflex arteries. LAD = left anterior descending coronary artery, CIRC = left circumflex coronary artery, RCA = right coronary artery. (Reprinted from Ref. 5.)

C. Translesional Velocity Measurements

After diagnostic angiography or during angioplasty, the Doppler guidewire is passed through a standard angioplasty Y-connector attached to either a 6-French or 8-French guiding catheter. Heparin (5000–10,000 units intravenously) is always administered before inserting the wire into the coronary artery. The guidewire is then advanced into the artery. Baseline flow velocity data are acquired at least 1 cm proximal to the lesion in question. This location was selected to avoid a falsely high signal in the convergence acceleration zone of the arterial narrowing. The wire is then advanced at least 5–10 artery-diameter lengths (≈ 2 cm) beyond the stenosis, avoiding placement in any side branches. At this distance, laminar flow has been reconstituted and accurate distal velocity values can be obtained. Diffuse disease, serial lesions, or tandem lesions will elevate distal velocity. Simultaneous electrocardiogram and aortic pressure are displayed on the video monitor to assist in phasic cycle timing and to identify guide catheter damping that may obstruct normal flow. The translesional velocity assessment requires approximately 10 min. Coronary hyperemia is induced with intracoronary adenosine (6–18 μg) as described (6). In more than 500 patients studied in our laboratory, no heart block or hypotension has been observed with the use of adenosine in these doses. The effect of intracoronary adenosine is approximately 30–45 s, making this drug the hyperemic agent of choice for repetitive studies.

On traversing a lesion, an intralesional high jet velocity may be observed, but is not routinely sought because of the difficulty in obtaining a stable signal and potential for excessive lesion manipulation and activation in a critical area. In more than 200 studies performed in our laboratory with normal or mildly diseased vessels, no patient has had a Doppler guidewire complication (8). Nationwide, only 1 of 3000 cases has produced serious artery injury reported to the manufacturer or FDA.

D. Limitations and Assumptions

The measurement of Doppler velocity is a rapid, easy, and safe technique to assess the hemodynamically significant lesion with or without associated ischemic stress testing. However, despite the ease of application in daily use, the Doppler guidewire has several limitations. As with all ultrasound-based technology, placement of the transducer as near to parallel to blood flow as possible facilitates accurate peak velocity measurements (9). The position-dependent component of signal acquisition is minimized by utilizing a broad beam spread (27°), which makes most wire positions satisfactory for detecting the highest flow velocities. In tortuous arterial segments, further manipulation may be required to achieve satisfactory signals.

Considerable overlap exists in absolute velocity values, particularly in proximal abnormal arteries where signal contamination by high lesional jet velocities may result in falsely elevated or pseudonormalized proximal velocities. Although more complete velocity information is obtained with the spectral guidewire, which theoretically permits more accurate calculations of absolute flow, the variety of conditions in which true velocity values may be impaired is still under investigation (4,5).

IV. CLINICAL AND RESEARCH APPLICATIONS FOR DOPPLER FLOW VELOCITY

Measurement of coronary flow velocity has a great variety of routine clinical and research applications (Table 1). The versatility and ease of flow velocity signal acquisition provides an excellent opportunity to explore areas of the coronary circulation previously unobtainable in humans. Three major clinical uses have been the focus of current research and include angioplasty endpoint assessment, procedural flow monitoring, and physiological assessment of angiographically intermediately severe lesions.

A. Angioplasty Endpoint Assessment

During routine angioplasty, the Doppler guidewire can be used as the primary wire in >85% of attempts. The setup time of the flowire system is usually <10 min. It is easily incorporated into routine angioplasty procedures, provides additional physiological information on lesion severity and responses to balloon occlusions, and continuously monitors flow in the postprocedural period without frequent contrast injections. Flow velocity signals may be suboptimal in vessels that are severely angled or highly complex. In these vessels, the flowire (and other angioplasty wires as well) will have the most difficulty. In the highly tortuous artery, a 0.012–0.014-in. softer angioplasty guidewire can be used to position a small tracking catheter in the distal part of the vessel across the stenosis in question. The initial guidewire is then exchanged for the 0.018-in. flowire through the tracking catheter, and then the tracking catheter is withdrawn before velocity is measured. This method also provides the ability to obtain pressure gradient through the tracking catheter.

Angioplasty is performed routinely using the flowire. A wire-steering tool can be advanced over the distal end of the guidewire and then the wire is reconnected to its preamplifier cable connector. Rapid exchanges or guidewire trapping techniques for balloon catheter upsizing are recommended. A "dock" extension capability does exist for the long wire exchange technique. During angioplasty, monitoring of flow velocity demonstrates gratifying physiological responses to coronary occlusion, recanalization, and potential flow-limiting complications (4,5,10–13).

1. Flow Velocity Distal to Severe Lesions

The flow velocity findings distal to severe coronary stenoses demonstrate four common findings (4,10): (1) a decrease in mean velocity, usually <20 cm/s; (2) a mean proximal:distal flow velocity ratio >1.7; (3) an impaired diastolic/systolic phase pattern of coronary flow; and (4) an impaired distal coronary hyperemia (<2.0 × basal values).

Normally, the diastolic component of phasic flow velocity is nearly two times the systolic component. A normal DSVR is usually >1.8 for the left coronary artery (10). This value may vary normally among vessels, but in severe lesions, a DSVR <1.4 is common.

Although most studies report a coronary vasodilatory reserve ratio of 3.5–5 in normal patients (14) and experimental animal models, in our and other laboratories, lower values (≤2.5) have commonly been observed in patients with chest pain and angiographically normal arteries. It should be noted that in severe coronary lesions, proximally measured flow velocity can produce nearly normal hyperemia (and hence coronary reserve) due to augmentation of branch vessel flow (15). Flow velocity beyond severe stenoses is universally impaired (Figs. 8 and 9).

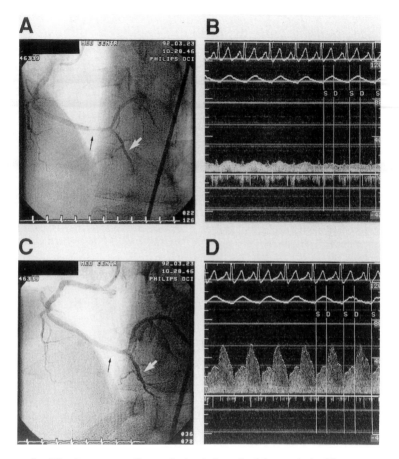

Figure 8 Distal coronary flow velocity is impaired beyond significant stenoses. (A) The right coronary artery (left anterior oblique projection) shows severe narrowing (small black arrow). Distal velocity is measured in the posterior descending branch (white arrow). (B) Abnormal distal flow with blunted diastolic/systolic velocity ratio and low mean velocity (10 cm/s). (C) Post-PTCA angiogram with minimal RCA lesion (black arrow). (D) Normal distal RCA velocity measured at location on panel (C) at white arrow. Phasic diastolic/systolic velocity ratio is now normal and mean velocity is increased to 30 cm/s.

During coronary balloon occlusion, flow velocity rapidly falls to near zero with an occasional low-frequency (wall thump) artifact visible. If persistent antegrade flow occurs, the balloon is undersized or there is collateral input distal to the balloon but proximal to the wire tip. If flow velocity initially falls to zero and then becomes visible below the baseline (negative), retrograde collateral flow is occurring (Fig. 10). The presence of retrograde

LAO   RAO

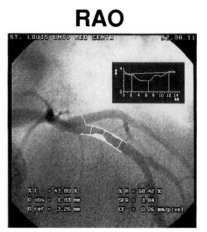
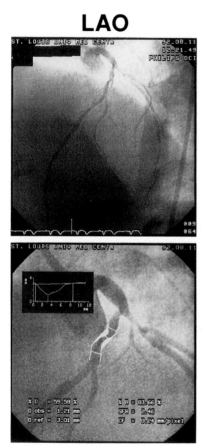

(A)

Figure 9 (A) Coronary cineangiogram in the left anterior oblique projection (LAO) and right anterior oblique projection (RAO) of the left anterior descending artery demonstrating a 60% diameter narrowing of the proximal segment by quantitation coronary angiography in the "worst" projections. (B) Coronary cineangiogram in the left anterior oblique projection (LAO) and right anterior oblique projection (RAO) of the right coronary artery also demonstrating a 63% diameter narrowing of an eccentric lesion. (C) Left anterior descending coronary blood flow velocity proximal and distal to the stenosis at baseline and during maximal hyperemia with 12 μg of intracoronary adenosine (flow velocity scale = 0–200 cm/s) before angioplasty. The distal flow velocity is abnormal. The phasic DSVR pattern is 1.1 (normal >1.7). The ratio of proximal to distal flow velocity is 1.9 (normal <1.7). Distal hyperemia was impaired with a flow reserve ratio of approximately 1.42 (normal >2.0). Note the *normal* proximal hyperemia that does not reflect flow limitation beyond the stenosis. (D) (top) Translesional pressure gradient before and after left anterior descending angioplasty at baseline and during maximal hyperemia with adenosine.

LAO RAO

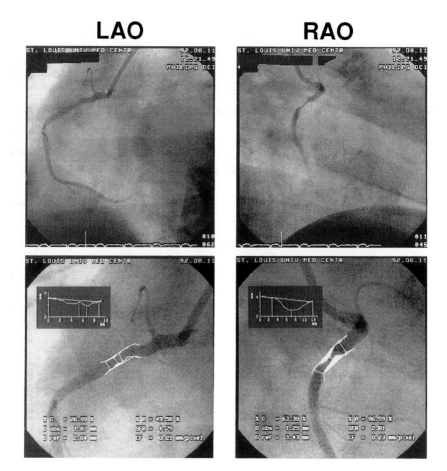

(B)

Hemodynamic tracings show electrocardiogram, aortic pressure, and distal coronary pressure (from the top down, 0–200 mm Hg scale). Resting gradient is 40 mm Hg, which widens to approximately 50 mm Hg at maximal hyperemia. Following angioplasty, baseline gradient is 8 mm Hg, which widens to approximately 20 mm Hg during maximal hyperemia. (bottom) Distal velocity shows equivalent values to proximal velocity before angioplasty with restoration of the phasic DSVR. Distal hyperemia is 2.1 times basal flow velocity in association with the reduction in the translesional gradient and angiographic stenosis. (E) Flow velocity data for the right coronary artery, proximal and distal to the eccentric stenosis. The DSVR is normal for a proximal right coronary artery. Proximal to distal flow velocity ratio was 0.9. Distal hyperemia was 2.9 times baseline flow. There was no translesional gradient at rest or during hyperemia in this artery. Angioplasty was not performed. (Reprinted with permission from Ref. 11.)

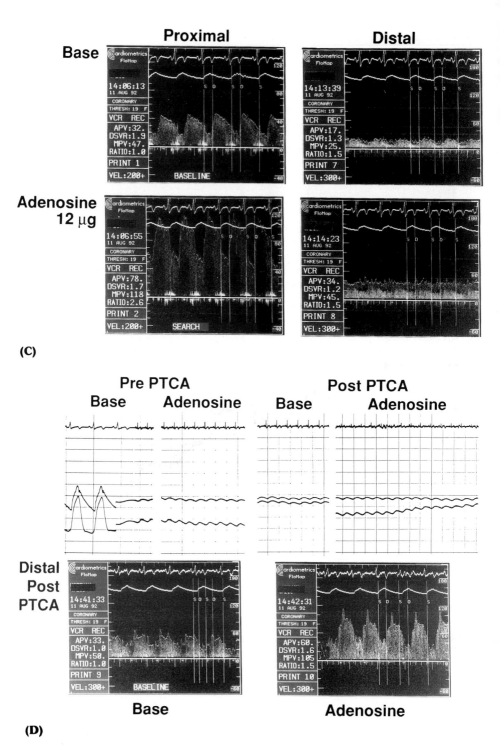

Figure 9 Continued

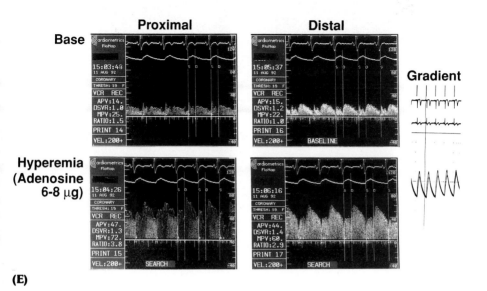

(E)

collateral flow velocity occurs in 10–15% of cases and may be a useful indicator of the patient's potential tolerance for prolonged balloon occlusions (13,16,17).

2. Flow Velocity After Angioplasty

A satisfactory angioplasty result is demonstrated by normalization of the four features described above. In addition, an immediate postischemic hyperemic velocity, usually >2 times basal flow, that equilibrates over the next 3–4 min to the new post-PTCA basal level, is often seen. Failure to observe post-PTCA balloon hyperemia likely indicates continued obstruction to flow at or below the level of the angioplasty site. To assure proper velocity assessment after PTCA, the guidewire tip should be free in the major vessel and not in a side branch. The guiding catheter should not obstruct flow into the vessel.

After successful angioplasty, the distal mean velocity is increased (usually >20–30 cm/s), or at least equal to the proximal preprocedural basal flow velocity. In a study by Segal et al. (10), the distal coronary velocity appeared to be more predictive of successful angiographic outcome of balloon angioplasty than did velocity found proximal to the stenosis. Average peak velocity (mean velocity) increased significantly from 19 ± 12 to 35 ± 16 cm/s ($p < 0.01$) in the distal vessel following angioplasty, whereas changes in proximal average peak velocity were increased but to a lesser degree (preangioplasty 34 ± 18 cm/s versus postangioplasty 41 ± 14 cm/s, $p = 0.04$) (Figs.

LAD with Collaterals

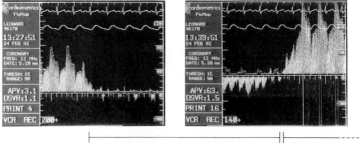

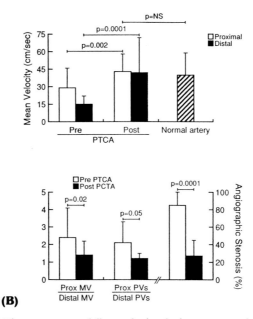

(B)

Figure 10 (A) Time sequence of flow velocity during coronary balloon occlusion in a patient with left anterior descending filled with collaterals originating from the right coronary artery. Note: retrograde collateral flow velocity below the baseline in a phasic pattern appearing after 15 s of coronary occlusion. On release of balloon occlusion, immediate antegrade hyperemia can be observed in the distal bed with loss of the retrograde flow pattern corresponding with successful angioplasty. LAD = left anterior descending coronary artery. (Reprinted with permission from Ref. 17.) (B) Mean velocity before and after angioplasty in proximal and distal regions (top). The reduction of the proximal to distal flow velocity ratio corresponds to traditional angiographic improvement (bottom). PVs = peak systolic velocity. PTCA = percutaneous transluminal angioplasty; MV = mean velocity. (From Ref. 4.)

10A, 11) (4). Coronary flow reserve was unchanged after angioplasty whether measured in the distal or proximal coronary artery.

3. Alterations of Phasic Coronary Flow After Angioplasty

Patent human vein grafts and occluded normal dog coronary arteries have demonstrated diastolic predominant flow, with mean diastolic to systolic flow ratios of >2.0. Occluded vein grafts and stenosed coronary arteries are different, demonstrating a decrease in diastolic flow compared to systolic flow, with a decrease in mean diastolic to systolic flow ratios to <1.3. Similar data were obtained in patients using an 80-channel pulsed Doppler velocimeter and surgically placed coronary artery probes (1,18,19).

A multicenter trial has been reported (10), showing coronary balloon angioplasty improved abnormal distal coronary artery flow velocity and normalized diastolic/systolic flow velocity patterns. In 38 patients undergoing balloon angioplasty and 12 patients without significant coronary artery disease serving as controls, velocity measurements were performed. Luminal stenosis diameter was reduced from $80 \pm 17\%$ to $33 \pm 23\%$. During this reduction in angiographic stenosis, flow velocity signals demonstrated a marked improvement in the diastolic to systolic average velocity ratio from 1.9 ± 0.6 to 2.8 ± 1.1, a 46% increase from preangioplasty values (normal ratios >2.0) (Fig. 11). The diastolic/systolic integral ratios also improved 48% over angioplasty values. Following relief of stenosis with angioplasty, the diastolic flow increased significantly with a limited increase in systolic flow. When measured distal to significant stenoses (>70%), the diastolic/systolic flow patterns were noted to be abnormal with low diastolic to systolic flow ratios (1.3 ± 0.5) when compared to patterns measured in coronary arteries of patients without significant stenoses (diastolic to systolic flow ratio = 1.8 ± 0.5, $p < 0.01$). Phasic velocity patterns were noted to normalize with significant increases in diastolic to systolic flow ratios within 10–15 min following successful balloon angioplasty. When measurements were performed in the proximal vessel, phasic diastolic/systolic flow patterns were not significantly different from those seen in normal vessels (diastolic to systolic flow ratios = 1.8 ± 0.8 vs 1.8 ± 0.5, $p = $ NS) and diastolic to systolic flow ratios did not increase significantly following angioplasty.

B. Monitoring Postprocedural Flow Velocity

The period immediately following a coronary intervention offers a unique opportunity to study important features of fluctuations in coronary blood flow. Methods to assess the stability of coronary flow following interventions have not been widely available. Periodic flow velocity measurements obtained over several minutes following interventional procedures were limited to proximal locations. These observations suggested coronary flow responses remained constant during this time period. However, coronary

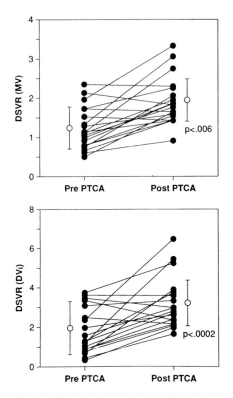

Figure 11 Diastolic/systolic velocity ratio (DSVR) before and after angioplasty. DVi=diastolic velocity integral; MV=mean velocity. (Modified from Ref. 10.)

flow can change, sometimes abruptly, in the minutes following an intervention as noted by Sinclair et al. (20). Approximately 50% of all in-lab abrupt closure events occurred during a 15-min monitoring period following completion of angioplasty. Redd et al. (21) monitored transstenotic pressure gradients for 1 to 2 min in 463 patients following angioplasty. A stable pressure gradient (stable flow) was associated with a lower risk of later abrupt closure, while a rising pressure gradient trend (declining flow) was associated with a much higher risk of later abrupt closure (4% vs. 17%). Based on these reports, coronary flow monitoring following coronary interventions appears to be useful (22–25).

The time course of hyperemia, changing vasomotor tone, coronary spasm, and abrupt closure may be elucidated. Cyclic flow variations, caused by repetitive accumulation and dislodgement of platelet aggregates and release of platelet-derived mediators at sites of coronary stenosis with endothelial injury, have been found to occur following angioplasty both in experimental animal models as well as in humans (22,23).

Anderson et al. (24) examined postprocedure flow velocity in patients treated by coronary balloon angioplasty or directional coronary atherectomy. The patients received standard doses of aspirin, heparin, nitrates, and calcium channel antagonists. Studies were conducted with a 0.018-in. flowire. Flow velocity measurements were obtained in patients with single, discrete lesions in one or more coronary arteries. Continuous flow monitoring was always performed with the Doppler guidewire distal to the subject lesion. The data were displayed on a video screen that contained separate channels for electrocardiogram and blood pressure from the physiological monitor, as well as the phasic velocity waveform and 15-min trend plot of the average peak velocity.

Two patterns of postprocedural coronary flow velocity monitoring have been associated with abrupt in-laboratory coronary occlusion (25).

1. Cyclic Flow Variations

The first cyclic flow variations were initially described by Folts et al. (26) and are now a well-characterized phenomenon in experimental animal models (27–29). The accumulation of platelet aggregates at sites of coronary arterial stenosis with endothelial injury over several minutes causes coronary flow to decline. A pressure gradient across the platelet mass develops and, once it is sufficiently great, the mass suddenly dislodges with an abrupt increase in flow. Agents that interfere with platelet function can abolish or attenuate cyclic flows (30,31). Cyclical coronary flow velocity variations have been associated with thrombus and abrupt closure during angioplasty (Fig. 12).

2. Downward Flow Velocity Trends

The second important abnormal flow pattern is a downward flow velocity trend first seen during rescue angioplasty for acute myocardial infarction. It was related to abrupt but symptomatically silent vessel closure occurring before angiography and was helpful to show vessel abnormality (Fig. 13).

Using flow velocity trend monitoring, adverse coronary flow phenomena that occur following coronary interventions can be documented and correlated to clinical events. In most patients, coronary flow velocity monitored for 30 min following an intervention remains stable at a higher value than that which is measured before intervention (24).

C. Assessing Lesions of Intermediate Severity

Although coronary angiography is the standard in diagnosing coronary artery disease, numerous studies have documented high inter- and intraobserver variability in judging the severity of coronary lesions (15,32). Angiography cannot distinguish the physiological significance of lesions, espe-

Pre

Post
During Flow Monitoring

Trend

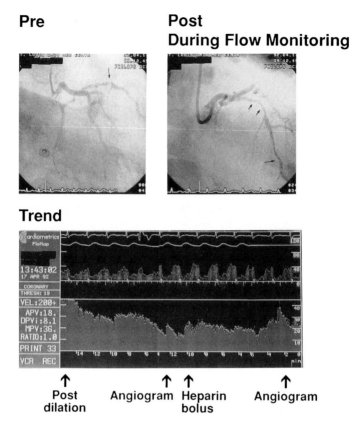

↑   ↑   ↑   ↑
Post   Angiogram Heparin   Angiogram
dilation   bolus

Figure 12 Cineangiographic frames of lesion in left anterior descending (LAD) artery stent/stenosis (top left panel, arrow) before (Pre) angioplasty. After (post) angioplasty (top right panel) during flow velocity monitoring, angiographic haziness and mottling (two arrows) at angioplasty site was associated with cyclical flow variations measured at tip of Doppler guidewire (distal arrow) as shown on lower panel flow velocity trend plot. Trend plot displays the following signals (from top to bottom): ECG, aortic pressure, phasic velocity (0–200 cm/s scale) and continuous plot of average velocity (APV) (0–50 cm/s scale). Events at arrows are described in text. (Reprinted with permission from Ref. 12.)

cially those of intermediate severity (>40% and <70–80% diameter stenosis). The relationship between the angiographic measurement of stenosis severity (including quantitative angiographically determined minimal lumen diameter) and the effect of a lesion on blood flow (15,33,34) has a high variable correlation depending on the model and techniques employed. In humans, a weak relationship exists between coronary flow reserve, as measured by Doppler techniques, and percent diameter stenosis (34).

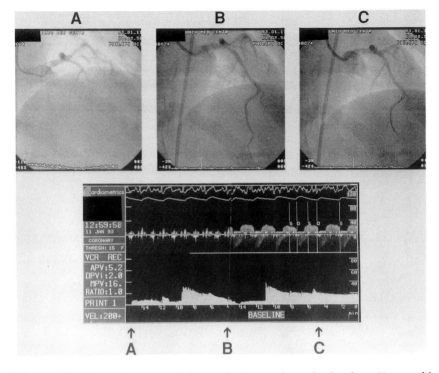

Figure 13 Cineangiogram and flow velocity trend monitoring in a 41-year-old woman during angioplasty for acute anterior myocardial infarction. (top) Cineangiographic frames obtained (A) before angioplasty, (B) after the initial balloon inflations, and (C) after the final inflations. (bottom) Composite average peak velocity trend plot (time scale is 15 min with 2-min time marks; velocity scale is 0–100 cm/s). Velocity at locations (A), (B), and (C) correspond to angiographic frames above. Note (A) immediately after guidewire advancement to the distal left anterior descending coronary artery, flow velocity near zero was recorded. (B) After the first dilatation, hyperemia was observed with a continued declining flow velocity trend to near zero, predicting vessel occlusion. (C) After the final dilation, hyperemia and flow velocity stabilized and vessel patency was maintained. The declining flow trend was one of the two abnormal trend patterns associated with abrupt in-laboratory vessel occlusion.

During diagnostic angiography, the flowire can be easily inserted into a 5- or 6-French diagnostic catheter through a standard angioplasty Y connector. The flowire can then be carefully advanced proximal to and then distal to the coronary lesion in question to confirm the physiological significance of these lesions.

After obtaining proximal velocity, distal basal velocity and adenosine-induced hyperemic velocity data are recorded. Ninety-eight percent of coronary

(A)

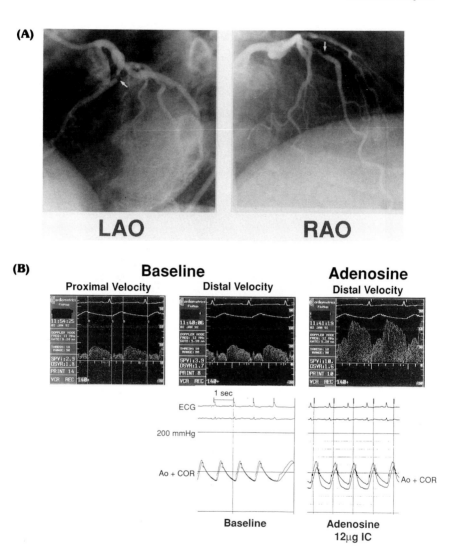

Figure 14 (A) Single vessel coronary artery disease with eccentric left anterior descending lesion (80% in the left anterior oblique view, 40% in the right anterior oblique view). White arrow is lesion. (Modified with permission from the American College of Cardiology (J Am Coll Cardiol 1993;22:449–458). (B) Flow velocity proximal and distal to the left anterior descending lesion in Figure 14A shows normal proximal flow, distal flow and distal hyperemic flow velocity. The translesional gradient, shown below the velocity panels, indicates 0 gradient at rest and 10 mm Hg gradient during peak hyperemia. No angioplasty was performed. This patient has done well at 12-month follow-up. (Reprinted with permission from Ref. 35.)

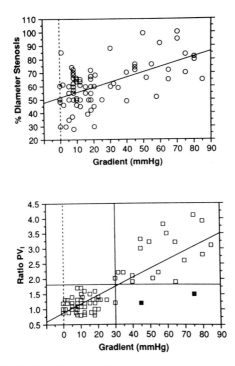

Figure 15 Individual patient correlations for translesional gradient and percent diameter stenosis (top panel) and gradient and proximal to distal flow velocity integral ratio (PVi) (bottom panel). There is a weak correlation with the translesional gradient and percent diameter stenosis. In the intermediate (40–70%) lesions, the correlation was poor. A proximal to distal velocity integral ratio of < 1.7 is associated with translesional gradients of < 30 mm Hg in all but two cases. The two dark squares indicate two patients with proximal right coronary arteries in whom the continuity equation applies but the branched model of flow does not. See text for discussion. (Reprinted with permission from Ref. 35.)

narrowings with translesional gradients of ≥30 mm Hg are associated by a proximal/distal total velocity integral ratio >1.7 (35) (Figs. 14, 15). The clinical characteristics of patients with intermediate lesions and translesional gradients are shown in Table 3. The flow velocity data for these two groups with translesional pressure gradients >20 mm Hg or <20 mm Hg separated significant differences in distal, but not proximal, flow velocity (Table 4).

The decremental distal flow relative to proximal flow velocity is predicted on a branched tube model, wherein flow is diverted away from the branch(es) with a high resistance (stenosis) to branches with lower resistances. As described earlier, normal coronary volumetric flow decreases over the proximal

Table 3 Clinical Data in Patients with Intermediate Lesions

	Group 1 (<20 mm Hg) (n = 56)	Group 2 (≥20 mm Hg) (n = 28)	p value
Male (%)	82	74	NS
Age, mean (range)	57 (28–78)	59 (31–80)	NS
History of MI (%)	26	18	NS
History of prior CABG (%)	5	2	NS
History of prior PTCA (%)	29	37	NS
Diabetes (%)	23	39	NS
Smoking (%)	57	53	NS
Hypertension (%)	79	53	NS
Medications (% of patients receiving)			
Calcium channel blocker	83	91	NS
Nitrates	61	44	NS
Beta blocker	35	35	NS

CABG = coronary artery bypass graft surgery; PTCA = percutaneous transluminal coronary angioplasty; MI = myocardial infarction.
Source: Reproduced with permission from Ref. 35.

Table 4 Flow Velocity for Patients with Intermediate Lesions

	Systolic integral (units)	Peak systolic velocity (cm/s)	Diastolic velocity integral (units)	Peak diastolic velocity (cm/s)	Total flow integral (units)	Mean velocity (cm/s)	Systolic to diastolic ratio
Proximal							
Gradient ≤20 mm Hg	8.7 ± 6.0	34 ± 19	22 ± 13	55 ± 25	31 ± 18	35 ± 16	0.7 ± 0.3
Gradient ≥20 mm Hg	8.9 ± 5.5	38 ± 21	38 ± 21	65 ± 35	38 ± 20	45 ± 23	0.6 ± 0.2
p value	0.873	0.483	0.0578	0.175	0.121	0.062	0.579
Distal							
Gradient ≤20 mm Hg	7.7 ± 5.4	31 ± 18	21 ± 14	49 ± 23	29 ± 18	33 ± 16	0.6 ± 0.2
Gradient ≥20 mm Hg	4.6 ± 6.5	17 ± 9	11 ± 8	26 ± 13	14 ± 9	17 ± 9	—
p value	0.038	0.0001	0.0001	0.0001	0.0001	0.0001	0.233
PVD							
Gradient ≤20 mm Hg	0.0628	0.085	0.449	0.032	0.118	0.075	0.435
Gradient ≥20 mm Hg	0.002	0.001	0.001	0.0001	0.0001	0.0001	0.202
Proximal to Distal Ratios							
Intermediate vs. severe							
Gradient ≤20 mm Hg	1.2 ± 0.4	1.1 ± 0.3	1.1 ± 0.2	1.1 ± 0.3	1.1 ± 0.2	1.1 ± 0.3	1.0 ± 2.3
Gradient ≥20 mm Hg	2.8 ± 1.9	2.5 ± 1.4	3.6 ± 3.7	2.7 ± 1.3	3.2 ± 1.9	3.9 ± 1.7	1.0 ± 0.6
t value	0.0001	0.0001	0.0001	0.0001	0.0001	0.0297	0.823

Source: Reprinted with permission from Ref. 2.

to distal course of the epicardial arteries. As the volume is distributed to the branches, the major coronary conduit vessels gradually decrease in the cross-sectional area. Since volume flow can be estimated from the product of mean flow velocity and cross-sectional area, velocity is maintained with a proximal to distal flow velocity ratio $= 1$ (5). The proximal/distal ratio will not apply in single tubes without branches where the continuity equation mandates equality of flow at any point along the circuit (Fig. 16). In arteries that are single tube conduits without branches, such as in very proximal segments of the right coronary artery or in bypass grafts, the proximal and distal blood flow velocities will be affected equally as determined by the continuity equation. Hence, the transstenotic velocity ratio is not useful for predicting stenosis severity. The proximal/distal flow velocity ratio cannot be used in three common conditions: (1) nonbranching conduits (i.e., saphenous vein grafts, left internal mammary artery (IMA), proximal right coronary artery); (2) ostial lesions without a proximal velocity; and (3) diffuse distal disease with increases in the distal velocity out of proportion to proximal vessel flow.

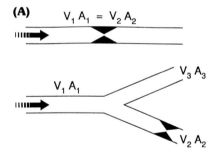

Figure 16 (A) Diagram of the single tube (top) and the branching tube (bottom) flow models. As stated by the continuity equation, volumetric flow is equivalent at any point along the single tube model. [Volume flow = cross-sectional area (A) × velocity (V)]. The continuity relationship is not applicable in the branching tube model where flow is diverted to regions of lower resistance. The velocity-area product at any point in the single tube model equals velocity-area at any other point along its course, whereas in the branching model the velocity × area$_1$ will not equal velocity × area$_2$ when a significant stenosis occurs. (B) The alterations in the flow in the branched tube model were validated in vitro, measuring directly the transstenotic gradient and instantaneous peak velocity (IPV) (top). Flow in the normal (nonstenotic) segment increases while flow beyond the stenosis (distal) is diminished since total flow must remain constant. The single tube model (bottom) shows equal average peak velocity (APV), despite a large translesional gradient due to the tube narrowing. (C) Data recorded for in vitro branching tube model. As the pressure gradient between proximal and distal regions increases, average peak flow velocity (APV) in the two branches are changed, consistent with increasing flow to the branch(es) of lowest resistance.

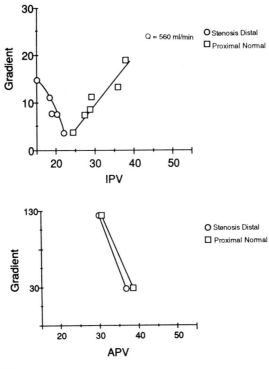

(B)

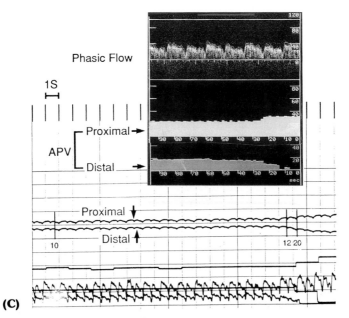

(C)

Figure 16 Continued

D. Quantification of Collateral Flow During Angioplasty

Only a qualitative and subjective angiographic determination of mature epicardial collateral vessels (37,38) or acutely recruitable collateral vessels during angioplasty (39–42) has been achieved. Although acutely recruitable and mature collateral flow has been shown during angioplasty by both hemodynamic (coronary occlusion wedge pressure) (42–44) and angiographic methods (37–42), neither technique is sufficiently quantitative to assess collateral function during hemodynamic or pharmacological perturbations. Detection of continued antegrade or newly appearing retrograde flow velocity can be observed by an angioplasty guidewire with a Doppler flowire that permits quantitative measurement of coronary blood flow velocity beyond severe and totally occluded arterial segments (5,16,17) (Fig. 17). During routine coronary angioplasty, retrograde collateral flow velocity during coronary balloon inflation may be observed in 10–20% of patients. When present, retrograde flow, seen as an inverted signal below the baseline, is a reproducible phenomenon. Retrograde flow velocity is associated with mature and acutely recruited angiographic collateral supply (5,16,17). In a recent multicenter study, quantitative coronary collateral flow velocity data were obtained during angioplasty to compare both angiographic grade and the spectrum of coronary collateral flow velocity relative to normal ante-

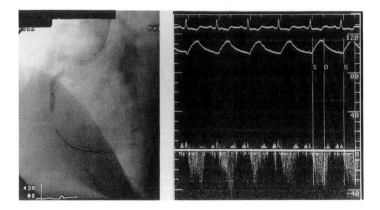

Figure 17 Balloon occlusion of a right coronary artery stenosis showing acutely recruited collateral flow velocity reversal. This acutely recruited collateral flow pattern is monophasic. Mature collateral flow via epicardial arteries is usually biphasic.

grade flow patterns (16). The spectral velocity signal was analyzed using the area beneath the diastolic and systolic velocity signals (flow velocity integral). If the direction of collateral flow was retrograde (coming toward) to the Doppler source (guidewire tip), the signal was assigned a negative value and displayed below baseline. Normal antegrade flow was computed in a similar fashion. Systolic and diastolic periods were demarcated by the upstroke and dicrotic notch of the simultaneous recorded aortic pressure. When feasible, coronary collateral pressure was measured with a 2.2 French tracking catheter and fluid-filled transducers.

In 22 patients undergoing routine coronary angioplasty for typical clinical indications, 10 patients had angiographic evidence of established collateral flow and 12 patients had acutely recruitable collateral flow velocity (17) (Table 5). All patients received 10,000 U intravenous bolus heparin with 1000 U/h infusion and 25 mg intravenous Demerol.

1. Collateral Appearance Time

The mean time of appearance of retrograde collateral flow velocity was 18 ± 7 s. Acutely recruitable collateral flow occurred in 11 patients: left-to-right collaterals in 5 patients, right-to-left collaterals in 5 patients, and ipsilateral collateral flow in 1 patient. Left-dominant and right-dominant circulations were present in 7 patients in both the acutely recruitable and mature collateral groups.

2. Retrograde Collateral Flow

Retrograde collateral flow was observed in 17 patients. Mean diastolic flow and diastolic and systolic velocity integrals were 13 ± 6 cm/s, 4.4 ± 4.8 U, and 3.7 ± 2.2 U, respectively (Table 6). These values were approximately 25% of corresponding antegrade flow velocity after angioplasty (all $p < 0.001$).

Table 5 Anatomical Characteristics of Collateral Flow in 21 Patients

Patients	(21)			
Men	(17)	Right coronary	Circumflex	Left anterior
Women	(4)	artery	artery	descending artery
PTCA artery		6	5	10
Angiographic collateral source artery		5	1	4

Angiographic collateral grade	(n)
0	11
1	3
2	5
3	2

Source: Reprinted with permission from Ref. 16.

Table 6 Characterization of Retrograde Coronary Collateral Flow Velocity During Angioplasty to Postprocedural Antegrade Flow

	Heart rate (beats/min)	Mean velocity (cm/s)	Diastolic flow velocity integral (units)	Systolic flow velocity integral (units)	D_i/S_i
Antegrade proximal	71 ± 10	35 ± 17	19.9 ± 11.3	8.3 ± 4.6	2.8 ± 1.3
Retrograde collateral	77 ± 11	13 ± 6	4.4 ± 4.8	3.7 ± 2.2	1.3 ± 1.4
p value	NS	.001	.001	.001	.02

D_i/S_i = diastolic/systolic velocity integral ratio.
Source: Reproduced with permission from Ref. 16.

The collateral data demonstrated that there were no differences between left-to-right collateral flow patterns with respect to mean velocity (MV), diastolic (D_1), or systolic (S_1) velocity integrals or the ratio of the diastolic to systolic flow integrals. In two patients, contralateral supply artery injection of nitroglycerin (20 μg) failed to increase coronary collateral flow. There was no difference between systolic or diastolic velocity between the right or left coronary artery. These data demonstrated a new method to quantitate collateral flow in patients during angioplasty and examine interventions postulated to alter human collateral supply.

E. Assessing Coronary Vasodilatory Reserve

Determination of coronary vasodilatory reserve has significant clinical importance in patients with coronary artery disease, syndrome X, follow-up responses after cardiac transplantation (especially during episodes of rejection), other atypical chest pain syndromes, and microvascular disorders (14,49-55). Coronary vasodilatory reserve is calculated as the ratio of hyperemic velocity to basal mean flow velocity and can be normalized for arterial pressure by dividing each flow value by the corresponding mean arterial pressure producing the reserve ratio (14,56).

Hyperemic blood flow velocity can be induced with a variety of vasodilatory agents, such as nitroglycerin (56,57), papaverine (58), adenosine (6,59), and contrast media (60). Only adenosine and papaverine produce maximal hyperemia. When assessing coronary artery disease, proximal and distal coronary flow reserve measurements are obtained at baseline and after intracoronary adenosine (6-8 μg in the right coronary artery and 12-18 μg in the left coronary artery) (6). Diminished distal basal arterial flow and hyperemia beyond lesions in question reflect significant translesional gradients and stenotic flow resistance as discussed earlier.

Coronary vasodilatory reserve has not been used to assess intermediate lesions or postinterventional procedure results for several reasons. First, improvement in coronary reserve has not been consistently demonstrated after angioplasty (56,61,62). Coronary flow reserve has not been accepted as a determinant of lesion significance in humans because of the wide range of base and hyperemic values and lack of angiographic correlations. Factors such as infarcted myocardium, hypertension, and microvascular disease impair normal hyperemia. Basal flow may be increased with tachycardia or hypertension, also reducing the coronary vasodilatory reserve ratio (Fig. 18). In addition, prior studies of coronary reserve used measurements of proximal vessel hyperemia. These results would not differentiate diversion of flow to small proximal branches from a flow-limiting stenosis, and thus hyperemia obtained in the proximal location would not necessarily reflect the significant flow-limiting nature of a stenosis. Using the distal velocity data after angioplasty, coronary vasodilatory reserve ratios obtained with the flowire, as in other similar studies (56,61,62), were not significantly increased after angioplasty, averaging 2.3 ± 0.8 both before and after the procedure (10).

F. Assessing Flow Velocity After Atherectomy and Stent Placement

Studies are under way to provide comparisons of atherectomy, laser, and Rotablator influences on postprocedural flow characteristics (43,45–48). Preliminary studies by Deychak et al. (47,48) suggest suboptimal improvement

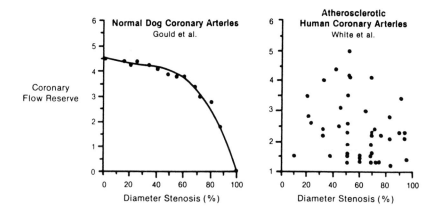

Figure 18 Comparison of coronary flow reserve in experimental canine model (left) and in patients (right). (Reprinted with permission from Ref. 50.)

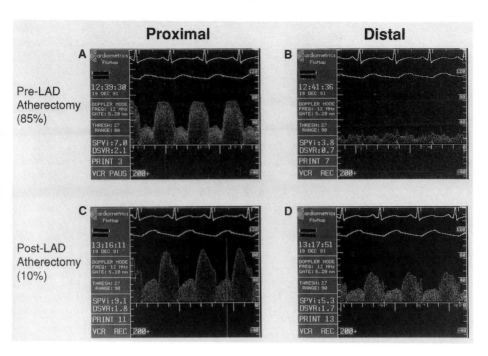

(A)

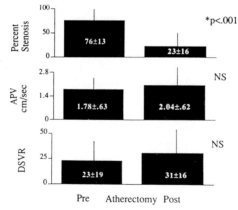

(B)

Figure 19 (A) Flow velocity proximal and distal to the left anterior descending (85%) lesion before (top) and after (bottom) directional coronary atherectomy. Although angiographic result was excellent, distal flow did not achieve equalization to proximal preprocedural flow values. (B) Increases in average peak velocity (APV) and diastolic/systolic velocity ratio (DSVR) after directional atherectomy. (Reprinted from Ref. 2.) (C) Increases in average peak velocity (APV) diastolic/systolic velocity ratio (DSVR) and after excimer laser and laser + angioplasty. (Reprinted from Ref. 2.)

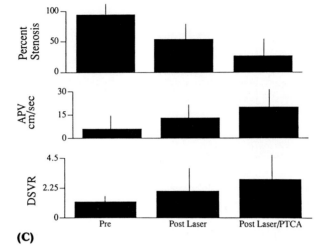

(C)

Figure 19 Continued

in flow after atherectomy and laser angioplasty compared to standard balloon angioplasty (Fig. 19).

V. THALLIUM SCINTIGRAPHIC CORRELATIONS WITH FLOW VELOCITY FINDINGS

In a preliminary study by Donohue et al. (36), resting translesional flow velocity measurements made with a Doppler guidewire were compared to translesional pressure gradients and perfusion defects measured by exercise or adenosine thallium scintigraphy. Among 23 patients with negative thallium tests, 22 (96%) also had normal flow velocity and pressure gradient criteria derived from a previous study of translesional gradient correlations (35). Among 26 patients with positive thallium tests, 15 (42%) had normal translesional flow velocity (and pressure) criteria. Hyperemic flow responses improved the specificity of thallium results (Fig. 20), but still yielded 20% falsely positive scans in lesions with translesional pressure gradients < 15 mm Hg. More interesting was the fact that 14 of the 15 patients who had positive thallium scans but who did not have impaired flow by flow velocity criteria had insignificant translesional pressure gradients, with an average gradient of 10 ± 8 mm Hg. None of the 15 patients underwent angioplasty and all have done well clinically at 7 ± 5 months (2–12 months) follow-up (8). Although thallium scintigraphy is currently the standard for determining lesion significance, direct assessment of postlesional flow responses may

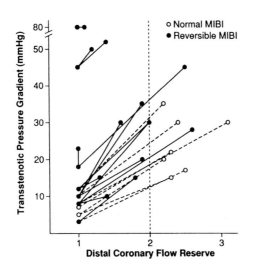

Figure 20   Correlations for adenosine sestamibi, translesional gradient, and flow velocity. Flow velocity reserve >2.0 is associated with normal perfusion studies. Flow reserve <2.0 is associated with positive scans, despite many patients with translesional gradients <20 mm Hg.

prove to be equivalent or superior and can be easily obtained at the time of diagnostic study.

VI. CONCLUSIONS

The goal of interventions in coronary artery disease is to relieve ischemia by restoration of coronary blood flow. However, angiography is a poor predictor of lesion physiology for intermediate narrowings and is limited in its ability to assess postprocedure flow results. Similarly, stress scintigraphy is an indirect, noninvasive method to assess blood flow with a substantial but unavoidably low specificity. Translesional pressure gradients are difficult to measure, especially during diagnostic studies, are prone to error in tortuous vessels, and provide minimal information about microcirculatory vasodilator capacity. The Doppler guidewire flow velocity technology can assess the blood flow responses distal to coronary lesions. Numerous studies have shown that neither thallium testing nor angiography is sufficiently reliable to distinguish the physiological significance of "marginal" coronary lesions. In such cases, flow velocity measured distal to a coronary stenosis can physiologically distinguish intermediate and severe coronary lesions.

During and after coronary interventions, monitoring flow velocity can assist the operator in selecting more vigorous mechanical strategies or in recognizing limited flow and preparing for surgery or stent placement to avoid abrupt vessel closure. Incorporation of flow velocity studies into clinical practice will provide an objective measurement on which to base decisions for coronary interventions and will quantitatively assess results of new procedures.

ACKNOWLEDGMENTS

The authors wish to thank the J.G. Mudd Cardiac Catheterization Laboratory and Donna Sander for manuscript preparation.

REFERENCES

1. Kern MJ. Intracoronary flow velocity: current techniques and clinical applications of Doppler catheter methods. In: Tobis JM, Yock PG, eds. Intravascular Ultrasound Imaging. New York: Churchill Livingstone, 1992:93–111.
2. Kern MJ, Anderson HV (eds). A symposium: the clinical applications of the intracoronary Doppler guidewire flow velocity in patients: understanding blood flow beyond the coronary stenosis. Am J Cardiol 1993;71:1D–86D.
3. Doucette JW, Corl PD, Payne HM, et al. Validation of a Doppler guide wire for intravascular measurement of coronary artery flow velocity. Circulation 1992;85:1899–1911.
4. Ofili EO, Kern MJ, Labovitz AJ, St. Vrain JA, Segal J, Aguirre F, Castello R. Analysis of coronary blood flow velocity dynamics in angiographically normal and stenosed arteries before and after endoluminal enlargement by angioplasty. J Am Coll Cardiol 1993;21:308–316.
5. Ofili EO, Labovitz AJ, Kern MJ. Coronary flow velocity dynamics in normal and diseased arteries. In: Kern MJ, Anderson HV (eds): A symposium: the clinical applications of the intracoronary Doppler guidewire flow velocity in patients: understanding blood flow beyond the coronary stenosis. Am J Cardiol 1993;71: 3D–9D.
6. Wilson RF, Wyche K, Christensen BV, Zimmer S, Laxson DD. Effects of adenosine on human coronary arterial circulation. Circulation 1990;82:1595–1606.
7. Heller LI, Villegas BJ, Weiner BH. Phasic coronary artery flow following right coronary artery PTCA (abstr). Cathet Cardiovasc Diagn 1993;29:89.
8. Mechem CJ, Kern MJ, Aguirre F, Cauley M, Stonner T. Safety and outcome of angioplasty guidewire Doppler instrumentation in patients with normal or mildly diseased coronary arteries (abstr). Circulation 1992;86:I-323.
9. Hatle L, Angelsen B. Flow velocity and volumetric principle. In: Doppler Ultrasound in Cardiology. Philadelphia: Lea & Febiger, 1985:15.
10. Segal J, Kern MJ, Scott NA, King SB III, Doucette JW, Hueser RR, Ofili E, Siegel R. Alterations of phasic coronary artery flow velocity in man during percutaneous coronary angioplasy. J Am Coll Cardiol 1992;20:276–286.

11. Kern MJ, Flynn MS, Caracciolo EA, Bach RG, Donohue TJ, Aguirre FV. Use of translesional coronary flow velocity for interventional decisions in a patient with multiple intermediately severe coronary stenoses. Cathet Cardiovasc Diagn 1993;29:148–153.

12. Kern MJ, Dononue T, Bach R, Aguirre F, Bell C. Monitoring cyclical coronary blod flow alterations after coronary angioplasty for stent restenosis with a Doppler guidewire. Am Heart J 1993;125:1159–1161.

13. Ofili E, Kern MJ, Tatineni S, et al. Detection of coronary collateral flow by a Doppler-tipped guidewire during coronary angioplasty. Am Heart J 1991;122:221–225.

14. Wilson RF, Laughlin DE, Ackell PH, et al. Transluminal subselective measurement of coronary artery blood flow velocity and vasodilator reserve in man. Circulation 1985;72:82–92.

15. Gould KL, Lipscomb K, Hamilton GW. Physiologic basis for assessing critical coronary stenosis: instantaneous flow response and regional distribution during coronary hyperemia as measures of coronary flow reserve. Am J Cardiol 1974;33:87–94.

16. Donohue TJ, Kern MJ, Aguirre FV, Bell C, Penick D, Ofili E. Comparison of hemodynamic and pharmacologic perturbations of coronary collateral flow velocity in patients during angioplasty (abstr). J Am Coll Cardiol 1992;19:383A.

17. Kern MJ, Dononue TJ, Bach RG, Aguirre FV, Caracciolo EA, Ofili EO. Quantitating coronary collateral flow velocity in patients during coronary angioplasty using a Doppler guidewire. In: Kern MJ, Anderson HV, eds, A Symposium: The Clinical Applications of the Intracoronary Doppler Guidewire Flow Velocity in Patients: Understanding Blood Flow Beyond the Coronary Stenosis. Am J Cardiol 1993;71:34D–40D.

18. Kajiya F, Ogasawara Y, Tsujioka K, et al. Evaluation of human coronary blood flow with an 80 channel 20 MHz pulsed Doppler velocimeter and zero-cross and Fourier transform methods during cardiac surgery. Circulation 1986;74(suppl III):III 53–III 60.

19. Kajiya F, Tsujioka K, Ogasawara Y, et al. Analysis of flow characteristics in post-stenotic regions of the human coronary artery during bypass graft surgery. Circulation 1987;76:1092–1100.

20. Sinclair IN, McCabe CH, Sipperly ME, Baim DS. Predictors, therapeutic options and long-term outcome of abrupt reclosure. Am J Cardiol 1988;61:61G–66G.

21. Redd DCB, Roubin GS, Leimgruber PP, Abi-Mansour P, Douglas JS, King SB. The transstenotic pressure gradient trend as a predictor of acute complications after percutaneous transluminal coronary angioplasty. Circulation 1987;76:792–801.

22. Anderson HV, Yao S-K, Murphree SS, Buja LM, McNatt JM, Willerson JT. Cyclic coronary artery flow in dogs after coronary angioplasty. Coronary Artery Disease 1990;1:717–723.

23. Eichhorn EJ, Grayburn PA, Willard JE, et al. Spontaneous alterations in coronary blood flow velocity before and after coronary angioplasty in patients with severe angina. J Am Coll Cardiol 1991;17:43–52.

24. Anderson HV, Kirkeeide RL, Stuart Y, Smalling RW, Heibig J, Willerson JT. Coronary artery flow monitoring following coronary interventions. In: Kern MJ, Anderson HV, eds. A Symposium: The Clinical Applications of the Intracoronary Doppler Guidewire Flow Velocity in Patients: Understanding Blood Flow Beyond the Coronary Stenosis. Am J Cardiol 1993;71:62D–69D.

25. Kern MJ, Aguirre FV, Donohue TJ, Bach RG, Caracciolo EA, Flynn MS. Coronary flow velocity monitoring after angioplasty associated with abrupt reocclusion. Am Heart J 1994;127:436–438.

26. Folts JD, Crowell EB, Rowe GG. Platelet aggregation in partially obstructed vessels and its elimination with aspirin. Circulation 1976;54:365–370.

27. Eidt JF, Ashton J, Golino P, McNatt J, Buja LM, Willerson JT. Thromboxane A2 and serotonin mediate coronary blood flow reductions in unsedated dogs. Am J Physiol 1989;257:H873–H882.

28. Yao S-K, Rosolowski M, Anderson HV, Golino P, McNatt JM, DeClerck F, Buja LM, Willerson JT. Combined thromboxane A2 synthetase inhibition and receptor blockade are effective in preventing spontaneous and epinephrine-induced canine coronary cyclic flow variations. J Am Coll Cardiol 1990;16: 705–713.

29. Yao S-K, Ober JC, McNatt J, et al. ADP plays an important role in mediating platelet aggregation and cyclic flow variations in vivo in stenosed and endothelium-injured canine coronary arteries. Circ Res 1992;70:39–48.

30. Ashton JH, Schmitz JM, Campbell WB, et al. Inhibition of cyclic flow variations in stenosed canined coronary arteries by thromboxane A2/prostaglandin H2 receptor antagonists. Circ Res 1986;59:568–578.

31. Anderson HV, Revana M, Rosales O, et al. Intravenous administration of monoclonal antibody to the platelet GPIIb/IIIa receptor to treat abrupt closure during coronary angioplasty. Am J Cardiol 1992;69:1373–1376.

32. White CW, Wright CB, Doty DB, et al. Does visual interpretation of the coronary arteriogram predict the physiologic importance of a coronary stenosis? N Engl J Med 1984;310:819–824.

33. Gould KL, Kelley KO. Physiological significance of coronary flow velocity and changing stenosis geometry during coronary vasodilation in awake dogs. Circ Res 1982;50:695–704.

34. Wilson RF, Marcus ML, White CW. Prediction of the physiologic significance of coronary arterial lesion by quantitative lesion geometry in patients with limited coronary artery disease. Circulation 1987;75:723–732.

35. Donohue TJ, Kern MJ, Aguirre FV, Bach RG, Wolford T, Bell CA, Segal J. Assessing the hemodynamic significance of coronary artery stenoses: analysis of translesional pressure-flow velocity relationships in patients. J Am Coll Cardiol 1993;22:449–458.

36. Donohue T, Kern MJ, Miller DD, et al. Improved decision making for coronary interventions: comparison of intracoronary lesion flow dynamics versus ischemic stress testing (abstr). J Am Coll Cardiol 1993;21:152A.

37. Gensini GG, DaBruto Costa BC. The coronary collateral circulation in living man. Am J Cardiol 1969;24:393–400.

38. Helfant RH, Vokonas PS, Gorlin R. Functional importance of the human coronary collateral circulation. N Engl J Med 1971;2384:1277–1281.

39. Cohen M, Rentrop KP. Limitation of myocardial ischemia by collateral circulation during sudden controlled coronary artery occlusion in human subjects: a prospective study. Circulation 1986;74:469–476.
40. Khaja F, Sabbah HN, Brymer JF, Stein PD. Influence of coronary collaterals on left ventricular function in patients undergoing coronary angioplasty. Am Heart J 1988;116:1174–1180.
41. Rentrop KP, Thornton JC, Feit F, Van Buskirk M. Determinants and protective potential of coronary arterial collateral as assessed by an angioplasty model. Am J Cardiol 1988;61:677–684.
42. Rentrop KP, Cohen M, Blanke H, Phillips RA. Changes in collateral channel filling immediately after controlled coronary artery occlusion by an angioplasty balloon in human subjects. J Am Coll Cardiol 1985;5:587–592.
43. Dervan JP, McKay RG, Baim DS. Assessment of the relationship between distal occluded pressure and angiographically evident collateral flow during coronary angioplasty. Am Heart J 1987;114:491–497.
44. Probst P, Zangl W, Pachinger O. Relation of coronary arterial occlusion pressure during percutaneous transluminal coronary angioplasty to presence of collaterals. Am J Cardiol 1985;55:1264–1269.
45. Younis L, Kern MJ, Bach R, et al. Post-procedural normalization of coronary flow dynamics following successful atherectomy, PTCA and stenting: analysis by intracoronary spectral Doppler. J Am Coll Cardiol 1993;21:79A.
46. Bach RG, Kern MJ, Bell C, Donohue T, Aguirre F. Clinical application of coronary flow velocity for stent placement during coronary angioplasty. Am Heart J 1993;125:873–877.
47. Deychak YA, Thompson MA, Rohrbeck SC, et al. A Doppler guidewire used to assess coronary flow during directional coronary atherectomy (abstr). Circulation 1992;86:I-122.
48. Segal J. Applications of coronary flow velocity during angioplasty and other coronary interventional procedures. In: Kern MJ, Anderson HV, eds. A Symposium: The Clinical Applications of the Intracoronary Doppler Guidewire Flow Velocity in Patients: Understanding Blood Flow Beyond Coronary Stenosis. Am J Cardiol 1993;71:17D–25D.
49. Treasure CB, Vita JA, Ganz P, Ryan TJ Jr, Schoen FJ, Vekshtein VI, Yeung AC, Mudge GH, Alexander W, Selwyn AP, Fish RD. Loss of the coronary microvascular response to acetylcholine in cardiac transplant patients. Circulation 1992;86:1156–1164.
50. Wilson RF. Assessment of the human coronary circulation using a Doppler catheter. In: Parmely WW, ed. A Symposium: Proceedings of the Second International Heart Failure Workshop. Am J Cardiol 1991;67:44D–56D.
51. Marcus ML, White CW. Coronary flow reserve in patients with normal coronary angiograms. (Editorial) J Am Coll Cardiol 1985;6:1254–1256.
52. McGinn AL, Wilson RF, Olivari MT, Homans DC, White CW. Coronary vasodilator reserve after human orthotopic cardiac transplantation. Circulation 1988;78:1200–1209.
53. Cannon RO, Leon MB, Watson RM, Rosing DR, Epstein SE. Chest pain and "normal" coronary arteries—role of small coronary arteries. Am J Cardiol 1985;55:50B–60B.

54. Nitenberg A, Tavolaro O, Benvenuti C, et al. Recovery of a normal coronary vascular reserve after rejection therapy in acute human cardiac allograft rejection. Circulation 1990;81:1312–1318.
55. Klocke FJ. Measurements of coronary blood flow and degree of stenosis: current clinical implications and continuing uncertainties. J Am Coll Cardiol 1983;1:31–41.
56. Kern MJ, Deligonul U, Vandormael M, et al. Impaired coronary vasodilator reserve in the immediate postcoronary angioplasty period: analysis of coronary artery flow velocity indexes and regional cardiac venous efflux. J Am Coll Cardiol 1989;13:860–872.
57. Kern MJ, Presant S, Deligonul U, Vandormael M, Kennedy HL. The effects of coronary angioplasty on nitroglycerin-induced augmentation of regional myocardial blood flow. J Interventional Cardiol 1988;1:121–130.
58. Wilson RF, White CW. Intracoronary papaverine: an ideal coronary vasodilator for studies of the coronary circulation in conscious humans. Circulation 1986; 73:444–451.
59. Kern MJ, Deligonul U, Tatineni S, Serota H, Aguirre F, Hilton TC. Intravenous adenosine: continuous infusion and low dose bolus administration for determination of coronary vasodilatory reserve in patients with and without coronary artery disease. J Am Coll Cardiol 1991;18:718–729.
60. Hodgson JM, Williams DO. Superiority of intracoronary papaverine to radiographic contrast for measuring coronary flow reserve in patients with ischemic heart disease. Am Heart J 1987;114:704–710.
61. Wilson RF, Johnson MR, Marcus ML, Aylward PEG, Skorton DJ, Collins S, White CW. The effect of coronary angioplasty on coronary flow reserve. Circulation 1988;77:873–885.
62. Laarman GJ, Serruys PW, Suryapranata H, et al. Inability of coronary blood flow reserve measurements to assess the efficacy of coronary angioplasty in the first 24 hours in unselected patients. Am Heart J 1991;122:631–639.
63. Donohue T, Kern MJ, Wolford T, Bach R, Aguirre F, Miller L. The effects of epicardial coronary spasm in intracoronary flow velocity and pressure gradient in a patient after cardiac transplantation. Am Heart J 1992;124:1645–1648.
64. Di Mario C, de Feyter PJ, Gil R, de Jaegere P, Strikwerda S, Serruys PW. Intracoronary blood flow velocity and transstenotic pressure gradient simultaneously assessed with sensor-tip Doppler and pressure guidewires. Circulation 1992;86:I-122.
65. Al-Joundi B, Kern MJ, Donohue T, Bach R, Aguirre FV, Chaitman BR, Miller DD. Is intravenous dipyridamole coronary hyperemia reversal by aminophylline equivalent to adenosine cessation? Comparison using continuous intracoronary spectral flow velocity measurements (abstr). J Am Coll Cardiol 1993;21:420A.
66. Kern MJ, Aguirre F, Tatineni S, et al. Enhanced coronary blood flow velocity during intra-aortic balloon counterpulsation in critically ill patients. J Am Coll Cardiol 1993;21:359–368.
67. Kern MJ, Aguirre F, Bach R, Donohue T, Segal J. Augmentation of coronary blood flow by intra-aortic balloon pumping in patients after coronary angioplasty. Circulation 1993;87:500–511.
68. Bach RG, Kern MJ, Donohue T, Aguirre F, Penick D. Comparison of arterial and venous coronary bypass conduits: analysis of intravessel blood flow velocity characteristics (abstr). Circulation 1992;86:I-181.

4

The Practical Application of Quantitative Angiographic Methods for Investigating Newer Coronary Interventions and Balloon Angioplasty

Jeffrey J. Popma
Washington Hospital Center, Washington, DC

Richard E. Kuntz
Harvard Medical School and Beth Israel Hospital, Boston, Massachusetts

I. INTRODUCTION

Over the past several years, coronary angioplasty has subsumed a wide variety of mechanical techniques, and analytical methods used to assess their results have become increasingly sophisticated. Accordingly, our understanding of both the mechanism of lumen improvement and the underlying factors responsible for the eventual angiographic and clinical outcomes has become more complex. Angiographic restenosis, once conceptually described as a fairly unpredictable "all or none" phenomenon (1), is now thought to be a continuous and ubiquitous process, largely dependent upon the acute procedural result (2,3). Along with such shifts toward more quantitative conceptual frameworks used to describe restenosis (models or paradigms) (4) comes the need to measure precisely the acute result rather than rely on the definitions of whether or not a residual diameter stenosis <50% was achieved or to categorically estimate deciles of visually determined final % diameter stenoses (10, 20, 30%, etc). Consequently, the current analysis of balloon angioplasty and newer devices will rely increasingly upon computer-assisted quantitative measuring systems for the angiogram (and possibly the intravascular ultrasound videotape) that maximize precision and reproducibility, while minimizing bias and measurement error. Moreover, such desirable accurate data will be further analyzed by using statistical models in order to control the multitude of new technology variables that introduce noise and confounding. In essence, the days of simple comparisons among competing devices are likely gone as the complete arena of coronary angioplasty expands to include lesion-specific devices, and devices with minimal inherent differences. On the other hand, a vigilant approach toward the practical applications of these methods will help to assure that the analytical "tail" will not wag the "dog" of coronary angioplasty.

For the clinician, a basic understanding of the angiographic tools currently used to evaluate balloon and new device angioplasty is of critical importance, since the results and clinical interpretations of randomized trials, such as CAVEAT, CCAT, and STRESS, are based on different quantitative angiographic systems and anatomical indices used in these trials (5–7). Likewise, the clinician must also be familiar with multivariable linear and logistic regression analyses that identify independent clinical and angiographic factors responsible for late outcome. Although these analytical methods appear formidable to those not trained in quantitative angiographic or statistical techniques, obtaining a practical understanding of their features is not difficult.

Given these issues, the purposes of this chapter are: (1) to review the tools available for the quantitative angiographic determination of lesion severity and their interventional result; (2) to outline the methodological and statistical considerations used to assess these outcomes; and (3) to develop a conceptual framework for the strategic evaluation of balloon and new device angioplasty in future randomized and nonrandomized studies.

II. QUALITATIVE AND QUANTITATIVE METHODS OF ASSESSING LESION SEVERITY

A. Qualitative Estimates of Lesion Severity

Although visual estimates of stenosis severity have been widely used in the clinical arena to assess the immediate angiographic result after coronary angioplasty, they have historically had poor inter- and intra-observer agreement (8–14). Compared with digital caliper or edge-detection methods, visual readings consistently overestimate preprocedural and underestimate postprocedural % diameter stenoses (8,15). It is not surprising, therefore, that angiographic success rates (< 50% diameter stenosis) are higher using clinical site angiographic readings than those reported using angiographic core laboratory determinations; these clinical site-core laboratory disagreements may account for a 10% difference in overall procedural success rates (6,16,17).

Visual readings are also unable to accurately estimate pre- and postprocedural lumen diameters, accounting for visual estimates of preprocedural %

diameter stenoses that are physiologically untenable (18,19). A 3.0-mm vessel with a 95% stenosis would have a minimal lumen diameter < 0.2 mm requiring such high coronary perfusion pressures that thrombosis and total occlusion would likely occur (19).

With continued exposure and feedback of quantitative angiographic readings to the clinician, it is possible that the investigator's eye can be "retrained" and provide more accurate and reproducible estimates of stenosis severity (20). Panel or consensus readings may also improve the reproducibility of visual readings (15). Despite these potential areas for improvement, visual estimates of stenosis severity should be considered suboptimal for research purposes, and more quantitative methods should be employed.

B. Caliper Methods

The use of digital or hand-held calipers is perhaps the simplest and most inexpensive method to quantitate lesion severity before and after coronary intervention (21–23). Using the injection catheter as the calibration standard, normal, and minimal lumen diameters may be estimated by adjusting the calipers to encompass the visually determined arterial borders. In general, it is recommended that the cineangiogram be magnified and projected upon a flat surface for quantitative measurements, although the arterial edges often become indistinct with higher magnifications. Properly applied, this method appears to be moderately correlated ($r = 0.89$) with relative diameter stenosis measurements obtained using automated-edge detection methods (22,23). The digital caliper method has been used in large-scale interventional trials, such as the Bypass Angioplasty Revascularization Investigation (BARI) (24).

Despite the clinical utility of digital calipers, several important limitations of this technique should be noted. If caliper measurements are obtained from nonmagnified images, the correlation with automated edge-detection algorithms may be less favorable ($r = 0.72$), potentially due to increased interobserver variability ($r = 0.63$ vs. $r = 0.95$ for quantitative angiography) (25). Absolute vessel dimensions (reference vessel and minimal lumen diameters) may also be systematically overestimated using digital caliper versus edge-detection methods (Fig. 1) (23,26). In one series, digital calipers overestimated edge-detection readings of vessel diameter by 0.44 ± 0.24 mm in those vessels > 2.5 mm (23); this systematic overestimation by the digital caliper method has also been shown using radiographic phantoms (27). Variabilities in estimates of % diameter stenosis have ranged from 7.4%–12.4% using digital calipers in validated angiographic core laboratories (22,23). Thus, studies using this approach must have sufficient sample size to be confident of neutral results (23), due to its reduced precision compared with automated edge-detection methods (22,23,25).

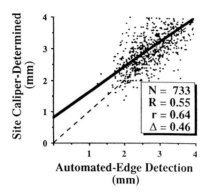

Figure 1 Clinical site digital-caliper readings were compared with angiographic core laboratory edge-detection (ARTREK) readings in a series of 733 lesions obtained from patients enrolled in the New Approaches to Coronary Intervention (NACI) Registry. Overall intraclass correlation (R) was 0.55 and the Pearson's correlation coefficient (r) was 0.64. The average overestimation of digital caliper readings compared with automated edge-detection readings (Δ) was 0.46 mm.

C. Quantitative Angiographic Methods

To allow more reproducible estimates of lesion severity, several computer-assisted methods have been used. These systems have sought: (1) to provide an accurate assessment of absolute and relative coronary artery dimensions; (2) to minimize the degree of observer interaction (thereby reducing operator variability); and (3) to shorten the time required for quantitative image processing and analysis (28–30). To these ends, a number of institutional and commercially available quantitative angiographic systems were developed, including the Cardiovascular Angiographic Analysis System (CAAS) (30), ARTREK (28), Cardiovascular Measurement System (CMS) (31), and the Duke University Quantitative/Qualitative Evaluation System (29), among others (32).

Quantitative arterial analysis may be divided into several separate processes, which include film digitization, image calibration, arterial contour detection, and report generation (diameter function curves). With the exception of recently available, on-line digital angiographic systems (33,34), the majority of quantitative angiographic series have been performed using off-line 35-mm cinefilm analysis. For most systems, a cine-video converter optically magnifies (2:1 to 8:1) and digitizes [512 × 512 (or 480) pixel matrix and an 8-bit gray scale] the image (27,30,35,36).

Image calibration is performed using the injection catheter as the reference standard. Because of differences in catheter composition, radiographic density, and size, the accuracy and reproducibility of image calibration may be dependent upon the type of injection catheter selected (37). Acceptable catheters for quantitative angiographic analysis are those with a mean difference between the angiographic and measured diameters $<3.5\%$ (37). In general, 6- to 8-French catheters are suitable calibration sources (31,38); 5-French catheters should not be used for image calibration (39–41) and the use of larger (>9 French) guiding catheters has not been validated. While noncontrast filled nylon catheters have previously been shown to increase observer variability due to lower catheter image gradients (42), more recent data have suggested that some 6- and 7-French nylon catheters are of sufficient radiographic quality to allow accurate image calibration (31).

After the automated edge-detection algorithm has identified the catheter contour, a scaling factor is entered to obtain the calibration factor. This scaling factor may be obtained from micrometer-determined measurements of the external catheter diameter, the outer or inner catheter diameter provided by the manufacturer, or by determination of the radiographic catheter diameter (43). Catheter calibration has been performed either without (44) or with (45) contrast within the injection catheter. Calibration factors ranging from 0.04–0.09 mm/pixel are recommended.

Most computer-assisted edge-detection algorithms use either the first derivative extremum or a weighted threshold of the first and second derivative extrema obtained from the linear density profile curves to identify the arterial edge (Fig. 2). Each angiographic system varies subtly with respect to the exact location of the arterial edge, construction of the arterial contours, required observer editing, identification of the reference segment, and method of reporting the quantitative results.

1. Cardiovascular Angiographic Analysis System (CAAS)

The CAAS-I system has been extensively validated using phantom and in vivo models (46,47) and has been the instrument for quantitative angiographic analysis for the past decade at the Thoraxcenter (30,48). Unique features of this PDP 11/44-based system include automated correction for pincushion distortion, an arterial edge-detection algorithm that uses a 50% weighted threshold between the first and second derivative extrema, arterial contour detection using a minimal cost matrix algorithm, and minimal observer editing. The "interpolated" reference vessel segment is reconstructed in the segment of interest using a second-degree polynomial function, which provides a reference arterial diameter in the region of the obstruction diameter (Fig. 3) (48). While this method is highly reproducible, it is difficult to apply in ostial stenoses, selected bifurcation lesions, and diffuse segments (49). Moreover, using currently applied methods, postprocedural ectasia, which may occur with the use of intracoronary stents, cannot be measured

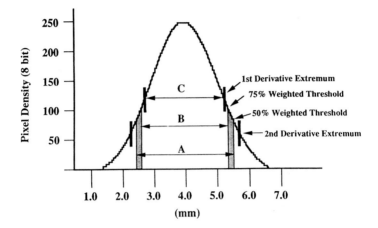

Figure 2 Schematic representation of a single density profile curve perpendicular to a centerline drawn through a reference segment. The solid bar represents the second derivative extrema and the shaded bar represents the first derivative extremum of the density profile curve. Different automated edge-detection algorithms use either a weighted threshold between the first and second derivative extrema [(A) and (B)] or the first derivative extremum itself (C) to measure the arterial diameters. The shaded area represents the difference in reference vessel diameters between those systems using a 50% weight toward the first derivative extrema (CAAS-I, CMS) and those that use a 75% weight toward the first derivative extrema (ARTREK), averaging 0.20–0.30 mm.

(49). Additional physiological parameters, including transstenotic pressure gradients, calculated coronary flow reserve, quantitative indices of symmetry, curvature, and plaque area, are also provided using the CAAS-I system (49,50). There are few limitations of the CAAS-I system, other than that abrupt changes in stenosis severity may be underestimated (29) and the lengthy time required for image analysis. Repeated analyses of reference and minimal lumen diameters using the CAAS-I system have demonstrated reproducibilities of ±0.06–0.13 mm and ±0.09–0.14 mm, respectively (35, 51). Reproducibilities of % diameter stenoses range from 3.5–5.3% (51). A Macintosh-based CAAS-II system has recently been introduced.

2. ARTREK

The ARTREK off-line 35-mm cineangiographic analysis system (QCS, Ann Arbor, MI) was derived from an on-line quantitative angiographic package developed at the University of Michigan (34). Although no correction for pincushion distortion is performed with this system, pincushion

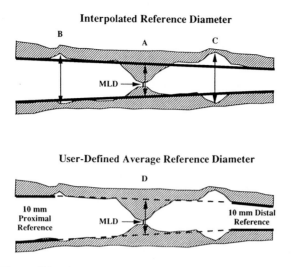

Figure 3 Two validated methods of measuring reference segment diameters. The interpolated normal segment uses a second-order polynomial to measure the estimated reference lumen diameter in the region of the minimal lumen diameter (MLD) (A). Using this method, focal areas of ecatasia [(B) and (C)] are not included in the reference segment calculations. Using the second method, a 10-mm reference segment without lumen irregularities is identified equidistant proximal and distal to the minimal lumen diameter. The reference vessel diameter in the region of the minimal lumen diameter is then estimated.

distortion accounts for an error < 5–8%, particularly when image acquisition is obtained using 4- to 7-in. magnifications (52,53). Arterial edges are identified using a 75% weighted threshold of the first and second derivative extrema (weighted toward the first derivative extremum) (34) and arterial edge contours are constructed using locally adaptive threshold methods applied to adjacent points (34). Observer editing is performed only to discard spatial outliers and arterial edges are reconstructed using linear interpolation. The reference segment is identified using an operator-defined 10-mm arterial segment proximal and distal to the lesion. The average of these two segments is used to calculate the reference diameter in the region of the stenosis (Fig. 3). This method has been validated using repeated intraobserver measurements (variable frame selection) with a reported variability of 0.15 mm (26). An "interpolated" normal determination is also available using ARTREK. Derived physiological measurements (transstenotic pressure gradients, coronary flow reserve) are provided. In vivo phantom validation studies have demonstrated standard errors of 0.23 and 0.21 mm for repeated measurements of minimal lumen diameter (28). Clinical validation studies have demonstrated observer variability of 0.16 mm before angioplasty and 0.23 mm after angioplasty (34,54). The interobserver variability for measuring percent diameter stenosis was 8.1–8.5% (54,55).

3. Cardiovascular Measurement System (CMS)

The Cardiovascular Measurement System (CMS, MEDIS, The Netherlands) is a PC-based quantitative angiographic system developed for off-line quantitative cineangiographic analysis (31,33,56). The edge-detection algorithm and methodology are similar to those developed for the CAAS-I system. Specific features of the CMS include two-point user-defined pathline (centerline) identification, arterial edge detection using a 50% weighted threshold between the first and second derivative extrema, arterial contour detection using a minimal cost matrix algorithm, and an "interpolated" reference vessel diameter (similar to that of the CAAS-I system described above). Physiological parameters, including transstenotic pressure gradients, calculated coronary flow reserve, quantitative indices of symmetry, curvature, and plaque area, are also provided. Repeated analyses of reference and minimal lumen diameters using the CMS system have demonstrated variabilities of 0.12–0.18 mm and 0.09–0.16 mm, respectively; reproducibilities are 3.7–5.8% for % diameter stenoses (51).

4. Other Automated Systems

Other commercially available and proprietary quantitative angiographic systems have also been validated and used for quantitative analysis (27,29, 32,53,57,58). In general, automated edge-detection algorithms have used either a weighted (66%) threshold of the first and second derivative extrema (weighted toward the first derivative extremum) or the first derivative extremum itself as the threshold for arterial edge identification. User-defined or hand-drawn arterial contours obtained from magnified images (with or without edge enhancement) have also been used. Clinical experience with these systems is less extensive by our group, but each has been validated with phantom or in vivo models.

5. Intersystem Comparisons

Over time, it has become apparent that there are important differences in the various quantitative angiographic systems with respect to the preferred method of calibration, location of the arterial border and construction of its contour, use of "smoothing" algorithms, and selection of normal "reference" segments. These identified systematic differences may affect the accuracy and precision of the absolute and relative angiographic measurements. Accordingly, the system-to-system variability may be substantial (59).

At least some of these intersystem differences may be explained by the individual edge-detection algorithm that has been designed and validated for for each analytical system. Edge-detection algorithms that identify the arterial edge using a 50% weighted threshold of the first and second derivative extrema may have systematically larger reference and obstruction diameters than those using a 75% weight (weighted toward the first derivative extremum) or the first derivative extremum (Fig. 2). Given similar reproducibilities for representative systems (± 0.09 mm for the CAAS system, 0.16 mm for the ImageComm system), little overall discriminatory differences between the two systems should be expected. Further intersystem validation studies will be needed to identify whether these intersystem variabilities will alter their ability to detect a difference between two treatment populations (48).

D. Other Sources of Error in the Quantitative Angiographic Method

Other factors may contribute to measurement error associated with quantitative angiography (Table 1). It should be apparent that the total variance [(standard deviation)^2] of minimal lumen and reference diameters within a particular study is a reflection of all the sources of variability contributing to differences in arterial dimensions (32). These sources of variability include: (1) the biological variability of lumen dimensions (e.g., intrinsic arterial size, vasomotor tone, thrombus); (2) inconsistencies in radiographic image acquisition parameters (quantum mottling, out-of-plane magnification, foreshortening); and (3) angiographic measurement variability (same frame, frame-to-frame, day-to-day). While some of these factors cannot be altered, precise control of those remaining factors will substantially improve overall angiographic reproducibility.

1. Biological Variability of Lumen Dimensions

The average diameter of reference vessels treated in balloon and new device angioplasty trials varies from 2.56 ± 0.52 mm to 3.23 ± 0.56 mm (5,60) (Table 2). Some new angioplasty devices (e.g., intracoronary stents, directional atherectomy) have been targeted for larger ($\geqslant 3.0$ mm) vessels, while others (i.e., rotational atherectomy, excimer laser) have been used in smaller (< 3.0 mm) ones (61). Studies that include a wide range of vessel sizes will have more biological variability in lumen diameters than those that are more restrictive in vessel sizing; edge-detection variance of the angiographic system may contribute to < 10–15% of total variability of vessel diameter in these studies (Table 2). Given the dependence of follow-up minimal lumen diameter on reference vessel size (48), the biological variability of vessel size alone may contribute importantly to the overall variance of late minimal lumen diameters.

Table 1 Sources of Imaging Error in Quantitative Coronary Angiography

Source of error	Potential corrections
Biological variation in lumen diameter	
Vessel size	Restrict entry criteria
Vasomotor tone	Standardize nitrate therapy
Intraluminal thrombus/dissection	Periprocedural anticoagulation
Variations in image acquisition	
Single studies	
Vessel motion	
Cardiac	End-diastolic/end-systolic cineframe
Respiration	Breath holding
Lesion eccentricity	Obtain multiple angiographic projections
Vessel foreshortening	As above
Insufficient contrast injection	Use large, high flow catheters
Branch vessel overlap	Obtain multiple angiographic projections
Out-of-plane magnification	—
Pincushion distortion	Image objects in center of image or correct for each
	Image intensifiers using computer-assisted methods
Sequential studies	
X-ray generator (pulse width/dose/beam quality)	Repeat study in same imaging laboratory
X-ray tube (focal spot/shape/tube current)	As above
Image intensifier (magnification/resolution)	As above
Differences in angles and gantry height	Record gantry height/angle/skew on worksheet
Image calibration	Use measured catheter diameter
Errors in image analysis	
Electronic noise	Recursive digitization and frame averaging
Quantum noise	Spatial filtering of digital image data
Automated edge-detection algorithm	Minimize observer interaction
Selection of reference positions	Interpolated or averaged normal segment
Identification of lesion length	Use of sidebranches, other landmarks
Frame selection	End-diastolic frame demonstrating sharpest and tightest view of the lesion

Source: Reprinted from Refs. 37, 45, 50.

Table 2 Contribution of Variance of QCA Measurements to Total Variance in Published Series

Series	PTCA method	QCA system	QCA system reproducibility ±SD (Reference[a])	Largest QCA system variance	Reference diameter		Follow-up MLD	
					mm	Total variance	mm	Total variance
Nobuyoshi (104)	Balloon	Digital calipers	±0.14 (23)	0.020	287±0.74	0.548	1.66±0.62	0.384
Serruys (103)	Balloon	CAAS	±0.06–0.14 (35,51)	0.020	2.81±0.66	0.536	1.69±0.55	0.303
Serruys (116)	Balloon	CAAS	±0.06–0.14 (35,51)	0.020	2.64±0.57	0.325	1.46±0.59	0.348
Adelman (5)	DCA	CMS	±0.09–0.18 (51)	0.032	3.13±0.47	0.221	1.55±0.60	0.360
	Balloon		±0.09–0.18 (51)	0.032	3.23±0.56	0.314	1.61±0.68	0.462
Kent (60)	Balloon	ARTREK	±0.16 (28)	0.026	2.56±0.52	0.270	1.35±0.66	0.435

[a]Reported from published series using repeated analysis of reference or obstruction diameters.

QCA = quantitative coronary angiography; MLD = minimal lumen diameter; SD = standard deviation; DCA = directional coronary atherectomy.

A second factor affecting variance in lumen diameter is the inadequate control of vasomotor tone. Humoral mediators and thrombus contribute to cyclic alterations in vasomotor tone during coronary intervention (62–65), resulting in distal vasoconstriction and vasospasm due to altered autoregulation (66). As pretreatment with oral calcium channel antagonists does not prevent postangioplasty coronary vasoconstriction (62), the use of sublingual, intravenous, or intracoronary calcium channel antagonists may be needed to prevent distal epicardial and arteriolar vasoconstriction. Maximum coronary vasodilation may also be achieved with intracoronary (50–200 μg) (67, 68) or intravenous (≥ 10 μg/min) nitroglycerin (62). Sublingual (5–10 mg) (69) or intracoronary (3 mg) (70,71) isosorbide dinitrate produces maximal coronary dilatation within 2–10 min of administration; its vasodilatory effects are unchanged 10–20 min later.

Nonionic contrast causes less coronary vasodilatation than ionic contrast agents, but the lower radiographic imaging quality and expense may limit its use, particularly when potent vasodilators are routinely used (68). The presence of intracoronary thrombus before the procedure may also affect the quantitative determination of lumen dimensions. Postprocedural intraluminal haziness creates indistinct arterial borders, attributable to varying degrees of dissections, flaps, and thrombus formation (49). These indistinct borders obscure the edge-detection gradients, particularly when a dissection comprises part of the arterial lumen (54,72).

2. Inconsistencies in Radiographic Acquisition Parameters

Accurate and reproducible angiographic analysis is dependent upon meticulous attention to high-quality cineangiogram acquisition (45). Limiting technical factors include motion artifact (cardiac and respiratory), vessel foreshortening, inadequate filling of the coronary artery (streaming) or overfilling of the aortic cusp (precluding analysis of proximal vessels) with contrast, failure to separate overlapping branch vessels from the stenosis, and vessel foreshortening (45). These factors may lead to either overestimation or underestimation of lesion severity. Out-of-plane magnification and pincushion distortion may also contribute to small errors in angiographic imaging (52).

Analysis of two orthogonal projections has been recommended to allow a more accurate assessment of the physiological significance of lesion severity, particularly in lesions with significant eccentricity (18,73). This approach is clearly preferable for angiographic restenosis, regression, and physiological studies (50); however, a second, technically suitable projection may not be available in many (14–53%) angiographic cases, due to vessel foreshortening, overlap, and poor image quality (53,74–76). If orthogonal projections are not available, analyses of the "worst-view" projection may provide sufficiently accurate information. A comparative analysis of 147 lesions using a single "worst" view and orthogonal view analysis was performed by Lesperance et al. (75). Identical "worst" view projections were analyzed before, after, and late after coronary angioplasty. The two methods were within ±0.2 mm for minimal lumen diameter in 96% of lesions and within ±10% in % diameter stenosis for over 97% of lesions (75). In general, % diameter stenoses were 3% higher for "worst view" versus two view analysis; pre-, post-, and follow-up minimal lumen diameters were 0.11–0.15 mm smaller for "worst" view analysis (15,45). Analysis of multiple (>2 projections) has also been recommended (48) but, in our opinion, the selection of >2 angiographic projections tends to underestimate preprocedural stenosis severity and late angiographic restenosis rates, particularly when projections that are foreshortened or with vessel overlap are used.

For sequential studies, replication of the x-ray generator, tube, and image intensifier parameters can be maintained by using the identical angiographic imaging laboratory. Differences in gantry height, angle, and skew can be minimized by using on-line registration or technician worksheets to record these parameters (45). Image calibration errors can be avoided by using identical catheters during sequential studies.

3. Angiographic Measurement Variabilities

Using the most precise angiographic systems, repeated analyses of the same frame demonstrate variabilities ranging from 0.07–0.10 mm for minimal lumen diameter and 2.7–5.1% for % diameter stenosis (32,35,45,51, 77,78). Variability is slightly higher when no attempt is made to match identical cineframes during repeated analysis (51) and highest when repeated analysis is performed on cineangiograms acquired on different days (35,45, 51). Frame-to-frame differences may result from out-of-plane magnification during the cardiac cycle, inadequate admixture of contrast, and lesion eccentricity (36), and day-to-day variabilities may result from incomplete control of vasomotor tone, calibration errors, or alterations in radiographic imaging parameters described above (32,35,45).

To assess the relative contributions of same frame, frame-to-frame, and day-to-day angiographic measurement variabilities, Herrington et al. (32) analyzed the cineangiograms of 20 patients undergoing diagnostic catheterization and coronary angioplasty 2.9 days later. Coefficients of variation for repeated analyses were highest for % diameter stenosis (14.0%) and lowest for average arterial diameter (8.1%). Using a components of variance model, the process of acquiring and analyzing quantitative angiography on selected cineframes (noise in the cine-video optical pathway, edge-detection algorithm) accounted for 57% of the total variability; day-to-day variations in the patient, procedure, and equipment accounted for 30% of total variability; frame selection accounted for the remaining 13% of total variability (32). When direct digital angiography is performed (avoiding the random errors associated with noise in the cine-video pathway), frame selection may be a much more important contributor to overall measurement variability (79).

Reproducibility studies performed after coronary angioplasty suggest that barotrauma-induced haziness and lumen disruption increase angiographic variability (54). No added variability has been noted with quantitative analysis of balloon versus new device angioplasty (26,80). Notably, most currently available quantitative angiographic systems have difficulty accurately assessing lumens < 1 mm (34,52,58,77), due to radiographic imaging limitations of small objects (e.g., veiling glare and point spread function) (81,82).

III. QUANTITATIVE ANGIOGRAPHIC OUTCOME AFTER CORONARY ANGIOPLASTY

To date, angiography has been the primary tool to assess procedural outcome after coronary angioplasty. Its principal role has been to provide a description of the relative changes in lumen dimensions occurring after coronary intervention and to identify major complications (dissections, thrombus) resulting from the procedure. Angiography provides little information regarding the mechanism of lumen improvement, particularly after the use of new devices (lumen dilatation versus atherectomy/ablation), or insight into the pathogenic processes contributing to late lumen renarrowing.

The use of quantitative angiographic methods has enhanced our understanding of the relative changes occurring after balloon and new device angioplasty, but remains inherently limited in its ability to provide insight into the morphological changes occurring after coronary angioplasty. Quantitative assessment of angiographic outcome can be divided into two phases: (1) relative and absolute changes that occur immediately after coronary angioplasty; and (2) relative and absolute changes that occur late (3–12 months) after the procedure.

A. Immediate Quantitative Angiographic Outcomes

Using quantitative methods, angiographic success rates (< 50% residual diameter stenosis) have ranged from 70–80% after standard balloon angioplasty (6,16,83). It has been somewhat disappointing that the immediate changes in lumen diameters achieved with balloon angioplasty have been modest (0.75–1.16 mm) (5,84,85); these notations have led to alternative approaches using new angioplasty devices designed to improve lumen dimensions, and, potentially, early procedural outcomes. In fact, randomized studies of balloon angioplasty versus intracoronary stents and directional atherectomy have demonstrated that larger initial lumen dimensions and higher angiographic success rates can be achieved with new devices (6,7,86).

The mechanism of this initial improvement in lumen dimensions after new device angioplasty appears related to its ability to alter lesion compliance (87,88). Some devices (intracoronary stents, thermal or physiological low-stress angioplasty) reduce the degree of elastic recoil by scaffolding or physiologically altering the arterial wall (89,90). Other devices (directional, rotational, or extraction atherectomy, excimer laser angioplasty) excise, ablate, or extract atherosclerotic plaque, which renders the lesion more amenable to adjunct balloon dilation and reduces the degree of passive elastic recoil (88).

1. Lesion Stretch

Some atherosclerotic lesions are extremely rigid during balloon angioplasty, resisting radial expansion and precluding full balloon inflation (residual "waist") even at high ($\geqslant$20 atm) inflation pressures. Concentric calcium rings or dense fibrosis demonstrated by intravascular ultrasound may partially account for this lesion rigidity. Rotational atherectomy and excimer laser angioplasty have been successful in "undilatable" lesions after standard balloon angioplasty (91,92), suggesting that partial plaque ablation may account for improved lesion compliance. Often, full balloon expansion is obtained at low inflation pressures after new device angioplasty in previously nondilatable lesions (91).

Lesion stretch $[[(Balloon_{MLD}-Pre_{MLD})/reference\ diameter]$, where MLD = minimal diameter], has been used as an index of the maximal gain in lumen diameter achieved during balloon angioplasty (87) (Fig. 4). Quantitative measurement of the largest balloon inflated at the highest pressure is the preferred method of determining lesion stretch (93). Balloon expansion is often incomplete and asymmetric, based upon a 0.59 ± 0.23-mm quantitative difference in maximal and minimal balloon diameters noted in one series (49,93). Accordingly, the diameter of the balloon should be measured at the most nondistensible portion (smallest diameter) of the segment (93). Using these criteria, lesion stretch averages 0.49 ± 0.18; the majority of lesion distensibility occurs at $\leqslant$2 atm of pressure (94).

2. Elastic Recoil

In contrast to rigid lesions, elastic lesions are those with excessive degrees of collapse (or recoil) of the arterial lumen despite full and unlimited balloon inflation (87). Elastic recoil, $[[(Balloon_{MDL}-Final_{MLD})/reference\ diameter]$, where MLD = minimal diameter], is an index of the maximal loss in lumen dimensions resulting from balloon deflation (93,95-98). Elastic

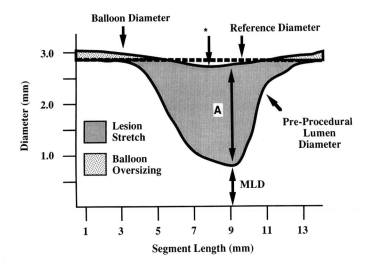

Figure 4 Lesion stretch can be schematically viewed as the overall dilatation that occurs within the diseased segment after balloon and new device angioplasty. The diameter function curve (Panel A), depicts the preprocedural lumen diameter (arrow) and minimal lumen diameter (MLD) before treatment. The reference segment diameter (dashed line) is shown. The inflated balloon diameter curve is superimposed on the arterial curve, demonstrating that balloon oversizing has occurred in the proximal and distal reference segments (light shading). The point of minimal balloon diameter is shown (*). The magnitude of lesion stretch (A) is demonstrated but incompletely reflects the overall dilatation that has occurred throughout the diseased segment (dark shading). Notably, significant balloon oversizing may result in complications and balloon undersizing may result in incomplete arterial dilatation. Lesion recoil can also be expressed using the diameter function curves (B). The postprocedural lumen diameter (arrow), residual MLD, and balloon diameter (dashed lines) are demonstrated. The amount of recoil that occurred from the time of balloon deflation is illustrated (B). Again, amount of recoil that has actually occurred within the lesion is incompletely reflected (dark shade). (Adapted from Ref. 93.)

recoil is preferably measured using the minimal balloon diameter (87,93). Elastic recoil averages 0.21 ± 0.15 after balloon angioplasty; lesions located in straight segments or in the distal vessel, with asymmetry or low plaque content, and dilated with an oversized balloon demonstrate larger degrees of elastic recoil (95–98). Virtually all elastic recoil occurs immediately after balloon deflation with little elastic recoil occurring in the hours to days following coronary angioplasty (95).

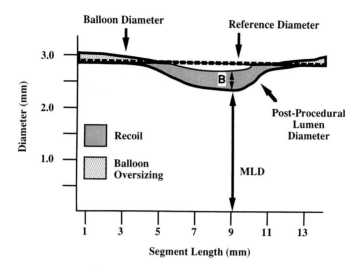

3. Residual Diameter Stenosis and Minimal Lumen Diameter

The net balance of lesion stretch and elastic recoil determines the postprocedural percent diameter stenosis and residual minimal lumen diameter. Despite comparable procedural success rates (>90%), it is apparent that new angioplasty devices result in lower postprocedural diameter stenoses and larger minimal lumen diameters than can be obtained after standard balloon angioplasty (5–7,86), due to their effect on lesion compliance and reduction in elastic recoil.

Whether early and late procedural success is best measured using % diameter stenosis (45,99,100) or minimal lumen diameter (3,4,48) is unsettled. It is well recognized that coronary atherosclerosis is a diffuse process, often involving the reference vessel segment, thereby severely underestimating the extent of atherosclerotic involvement (101). However, a major problem with the use of minimal lumen diameter is that it does not account for the large variability in vessel size (45). The physiological implications of a change in minimal lumen diameter of 1.5 mm as a result of coronary angioplasty will be markedly different, depending upon whether the vessel was 2.0 mm in reference diameter or 4.0 mm in reference diameter. Thus measures of angiographic success after coronary angioplasty should account for both the relative (% diameter stenosis) and absolute (minimal lumen diameter) changes in vessel dimensions and the reference vessel size. Both postprocedural % diameter stenosis and postprocedural lumen diameter have been correlated with late clinical outcome after new device angioplasty (2,102).

B. Lumen Renarrowing After Coronary Angioplasty

Sequential angiographic studies have formed the cornerstone of our understanding of the time-dependent pathophysiological responses after balloon angioplasty (4,103,104). The vast majority of treated lesions develop some degree of lumen renarrowing within 3–6 months after the procedure (103,104). Clinical events related to treatment site renarrowing generally occur within 8 months of the procedure (105), with further progression of lesion severity after 12 months uncommon (105). Progression of atherosclerotic disease at other sites is more common late (> 12 months) after coronary angioplasty, generally unrelated to treatment site lumen renarrowing (106–108).

Several biological factors have been identified which contribute to the overall magnitude of lumen renarrowing in the weeks to months following coronary angioplasty (48). These factors include: (1) myointimal hyperplasia occurring as a response to tissue injury (109); (2) platelet and thrombin deposition on the disrupted arterial surface, which may be proportional to the extent of vessel wall injury (110–112); (3) plaque remodeling with contraction of the external elastic lamina (113); and (4) elastic recoil which accounts for up to 30% loss of the maximal lumen diameter after balloon deflation (93,96,97,114), but probably contributes little to further lumen loss as assessed by angiographic studies 24 h after coronary angioplasty (95). Angiographically, these processes are indistinguishable; further insight into the mechanisms of restenosis may be possible using intravascular ultrasound studies.

1. Binary Restenosis Rates

A number of definitions have been used to calculate binary restenosis rates after coronary angioplasty (Table 3), resulting in angiographic recurrence rates ranging from 18–57% (6,16,115–117). The Emory definition of binary restenosis ($\geq$ 50% follow-up diameter stenosis) has been used most often in clinical restenosis trials, based upon the physiological reduction of coronary flow reserve in animal models with > 50% luminal narrowing (118). However, use of binary "cutoff" criteria for restenosis may be problematic, due to the perception by some that the restenosis process is an "all or none" phenomenon. In fact, the restenosis "process" is a near continuous biological one that occurs to some extent in virtually all patients (84,103,104). Similar limitations exist for the use of binary restenosis rates based on changes in late lumen dimensions (>0.72 mm) (119).

Table 3 Common Definitions of Binary Restenosis Rates After Coronary Angioplasty (PTCA)

Percent diameter stenosis
  National Heart, Lung, and Blood Institute (NHLBI) Criteria
  NHLBI 1—Loss of $\geq$ 30% diameter stenosis from pre-PTCA to follow-up (117)
  NHLBI 2—Final procedural % diameter stenosis < 50% and $\geq$ 70% follow-up
    diameter stenosis (117)·
  NHLBI 3—A return to with 10% of the pre-PTCA % diameter stenosis (117)
  NHLBI 4—Loss during follow-up $\geq$ 50% of the initial gain (117)
  $\geq$ 50% diameter stenosis at follow-up (1,125)
  An immediate % diameter stenosis < 50% that increases to $\geq$ 50% at follow-up
  (117)
  A diameter stenosis $\geq$ 70% at follow-up[a]
Minimal lumen diameter
  Loss $\geq$ 0.72 mm from post-PTCA to follow-up (48)
  Loss $\geq$ 0.50 mm from post-PTCA to follow-up (104)

[a]From Ref. 148.

2. Late Lumen Loss or the "Process" of Restenosis After Coronary Angioplasty

To surmount the difficulties determining serial changes in relative lumen reduction associated with the reporting of percent diameter stenosis (48), changes in the absolute lumen diameters have been used to assess the magnitude of lumen renarrowing after coronary angioplasty (103,104). The absolute reduction in lumen diameter, or late lumen loss, follows a near gaussian distribution after balloon angioplasty, averaging 0.27–0.50 mm (6,84,116, 120). The magnitude of late lumen loss after coronary angioplasty relates to clinical factors (e.g., recent onset angina, diabetes mellitus, serum cholesterol, male gender, prior restenosis) (121–124), lesion location and length (e.g., left anterior descending artery, saphenous vein grafts) (122,124–127), preprocedural lesion severity (125), and postprocedural results (e.g., initial gain, posttreatment lumen diameter) (3,125). Of these factors, postprocedural lumen diameter appears to be the most important (3). The understanding of the relative trade-off of acute gain and late loss has led to philosophical differences in the definitions of restenosis after coronary intervention (4,48). The process of restenosis (late lumen loss) may, in fact, be greater after new device angioplasty than after balloon angioplasty which is associated with smaller gain and smaller losses (119) (Fig. 5). However, the physiological consequence of proportional (0.4–0.6) loss/gain relationship may result in a larger lumen at follow-up in those lesions with larger initial gains (4).

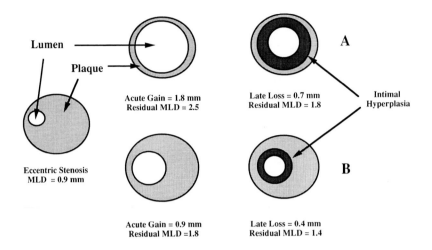

Figure 5 Schematic illustration of the proportional relationship between acute gain and late lumen loss after balloon and new device angioplasty. An eccentric stenosis may be treated with either directional atherectomy (A) or standard balloon angioplasty (B). The acute gain is larger in A than B, resulting in a large initial lumen diameter. During the follow-up period, the late lumen loss is also greater in A than B. Due to the proportional late loss/acute gain relationship (0.5), a larger minimal lumen diameter is noted at follow-up in A than B.

To further characterize the balance of initial gain and late loss, the loss index (late loss/acute gain) has been used (85). The loss index remains relatively constant after balloon and new device angioplasty, suggesting that late angiographic outcome relates to the initial angiographic result rather than to the device used for revascularization (85).

In 30% of lesions, an angiographic improvement in minimal lumen diameter has been noted during the follow-up period (84). Factors contributing to an improvement include resolution of intraluminal thrombus, remodeling of intimal flaps, and correction of preprocedural vasospasm. Intravascular ultrasound studies have noted that minimal lumen diameters and reference vessel size (external elastic lamina) also increase in 20% of patients after coronary angioplasty (113). These findings lend support to pathological studies that demonstrate compensatory enlargement of arterial diameters in early atherosclerosis (128).

Other continuous indices for restenosis have been proposed (48). These indices include the follow-up minimal lumen diameter, follow-up percent diameter stenosis, restenosis index (ratio between the decrease in lumen during follow-up and the initial gain [in millimeters] after the procedure), and the utility index (ratio between the final net gain at follow-up and the reference vessel diameter) (48).

3. Have Any Beneficial Restenosis Agents Been Overlooked?

The use of sophisticated angiographic and statistical methods in pharmacological restenosis trials has increased the ability of these studies to detect differences between two treatment populations (48). Although isolated clinical studies have demonstrated an angiographic benefit in the prevention of restenosis after coronary angioplasty, no agent thus far has been reproducibly shown to prevent restenosis in confirmatory series (60,116,120,125, 129). Many of these early studies have been limited by small sample sizes, inadequate preclinical testing, insufficient periprocedural dosing compared with animal models, and limited rigor of quantitative angiographic methods (129). In at least one study, a treatment benefit was identified using retrospective quantitative angiographic analysis that was not demonstrated using less reproducible, visual angiographic methods. Ciprostene, a prostacyclin analogue, failed to demonstrate a significant reduction in restenosis using site-determined visual angiographic endpoints (130); reanalysis of the cineangiograms using quantitative angiographic methods by an angiographic core laboratory demonstrated a significant reduction in angiographic restenosis (131). It is possible that other trials using less rigorous angiographic methods may also have overlooked a significant treatment effect (48).

IV. DEVELOPING A CONCEPTUAL FRAMEWORK FOR THE QUANTITATIVE EVALUATION OF BALLOON AND NEW DEVICE TECHNOLOGY

Quantitative angiographic and statistical methods developed over the past several years have allowed more rigorous comparisons of balloon and new device angioplasty in randomized (5–7,86) and nonrandomized (2,3, 114) clinical studies. One new device (i.e., tubular-slotted stent) has reduced the incidence of angiographic and clinical restenosis over balloon angioplasty in two preliminary reports (7,86), while another (i.e., directional atherectomy) has shown little benefit over balloon angioplasty in preventing angiographic or clinical recurrence (5,6,17). Accordingly, it would seem appropriate that generalized use of those therapies without demonstrated clinical advantage over balloon angioplasty should not be recommended, given that these modalities are often more expensive than standard balloon angioplasty (6,132). Closer scrutiny of one recently completed randomized trial of directional atherectomy and balloon angioplasty has suggested that directional atherectomy may have been committed to randomized study before the mechanism of its benefit over balloon angioplasty (i.e., the attainment of a larger initial lumen) was fully appreciated (6); in this study, site-to-site operator technique was an independent factor in determining late angiographic outcome (133). To the extent that "aggressive" atherectomy is associated with a larger initial lumen (134), the comparative advantage of directional atherectomy over balloon angioplasty might not have been realized. Given the important financial and public health implications of randomized device trials (135), it is imperative that the mechanisms of benefit of alternative treatment modalities be fully understood prior to subjecting new devices to randomized, comparative trials.

Further studies evaluating the quantitative benefit of alternative pharmacological and mechanical approaches to standard balloon angioplasty will focus on several critical issues: (1) acceptance of the limitations of angiographic criteria alone in assessing late outcome after coronary angioplasty; (2) identification of those clinical indices that represent failure due to treatment site renarrowing and those that represent progression of coronary atherosclerosis in other locations; and (3) incorporation of intravascular ultrasound into late angiographic studies to more fully understand the biological processes contributing to restenosis.

A. Limitations of Angiography in Assessing Late Clinical Benefit

In order for new therapies associated with relative improvements in quantitative angiographic indices to be clinically meaningful, the *biological* reduction in lumen renarrowing resulting from treatment should correlate with a *clinical* reduction in late cardiac events (e.g., a reduction in late recurrent ischemia). In the absence of this correlation, the benefit of a reduction in angiographic restenosis rates alone may be simply "cosmetic" with little clinical importance. At least one randomized trial has demonstrated a reduction in angiographic restenosis resulting from new device use without a similar reduction in composite late clinical outcome (136); others have suggested that asymptomatic restenosis may occur in 10–25% of patients after coronary angioplasty (117,137–139). These discrepancies in angiographic and clinical endpoints are explained, in part, by a clustering of late follow-up % diameter stenosis around 50–60%, the hesitation of physicians to act upon apparent borderline lesions in the absence of convincing symptoms, and the inability of isolated angiographic criteria (percent diameter stenosis, minimal lumen diameter) to fully predict functional decrements in coronary flow reserve after coronary angioplasty (18,140–143).

Given the expense of routine follow-up angiography ($1500–$2000), it is generally recommended that angiography only be performed in the event of recurrent ischemia. However, in the absence of near-complete ($>80\%$) ascertainment of 6-month angiographic follow-up studies, substantial referral biases based upon symptom status will affect the overall rates of restenosis and quantitative indices of late lumen loss (144,145), lessening their importance as biological markers for restenosis. Because of these limitations, identification of a simple, intuitive clinical surrogate for clinical restenosis after coronary angioplasty may be of value.

B. Identifying Clinically Useful Markers of Treatment Site Renarrowing

Major cardiac events (e.g., death, myocardial infarction, coronary bypass operation, or repeat coronary angioplasty) occur in approximately 25% of patients within 6–12 months after coronary angioplasty (60,120). The majority ($>85\%$) of these events occur as a result of repeat revascularization (i.e., coronary bypass operation or repeat coronary angioplasty) due to treatment site renarrowing; the greatest cumulative hazard for treatment-site revascularization is between 80–240 days, closely correlated with standard binary ($\geq 50\%$ diameter stenosis) restenosis criteria (kappa = 0.64) (146). Death and myocardial infarction occur much less often after coronary angioplasty (1% and 2%, respectively), showing an ongoing accumulation of these events unrelated to treatment site renarrowing (kappa = 0) (106,146,147). It is apparent from these important observations that the best clinical index of treatment-site renarrowing (the biological response) after coronary angioplasty may be treatment site revascularization.

C. Plaque Remodeling and Tissue Growth After Coronary Angioplasty

Late lumen loss after coronary angioplasty has been traditionally thought to be mediated by intimal hyperplasia, stimulated by balloon-induced arterial injury (109). Intravascular ultrasound may provide further insight into the pathogenesis of restenosis after coronary angioplasty (113). Sequential intravascular ultrasound studies of 74 patients after coronary angioplasty have shown that late lumen loss occurs as a result of both tissue growth (accounting for 40% of late lumen loss) and contraction of the external elastic lamina (accounting for 60% of late lumen loss). These relative contributions of plaque remodeling and tissue growth cannot be determined using standard angiography and can only be clinically determined using rigorously acquired intravascular ultrasound imaging.

V. CONCLUSIONS

In this chapter, we have reviewed the quantitative angiographic methods available for the comparative analysis of balloon and new device angioplasty. While important differences in the methodologies may exist between differing angiographic systems and core laboratories, standardization of the image acquisition, procedural, and analytical methods will substantially reduce observer variability, ultimately reducing the sample sizes required for statistical comparisons in randomized and nonrandomized series. Quantitative angiographic analysis has also yielded important insights into the mechanism and benefit of balloon and new device angioplasty, demonstrating that alterations in plaque compliance and recoil may be mechanistically responsible for the lower residual diameter stenosis shown with new device angioplasty. With the application of standard statistical methods to quantitative angiographic results, more appropriate interdevice comparisons can also be made. The use of target-site revascularization as an intuitive surrogate for the identification of treatment site renarrowing will undoubtedly be expanded. Finally, given the recognized limitations of angiography, further insights into the pathogenic processes leading to restenosis will be obtained using complementary imaging modalities, such as intravascular ultrasound.

REFERENCES

1. King SI, Weintraub W, Tao X, Hern J, Douglas JJ. Biomodal distribution of diameter stenosis 4 to 12 months after angioplasty: implications for definitions and interpretations of restenosis (abstr). J Am Coll Cardiol 1991;17:345A.
2. Kuntz R, Safian R, Levine M, Reis G, Diver D, Baim D. Novel approach to the analysis of restenosis after the use of three new coronary devices. J Am Coll Cardiol 1992;19:1493–1499.
3. Kuntz R, Gibson C, Nobuyoshi M, Baim D. A generalized model of restenosis following conventional balloon angioplasty, stenting and directional atherectomy. J Am Coll Cardiol 1993;21:15–25.
4. Kuntz R, Baims D. Defining coronary restenosis. Newer clinical and angiographic paradigms. Circulation 1993;88:1310–1323.
5. Adelman A, Cohen E, Kimball B, Bonan R, Ricci D, Webb J, Laramee L, Barbeau G, Traboulsi M, Corbett B, Schwartz L, Logan A. A comparison of directional atherectomy with balloon angioplasty for lesions of the left anterior descending coronary artery. N Engl J Med 1993;329:228–233.
6. Topol E, Leya F, Pinkerton C, Whitlow P, Hofling B, Simonton C, Masden R, Serruys P, Leon M, Williams D, King S, Mark D, Isner J, Holmes D, Ellis S, Lee K, Keeler G, Berdan L, Hinohara T, Califf R. A comparison of directional atherectomy with coronary angioplasty in patients with coronary artery disease. N Engl J Med 1993;329:221–227.

7. Schatz R, Penn I, Baim D, Nobuyoshi M, Colombo A, Ricci D, Cleman M, Goldberg S, Heuser R, Almond D, Fish D, Moses J, Gallup D, Detre K, Leon M. STent REstenosis Study (STRESS): Analysis of in-hospital results (abstr). Circulation 1993;88:1-594.
8. Fleming R, Kirkeeide R, Smalling R, Gould K. Patterns in visual interpretation of coronary arteriograms as detected by quantitative angioplasty. J Am Coll Cardiol 1991;18:945-951.
9. Zir L, Miller S, Dinsmore R, Gilbert J, Harthorne J. Interobserver variability in coronary angiography. Circulation 1976;53:627-632.
10. DeRouen T, Murray J, Owen W. Variability in the analysis of coronary arteriograms. Circulation 1977;55:324-328.
11. Fisher L, Judkins M, Lesperance J, Cameron A, Swaye P, Ryan T, Maynard C, Bourassa M, Kennedy J, Gosselin A, Kemp H, Faxon D, Wexler L, Davis K. Reproducibility of coronary arteriographic reading in the coronary artery surgery study (CASS). Cathet Cardiovasc Diagn 1982;8:565-575.
12. Detre K, Wright E, Murphy M, Takaro T. Observer agreement in evaluating coronary angiograms. Circulation 1975;52:979-986.
13. Goldberg R, Kleiman N, Minor S, Abukahil J, Raizner A. Comparison of quantitative angiography to visual estimates of lesion severity pre and post PTCA. Am Heart J 1990;119:178-184.
14. Schweiger M, Stanek E, Iwakoshi K, Hafer J, Jacob A, Tullner W, Gianelly R. Comparison of visual estimate with digital caliper measurement of coronary artery stenosis. Cathet Cardiovasc Diagn 1987;13:239-244.
15. Beauman G, Vogal R. Accuracy of individual and panel visual interpretations of coronary arteriograms: implications for clinical decisions. J Am Coll Cardiol 1990;16:108-113.
16. Bairati I, Roy L, Meyer F. Double-blind, randomized, controlled trial of fish oil supplements in prevention of recurrence of stenosis after coronary angioplasty. Circulation 1992;85:950-956.
17. The CAVEAT II Investigators. The Coronary Angioplasty Versus Excisional Atherectomy Trial (CAVEAT) II: Preliminary results (abstr). Circulation 1993; 88:1-594.
18. Kirkeeide R, Gould K, Parsel L. Assessment of coronary stenoses by myocardial perfusion imaging during pharmacologic coronary vasodilation — VII. Validation of coronary flow reserve as a single integrated functional measure of stenosis severity reflecting all its geometric dimensions. J Am Coll Cardiol 1986; 1986:103-113.
19. Gould K. Quantitative analysis of coronary artery restenosis after coronary angioplasty — Has the rose lost its bloom? J Am Coll Cardiol 1992;19:946-947.
20. Martinelli M, Deutsch E, Ferraro A, Bove A, Group MH. Comparison of angiographic center and local site analysis of PTCA results in a multicenter angioplasty-restenosis trial. Cathet Cardiovasc Diagn 1992;27:8-13.
21. Gensini G, Kelly A, DaCosta B, Huntington P. Quantitative angiography: The measurement of coronary vasomobility in the intact animal and man. Chest 1971;60:522-530.
22. Scoblionko D, Brown B, Mitten S, Caldwell J, Kennedy J, Bolson E, Doge H. A new digital electronic caliper for measurement of coronary arterial stenosis:

Comparison with visual estimates and computer-assisted measurements. Am J Cardiol 1984;53:689-693.

23. Uehata A, Matsuguchi T, Bittl J, Orav J, Meredith I, Anderson T, Selwyn A, Ganz P, Yeung A. Accuracy of electronic digital calipers compared with quantitative angiography in measuring coronary arterial diameter. Circulation 1993; 88:1724-1729.

24. Alderman E, Stadius M. The angiographic definitions of the Bypass Angioplasty Revascularization Investigation. Coronary Artery Disease 1992;3:1189-1207.

25. Kalbfleisch S, McGillem M, Pinto I, Kavanaugh K, DeBoe S, Mancini G. Comparison of automated quantitative coronary angiography with caliper measurements of percent diameter stenosis. Am J Cardiol 1990;65:1181-1184.

26. Popma J, Leon M, Keller M, Yeh W, DeFalco R, Ditrano C, Merritt A, Kennard E, Baim D, Detre K. Reproducibility of the angiographic Core Laboratory for the New Approaches to Coronary Intervention (NACI) Registry (abstr). Circulation 1993;88:I-653.

27. Uehata A, Davis S, Orav J, Yeung A. Validation of the accuracy of electronic digital calipers and quantitative angiography using calibrated phantoms (abstr). Circulation 1993;88:I-652.

28. Mancini G, Simon S, McGillem M, LeFree M, Friedman H, Vogal R. Automated quantitative coronary angiography: morphologic and physiologic validation of a rapid digital angiographic method. Circulation 1987;76:452-460.

29. Hermiller J, Cusma J, Spero L, Fortin D, Harding M, Bashore T. Quantitative and qualitative coronary angiographic analysis: Review of methods, utility, and limitations. Cathet Cardiovasc Diagn 1992;25:110-131.

30. Reiber J, Kooijman C, Slager C, Gerbrands J, Schuurbiers J, den Boer A, Wijns W, Serruys P, Hugenholtz P. Coronary artery dimensions from cineangiograms — Methodology and validation of a computer-assisted analysis procedure. IEEE Trans Med Imag 1984;M12:131-141.

31. Koning G, van der Zwet P, von Land C, Reiber J. Angiographic assessment of 6F and 7F Mallinckrodt Softtouch coronary contrast catheters from digital and cine arteriograms. Int J Card Imaging 1992;8:153-161.

32. Herrington D, Siebes M, Sokol D, Siu C, Walford G. Variability in measures of coronary lumen dimensions using quantitative coronary angiography. J Am Coll Cardiol 1993;22:1068-1074.

33. Reiber J, van der Zwet P, von Land C, Koning G, Loois G, Zorn I, van den Brand M, Gerbrands J. On-line quantification of coronary angiograms with the DCI system. Medicamundi 1989;34:89-98.

34. Mancini G. Quantitative coronary arteriography: Development of methods, limitations, and clinical applications. Am J Cardiac Imaging 1988;2(98-109).

35. Reiber J, Serruys P, Kooijman C, Wijns W, Slager C, Gerbrands J, Schuurbiers J, den Boer A, Hugenholtz P. Assessment of short-, medium-, and long-term variations in arterial dimensions from computer-assisted quantitation of coronary cineangiograms. Circulation 1985;71:280-288.

36. Reiber J, van Eldik-Helleman P, Visser-Akkerman N, Kooijman CJ, Serruys PW. Variabilities in measurement of coronary arterial dimensions resulting from variations in cineframe selection. Cathet Cardiovasc Diagn 1988;14:221-228.

37. Reiber J, den Boer A, Serruys P. Quality control in performing quantitative coronary arteriography. Am J Cardiac Imag 1989;3:172–179.
38. Ellis S, Pinto I, McGillem M, DeBoe S, LeFree M, Mancini G. Accuracy and reproducibility or quantitative coronary arteriography using 6 and 8 French catheters with cine angiographic acquisition. Cathet Cardiovasc Diagn 1991;22: 52–55.
39. Brown R, MacDonald A. Use of 5 French catheters for cardiac catheterization and coronary angiography: a critical review. Cathet Cardiovasc Diagn 1987; 13:214–217.
40. Molajo A, Ward C, Bray C, Dobson D. Comparison of the performance of superflow (5F) and conventional 8F catheter for cardiac catheterization by the femoral route. Cathet Cardiovasc Diagn 1987;13:275–276.
41. Ellis S, DeBoe S, Sanz M, Mancini G. Accuracy (A) and reproducibility (R) of 5 Fr catheter systems for outpatient use compared with 8 Fr systems (abstr). Circulation 1987;76:IV–369.
42. Reiber J, Kooijman C, den Boer A, Serruys P. Assessment of dimensions and image quality of coronary contrast catheters from cineangiograms. Cathet Cardiovasc Diagn 1985;11:521–531.
43. Fortin D, Spero L, Cusma J, Santoro L, Burgess R, Bashore T. Pitfalls in the determination of absolute dimensions using angiographic catheters as calibration devices in quantitative angiography. Am J Cardiol 1991;68:1176–1182.
44. di Mario C, Hermans W, Rensing B, Serruys P. Calibration using angiographic catheters as scaling devices — importance of filming the catheters not filled with contrast medium (letter). Am J Cardiol 1992;69:1377.
45. Lesperance J, Bourassa M, Schwartz L, Hudon G, Laurier J, Eastwood C, Kazim F. Definition and measurement of restenosis after successful coronary angioplasty: Implications for clinical trials. Am Heart J 1993;125:1394–1408.
46. Haase J, di Mario C, Slager C, van der Giessen W, den Boer A, de Feyter P, Versow P, Reiber J, Serruys P. In-vivo validation of on-line and off-line geometric coronary measurements using insertion of stenosis phantoms in porcine coronary arteries. Cathet Cardiovasc Diagn 1992;27:16–27.
47. di Mario C, Haase J, den Boer A, Reiber J, Serruys P. Edge detection versus videodensitometry in the quantitative assessment of stenosis phantoms: an invivo comparison in porcine coronary arteries. Am Heart J 1992;124:1181–1189.
48. Serruys P, Foley D, Kirkeeide R, King S. Restenosis revisited: Insights provided by quantitative coronary angiography. Am Heart J 1993;126:1243–1267.
49. Strauss B, Morel M-A, van Swijndredt E, Hermans W, Umans V, Rensing B, de Jaegere P, DeFeyter P, Serruys P. Methodologic aspects of quantitative coronary angiography (QCA) in interventional cardiology. Serruys PW, Strauss BH, Kings SB (eds) 1992;:11–50.
50. de Feyter P, Serruys P, Davies M, Richardson P, Lubsen J, Oliver M. Quantitative coronary angiography to measure progression and regression of coronary atherosclerosis. Value, limitations, and implications for clinical trials. Circulation 1991;84:412–423.
51. Lesperance J, Waters D. Measuring progression and regression of coronary atherosclerosis in clinical trials: problems and progress. Int J Cardiac Imaging 1992;8:165–173.

52. Popma J, Eichhorn E, Dehmer G. In vivo assessment of a digital angiographic method to measure absolute coronary artery diameters. Am J Cardiol 1989;64: 131–138.

53. Brown B, Bolson E, Frimer M, Dodge H. Quantitative coronary arteriography. Estimation of dimensions, hemodynamic resistance, and atheroma mas of coronary artery lesions using the arteriogram and digital computation. Circulation 1977;55:329–337.

54. Sanz M, Mancini G, LeFree M, Mickelson J, Starling M, Vogal R, Topol E. Variability of quantitative digital subtraction coronary angiography before and after percutaneous transluminal coronary angioplasty. Am J Cardiol 1987;55–60.

55. deCesare N, Williamson P, Moore N, DeBoe S, Mancini G. Establishing comprehensive quantitative criteria for detection of restenosis and remodeling after percutaneous transluminal coronary angioplasty. Am J Cardiol 1992;69:77–83.

56. van der Zwet P, Pinto I, Serruys P, Reiber J. A new approach for the automated definition of path lines in digitized coronary angiograms. Int J Card Imaging 1990;5:75–83.

57. Klein J, Gatlin S, Manoukian S, King S. Quantitative coronary angiography: An inexpensive and user friendly system (abstr). J Am Coll Cardiol 1993;21: 7A.

58. Spears J, Sandor T, Als A, Malagold M, Markis J, Grossman W, Serur J, Paulin S. Computerized image analysis for quantitative measurement of vessel diameter from cineangiograms. Circulation 1983;68:453–461.

59. Keane D, Montauban E, Haase J, diMario C, Serruys P. Multicentre validation of computerised quantitative coronary angiographic systems (abstr). Circulation 1993;88:I-653.

60. Kent K, Williams D, Cassagneua B, Broderick T, Chapekis A, Simpfendorfer C, Cote G, Bates E, Tauscher G, Kuntz R, Popma J, Foegh M. Double blind, controlled trial of the effect of angiopeptin on coronary restenosis following balloon angioplasty (abstr). Circulation 1993;88:I-506.

61. Popma J, Leon M. A lesion-specific approach to new device angioplasty. In: Topol E, ed. Interventional Cardiology. Vol. 2. Philadelphia: WB Saunders, 1993;973–985.

62. Fischell T, Derby G, Tse T, Stadius M. Coronary artery vasoconstriction routinely occurs after percutaneous transluminal coronary angioplasty. A quantitative arteriographic analysis. Circulation 1988;78:1323–1334.

63. Fischell T, Bausback K. Effects of luminal eccentricity on spontaneous coronary vasoconstriction after successful percutaneous transluminal coronary angioplasty. Am J Cardiol 1991;68:530–534.

64. Eichhorn E, Grayburn P, Willard J, Anderson H, Bedotto J, Carry M, Kahn J, Willerson J. Spontaneous alterations in coronary blood flow velocity before and after coronary angioplasty in patients with severe angina. J Am Coll Cardiol 1991;17:43–52.

65. El-Tamimi H, Davies G, Hackett D, Sritara P, Bertrand O, Crea F, Maseri A. Abnormal vasomotor changes early after coronary angioplasty: A quantitative arteriographic study of their time course. Circulation 1991;84:1198–1202.

66. Fischell T, Bausback K, McDonald T. Evidence of altered epicardial coronary artery autoregulation as a cause of distal coronary vasoconstriction after successful percutaneous transluminal coronary angioplasty. J Clin Invest 1990;86: 575–584.
67. Feldman R, Marx J, Pepine C, Conti C. Analysis of coronary responses to various doses of intracoronary nitroglycerin. Circulation 1982;66:321–327.
68. Jost S, Rafflenbeul W, Reil G, Trappe H, Gulba D, Hecker H, Gergardt U, Knop I. Elimination of variable vasomotor tone in studies with repeated quantitative coronary angiography. Int J Cardiac Imaging 1990;5:125–134.
69. Badger R, Brown B, Gallery C, Bolson E, Dodge H. Coronary artery dilatation and hemodynamic responses after isosorbide dinitrate therapy in patients with coronary artery disease. Am J Cardiol 1985;56:390–395.
70. Strauer B. Isosorbide dinstrate: Its action on myocardial contractility in comparison with nitroglycerin. Int J Clin Pharm Ther Toxicol 1982;66:321–327.
71. Lablanche J, Delforge M, Tilmant P, et al. Effects of hemodynamiques et coronaires du dinitrate di'isosorbide: Comparaison entre les voies d'injection intracoronaire en intraveineuse. Arch Mal Coeur 1982;75:303–316.
72. Serruys P, Reiber J, Wijns W, van der Brand M, Kooijman C, ten Katen H, Hugenholtz P. Assessment of percutaneous transluminal coronary angioplasty by quantitative coronary angiography: Diameter versus densitometric area measurements. Am J Cardiol 1984;54:482–488.
73. Thomas A, Davies M, Dilly S, Dilly N, Franc F. Potential errors in the estimation of coronary arterial stenosis from clinical arteriography with reference to the shape of the coronary arterial lumen. Br Heart J 1986;55:129–139.
74. Dehmer G, Popma J, van den Berg E, Eichhorn E, Prewitt J, Campbell W, Jennings L, Willerson J, Schmitz J. Reduction in the rate of early restenosis after coronary angioplasty by a diet supplemented with n-3 fatty acids. N Engl J Med 1988;319:733–740.
75. Lesperance J, Hudon G, White C, Laurier J, Waters D. Comparison by quantitative angiographic assessment of coronary stenoses of one view showing the severest narrowing to two orthogonal views. Am J Cardiol 1989;64:462–465.
76. Loaldi A, Polese A, Montorsi P, De Cesare N, Fabbiocchi F, Ravagnani P, Guazzi M. Comparison of nifedipine, propranolol and isosorbide dinitrate on angiographic progression and regression of coronary arterial narrowings in angina pectoris. Am J Cardiol 1989;64:433–439.
77. Brown B, Bolson E, Dodge H. Quantitative computer techniques for analyzing coronary arteriograms. Prog Cardiovasc Dis 1986;28:403–418.
78. Hudon G, Lesperance J, Waters D. Reproducibility of quantitative angiographic measurements under different conditions: in search of a gold standard (abstr). Circulation 1990;82:III–617.
79. Gurley J, Nissen S, Booth D, DeMaria A. Influence of operator- and patient-dependent variables on the suitability of automated quantitative coronary arteriography for routine clinical use. J Am Coll Cardiol 1992;19:1237–1243.
80. Umans V, Beatt K, Rensing B, Hermans W, de Feyter P, Serruys P. Comparative quantitative angiographic analysis of directional coronary atherectomy and balloon coronary angioplasty. Am J Cardiol 1991;68:1556–1563.

81. Seibert J, Nalcioglu O, Roeck W. Characterization of the veiling glare in x-ray image intensified fluoroscopy. Med Phys 1984;11:172-179.
82. Milne E. The role and performance of minute focal spots in roentgenology with special reference to magnification. CRC Crit Rev Radiol Sci 1971;2:269-310.
83. Parisi A, Frolland E, Hartigan P. A comparison of angioplasty with medical therapy in the treatment of single vessel coronary artery disease. N Engl J Med 1992;326:10-16.
84. Rensing B, Hermans W, Deckers J, de Feyter P, Tijssen J, Serruys P. Lumen narrowing after percutaneous transluminal coronary balloon angioplasty follows a near Gaussian distribution: A quantitative angiographic study in 1,445 successfully dilated lesions. J Am Coll Cardiol 1992;19:939-945.
85. Kuntz R, Foley D, Keeler G, Umans V, Berdan L, Simonton C, Holmes D. Relationship of acute luminal gain to late loss following directional atherectomy or balloon angioplasty in CAVEAT (abstr). Circulation 1993;88:I-495.
86. Serruys P, Macaya C, de Jaegere P, Kiemeneij F, Rutsch W, Heyndrickx G, Emaluelsson H, Marco J, Legrand V, Materne P, Belardi J, Buller N, Colombo A, Goy J, Delcan J, Morel M. Interim analysis of the benestent-trial (abstr). Circulation 1993;88:I-594.
87. Popma J, Bashore T. Qualitative and quantitative angiography. In: Topel E, ed. Interventional Cardiology. Vol. 2. Philadelphia: WB Saunders, 1993:1058-1062.
88. Brogan W, Popma J, Satler L, Pichard A, Kent K, Chuang Y, Keller M, Leon M. Determinants of luminal improvement after new device angioplasty in complex lesion subsets (abstr). J Am Coll Cardiol 1993;21:233A.
89. Haude M, Erbel R, Hassan I. Quantitative analysis of elastic recoil after balloon angioplasty and intracoronary implantation of balloon-expandable Palmaz-Schatz stents. J Am Coll Cardiol 1993;21:26-34.
90. Fram D, McKay R. "Hot" balloon angioplasty: Radiofrequency, neodynium: YAG, and microwave. In: Topol E, ed. Interventional Cardiology. Vol. 2. Philadelphia: WB Saunders, 1993:819-839.
91. Brogan WI, Popma J, Pichard A, Satler L, Kent K, Mintz G, Leon M. Rotational coronary atherectomy after unsuccessful coronary balloon angioplasty. Am J Cardiol 1993;71:794-798.
92. Israel D, Marmur J, Sanborn T. Excimer laser-facilitated balloon angioplasty of a nondilatable lesion. J Am Coll Cardiol 1991;18:1118-1119.
93. Hermans W, Rensing B, Strauss B, Serruys P. Methodological problems related to the quantitative assessment of stretch, elastic recoil, and balloon-artery ratio. Cathet Cardiovasc Diagn 1992;25:174-185.
94. Hjemdahl-Monsen C, Ambrose J, Borrico S, Cohen M, Sherman W, Alexopoulos D, Gorlin R, Fuster V. Angiographic patterns of balloon inflation during percutaneous transluminal coronary angioplasty: Role of pressure-diameter curves in studying distensibility and elasticity of the stenotic lesion and the mechanism of dilatation. J Am Coll Cardiol 1990;16:569-575.
95. Hanet C, Wijns W, Michel X, Schroeder E. Influence of balloon size and stenosis morphology on immediate and delayed elastic recoil after percutaneous transluminal coronary angioplasty. J Am Coll Cardiol 1991;18:506-511.

96. Rensing B, Hermans W, Beatt K, Laarman G, Suryapranata H, van den Brand M, de Feyter P, Serruys P. Quantitative angiographic assessment of elastic recoil after percutaneous transluminal coronary angioplasty. Am J Cardiol 1990;66:1039–1044.

97. Rensing B, Hermans W, Strauss B, Serruys P. Regional differences in elastic recoil after percutaneous transluminal coronary angioplasty: A quantitative angiographic study. J Am Coll Cardiol 1991;17:34B–38B.

98. Rensing B, Hermans W, Vos J, Beatt K, Bossuyt P, Rutsch W, Serruys P. Angiographic risk factors of luminal narrowing after coronary balloon angioplasty using balloon measurements to reflect stretch and elastic recoil at the dilatation site. Am J Cardiol 1992;69:584–591.

99. Gould K. Percent diameter stenosis: Battered gold standard, pernicious relic or clinical practicality? J Am Coll Cardiol 1988;11:886–888.

100. Vogel R. Assessing stenosis significance by coronary arteriography: Are the best variables good enough? J Am Coll Cardiol 1988;12:692–693.

101. Grondin C, Dyra I, Pasternac A, Campeau L, Bourassa M, Lesperance J. Discrepancies between cineangiographic and postmortem findings in patients with coronary artery disease and recent myocardial revascularization. Circulation 1974;49:703–708.

102. Popma J, Chuang Y, Sweet L, Syed R, Leon M. Clinical and angiographic predictors of target lesion revascularization after new device angioplasty (abstr). Circulation 1993;88:I-150.

103. Serruys P, Luijten H, Beatt K, Geuskens R, de Feyter P, van den Brand M, Reiber J, ten Katen H, van Es G, Hugenholtz P. Incidence of restenosis after successful coronary angioplasty: a time-related phenomenon. A quantitative angiographic study in 342 consecutive patients at 1, 2, 3, and 4 months. Circulation 1988;77:361–371.

104. Nobuyoshi M, Kimura T, Nosaka H, Mioka S, Ueno K, Yokoi H, Hamasaki N, Horiuchi H, Ohishi H. Restenosis after successful percutaneous transluminal coronary angioplasty: Serial angiographic follow-up of 229 patients. J Am Coll Cardiol 1988;12:616–623.

105. Gruentzig A, King S, Schlumpf M, Siegenthaler W. Long-term follow-up after percutaneous transluminal coronary angioplasty: the early Zurich experience. N Engl J Med 1987;316:1127–1132.

106. Weintraub W, Ghazzal Z, Cohen C, Douglas J, Liberman H, Morris D, King S. Clinical implications of late proven patency after successful coronary angioplasty. Circulation 1991;84:572–582.

107. Rosen D, Cannon R, Watson R, Bonow R, Mincemoyer R, Ewels C, Leon M, Lakatos E, Epstein S, Kent K. Three year anatomic, functional and clinical follow-up after successful percutaneous transluminal coronary angioplasty. J Am Coll Cardiol 1987;9:1–7.

108. Stone G, Ligon R, Rutherford B, McConahay D, Hartzler G. Short-term outcome and long-term follow-up following coronary angioplasty in the young patient: an 8 year experience. Am Heart J 1989;118:873.

109. Austin G, Ratliff N, Hollman J, Tabei S, Phillips D. Intimal proliferation of smooth muscle cells as an explanation for recurrent coronary artery stenosis

after percutaneous transluminal coronary angioplasty. J Am Coll Cardiol 1985; 6:369–375.

110. Schwartz R, Murphy J, Edwards W, Camrud A, Vleitstra R, Holmes D. Restenosis after balloon angioplasty. A practical proliferative model in porcine coronary arteries. Circulation 1991;82:2190–2200.

111. Schwartz R, Holmes DJ, Topol E. The restenosis paradigm revisited: An alternative proposal for cellular mechanisms. J Am Coll Cardiol 1992;20:1284–1293.

112. Schwartz R, Huber K, Murphy J, Edwards W, Camrud A, Vlietstra R, Holmes D. Restenosis and the proportional neointimal response to coronary artery injury: Results in a porcine model. J Am Coll Cardiol 1992;19:267–274.

113. Mintz G, Kovach J, Javier S, Ditrano C, Leon M. Geometric remodeling is the predominant mechanism of late lumen loss after coronary angioplasty (abstr). Circulation 1993;88:I-654.

114. Umans V, Strauss B, Rensing B, de Jaegere P, de Feyter P, Serruys P. Comparative angiographic quantitative analysis of the immediate efficacy of coronary atherectomy with balloon angioplasty, stenting, and rotational ablation. Am Heart J 1991;122:836–843.

115. Corcos T, David P, Val P, Renkin J, Dangiosse V, Rapold H, Bourassa M. Failure of diltiazem to prevent restenosis after percutaneous transluminal coronary angioplasty. Am Heart J 1985;109:926–931.

116. The Multicenter European Research Trial with Cilazapril After Angioplasty to Prevent Transluminal Coronary Obstruction and Restenosis (MERCATOR) Study Group. Does the new angiotensin converting enzyme inhibitor Cilazapril prevent restenosis after percutaneous transluminal coronary angioplasty? Results of the MERCATOR Study: A multicenter, randomized, double-blind placebo-controlled trial. Circulation 1992;86:100–110.

117. Holmes D, Vlietstra R, Smith H, Vetrovec G, Kent K, Cowley M, Faxon D, Gruentzig A, Kelsey S, Detre K, Van Raden M, Mock M. Restenosis after percutaneous transluminal coronary angioplasty (PTCA): a report from the PTCA Registry of the National Heart, Lung, and Blood Institute. Am J Cardiol 1984;53:77C–81C.

118. Gould K, Lipscomb K, Hamilton G. Physiological basis for assessing critical coronary stenosis: instantaneous flow response and regional distribution during coronary hyperemia as measures of coronary flow reserve. Am J Cardiol 1974;33:87–97.

119. Beatt K, Serruys P, Hugenholtz P. Restenosis after coronary angioplasty: New standards for clinical studies. J Am Coll Cardiol 1990;15:491–498.

120. Serruys P, Rutsch W, Heyndrickx G, Danchin N, Mast E, Eijns W, Rensing B, Vos J, Stibbe J. Prevention of restenosis after percutaneous transluminal coronary angioplasty with thromboxane A2-receptor blockade: A randomized, double-blind, placebo-controlled trial. Circulation 1991;84:1568–1580.

121. Carozza J, Kuntz R, Fishman R, Baim D. Restenosis following arterial injury in diabetics: an analysis of intimal hyperplasia following coronary stenting. Ann Intern Med 1993;118:344–349.

122. Bourassa M, Lesperance J, Eastwood C, Schwartz, Cote G, Kazim F, Hudon G. Clinical physiologic, anatomic and procedural factors predictive of restenosis after percutaneous transluminal coronary angioplasty. J Am Coll Cardiol 1991;18:368–376.

123. Fishman R, Kuntz R, Carrozza JJ, Miller M, Senerchia C, Schnitt S, Diver D, Safian R, Baim D. Long-term results of directional coronary athterectomy: Predictors of restenosis. J Am Coll Cardiol 1992;20:1101–1110.

124. Popma J, De Cesare N, Pinkerton C, Kereiakes D, Whitlow P, King SI, Topol E, Holmes D, Leon M, Ellis S. Quantitative analysis of factors influencing late lumen loss and restenosis after directional coronary atherectomy. Am J Cardiol 1993;71:552–557.

125. Hirshfeld J, Schwartz J, Jugo R, MacDonald R, Goldberg S, Savage M, Bass T, Vetrovec G, Cowley M, Taussig A, Whitworth H, Margolis J, Hill J, Pepine C. Restenosis after coronary angioplasty: A multivariate statistical model to relate lesion and procedure variables to restenosis. J Am Coll Cardiol 1991;18:647–656.

126. Kuntz R, Hinohara T, Robertson G, Safian R, Simpson J, Baim D. Influence of vessel selection on the observed restenosis rate after endoluminal stenting or directional atherectomy. Am J Cardiol 1992;70:1101–1108.

127. Carrozza JJ, Kuntz R, Levine M, Pomerantz R, Fishman R, Mansour M, Gibson C, Senerchia C, Diver D, Safian R, Baim D. Angiographic and clinical outcome of intracoronary stenting: Immediate and long-term results from a large single-center experience. J Am Coll Cardiol 1992;20:328–337.

128. Glagov S, Weisenberg E, Zarins C, Stankunacicius K, Kolettis G. Compensatory enlargement of various human atherosclerotic arteries. N Engl J Med 1987;316:1371–1375.

129. Popma J, Califf R, Topol E. Clinical trials of restenosis after coronary angioplasty. Circulation 1991;84:1426–1436.

130. Raizner A, Hollman J, Demke D, Wakefield L. Beneficial effects of ciprostene in PTCA: A multicenter, randomized, controlled trial (abstr). Circulation 1988;78:II-290.

131. Raizner A, Hollman J, Abukhalil J, Demke D. Ciprostene for restenosis revisited: Quantitative analysis of angiograms (abstr). J Am Coll Cardiol 1993;21:321A.

132. Dick R, Popma J, Muller D, Burek K, Topol E. In-hospital costs associated with new percutaneous coronary devices. Am J Cardiol 1991;68:879–885.

133. Lincoff A, Keeler G, Debowey D, Topol E. Is clinical site variability an important determinant of outcome following percutaneous revascularization with new technology? Insight from CAVEAT (abstr). Circulation 1993;88:I-653.

134. Popma J, Mintz G, Satler L, Pichard A, Kent K, Chuang Y, Matar F, Bucher T, Merritt A, Leon M. Clinical and angiographic outcome after directional coronary atherectomy: A qualitative and quantitative analysis using coronary arteriography and intravascular ultrasound. Am J Cardiol 1993;72:55E–64E.

135. Bittl J. Directional coronary atherectomy versus balloon angioplasty. N Engl J Med 1993;329:273–274.

136. Berdan L, Califf R. Restenosis: Does the six month angiogram tell the story? CAVEAT one year follow-up (abstr). Circulation 1993;88:I-595.

137. Popma J, van den Berg E, Dehmer G. Long-term outcome of patients with asymptomatic restenosis after percutaneous transluminal coronary angioplasty. Am J Cardiol 1988;62:1298-1299.

138. Hernandez R, Macaya C, Iniguez A, Alfonso F, Goicolea J, Fernandez-Ortiz A, Zarco P. Midterm outcome of patients with asymptomatic restenosis after coronary balloon angioplasty. J Am Coll Cardiol 1992;19:1402-1409.

139. Laarman G, Luijten H, van Zeyl L, Beatt K, Tijssen J, Serruys P, de Feyter P. Assessment of silent restenosis and long-term follow-up after successful angioplasty in single vessel coronary artery disease: the value of quantitative exercise electrocardiography and quantitative coronary angiography. J Am Coll Cardiol 1990;16:578-585.

140. Leimgruber P, Roubin G, Hollman J, Cotsnis G, Meier B, Douglas J, King S. Restenosis after successful coronary angioplasty in patients with single-vessel disease. Circulation 1986;73:710-717.

141. Vlay S, Chernilas J, Lawson W, Dervan J. Restenosis after angioplasty: don't rely on the exercise test. Am Heart J 1989;4:980-986.

142. Popma J, Dehmer G, Eichhorn E. Variability of coronary flow reserve obtained immediately after coronary angioplasty. Int J Card Imaging 1991;6:31-38.

143. Dietz W, Tobis J, Isner J. Failure of angiography to accurately depict the extent of coronary artery narrowing in three fatal cases of percutaneous transluminal coronary angioplasty. J Am Coll Cardiol 1992;19:1261-1270.

144. Kuntz R, Keaney K, Senerchia C, Baim D. Estimating late results of coronary intervention from incomplete angiographic follow-up. Circulation 1993;87:815-830.

145. Califf R, Fortin D, Frid D, et al. Restenosis after coronary angioplasty: An overview. J Am Coll Cardiol 1991;17:2B-13B.

146. Piana R, Kugelmass A, Moscucci M, Ho K, Mansour K, Kuntz R. Coronary restenosis rates defined by 6 month angiography compared to those defined by specific clinical events (abstr). Circulation 1993;88:I-654.

147. Kugelmass A, Piana R, Moscucci M, Leidig G, Senerchia C, Baim D. Optimal "clinical" endpoints for detecting coronary restenosis: Analysis using cumulative hazards for specific clinical events (abstr). Circulation 1993;88:I-655.

148. Reis G, Sipperly M, McCabe C, Sacks F, Boucher T, Silverman D, Baim D, Grossman W, Pasternak R. Randomized trial of fish oil for prevention of restenosis after coronary angioplasty. Lancet 1989;II:177-181.

5

Assessment of Myocardial Viability

Jorge Cheirif
Ochsner Medical Institutions, New Orleans, Louisiana

I. INTRODUCTION

The assessment of myocardial viability is one of the newest and most rapidly expanding areas of clinical and experimental research. A number of diagnostic techniques have been developed to help the clinician determine with a fair, and sometimes outstanding, degree of accuracy whether myocardial viability is present or absent in dyssynergic regions of the heart. This review is intended to be a summary of the accumulated clinical practical information regarding the need to detect the presence of myocardial viability, the existing methods used to diagnose it and their limitations, and finally the treatment strategies used in this entity.

A. History

The successful development of myocardial revascularization in the late 1960s opened a new era in modern cardiology. The number of aortocoronary bypass grafting (CABG) procedures grew in an almost exponential fashion in the ensuing years. This new form of treatment provided long-lasting relief of angina in most patients. The VA Cooperative study was the first to demonstrate the improved survival of patients with significant left main coronary artery stenosis treated with CABG in comparison to other medical therapies (1).

113

The Coronary Artery Surgery Study (CASS) and the European Cooperative Studies demonstrated an improved survival in patients with triple vessel coronary artery disease with and without depressed ejection fraction, respectively, when treated with CABG rather than medical therapy (2–4). No clear explanation has been provided for the improvement in survival demonstrated by CASS, but this finding is of interest to the present discussion.

B. Resting Wall Motion Abnormalities and Myocardial Viability

A potential explanation for improved survival could be that the patients with severe resting wall motion abnormalities could have had severely ischemic but yet viable myocardium that could have improved its function after myocardial revascularization. The following information supports this theory. To begin with, at autopsy, significant amounts of histologically normal myocardium have been observed in these types of patients with severe resting wall motion abnormalities (5). Some akinetic and even dyskinetic segments show the presence of enhanced glucose metabolism by positron emission tomography (PET) (6,7), sometimes even in the presence of "fixed" perfusion defects by thallium-201 (8). Furthermore, several reports in the literature (9–11) have demonstrated that these patients frequently show an improvement in regional wall motion after myocardial revascularization by CABG. More recently, the use of percutaneous transluminal angioplasty (PTCA) has also been found to improve resting wall motion abnormalities (12–14). Two potential underlying mechanisms for these resting wall motion abnormalities have been proposed. The first is known as myocardial "stunning," and the second as myocardial "hibernation."

1. Myocardial Stunning

Myocardial stunning is a state in which a severe but short-lasting episode (usually less than 15 min) of myocardial ischemia results in prolonged regional contractile dysfunction (up to 24 h) despite adequate reestablishment of coronary blood flow (15). Thus far, no definite structural abnormality has been identified as the cause of the impairment in contractility (16). This disruption might be mediated by oxygen-free radicals produced during myocardial reperfusion (15). Myocardial stunning is likely to occur in patients presenting with intense coronary vasospasm (17,18), after thrombolysis and/or PTCA in the acute phase of myocardial infarction (19–21), and in response to other noxious stimuli likely to cause temporary ischemia (i.e., CABG) (22–25).

2. Myocardial Hibernation

The second entity to consider is known as myocardial hibernation. Rahimtoola (26) was the first to coin the concept of myocardial hibernation to indicate a state of chronically depressed regional myocardial blood flow associated with depressed myocardial contractility. This abnormal contractility could be improved by successful myocardial revascularization. Rahimtoola (27) has suggested that hibernation may likely occur with unstable angina, chronic stable angina, left ventricular dysfunction of unknown causes, unrecognized coronary disease, and diabetes mellitus. It may also follow myocardial infarction, cardiac arrest, heart transplant, and myocardial revascularization.

II. CLINICAL IMPORTANCE OF ESTABLISHING MYOCARDIAL VIABILITY

Several studies (28,29) have highlighted the importance of a depressed ejection fraction in the long-term survival of patients with heart failure. Given the fact that coronary artery disease is a progressive disease and that ischemic damage will likely be cumulative over the life of the subject, it behooves us to determine if resting wall motion abnormalities are secondary to ischemic but viable myocardium that could improve function if adequate flow can be reestablished and/or if repeated episodes of ischemia can be prevented. Failing to recognize the presence of dysfunctional but viable myocardium could result in the refusal of a "muscle saving" procedure (i.e., revascularization). The following case report exemplifies the importance of detecting viable myocardium.

Case Report: The patient, MN, is a 67-year-old woman admitted with congestive heart failure. She had an inferior wall myocardial infarction with CPK elevations up to 2000. On physical examination, blood pressure was 90/60 with a pulse of 84. A JVP pressure of 8-10 cm was noted. Lungs showed bilateral basal crackles. Cardiac examination revealed a heaving apex with an S3 gallop. Abdomen was benign and there was no pedal edema. The EKG showed evidence of inferior and anteroseptal myocardial infarction. The right heart catheterization revealed the following hemodynamic data: RA: 11/11/8,; RV: 50/8; PA: 50/24; PCW: 30/28/28; AO: 100/44/66; LV: 100/30; LVEDP post: 30; Cardiac Output: 41/min (thermodilution), 3.51/min (Fick). Angiography was performed and the left ventriculogram showed a depressed left ventricular function with a measured ejection fraction of 30% and the following regional wall motion abnormalities: inferior and inferobasal segments were akinetic; the apex was hypokinetic, and the lateral and anterolateral walls were hypokinetic; the inferolateral wall was severely hypokinetic; and the best motion was noted in the anterobasal segment and the interventricular septum. There was 1 + mitral regurgitation, part of which was induced by the catheter. The left main coronary artery had an 80–90% stenosis at its distal portion. The left anterior descending artery was a long vessel of small diameter, with a tight stenosis noted in its proximal portion. The vessel filled slowly and emptied very late. A large ramus marginalis branch, which gave origin to a large branch at its proximal portion, was noted, and a 50% stenosis was noted at the proximal ramus.

The left circumflex artery was a very small vessel. There was a subtotal occlusion immediately after the origin of the first obtuse marginal branch. The second obtuse marginal branch of the left circumflex was very thin and filled very late. TIMI I flow was noted in this vessel. The right coronary artery was the dominant vessel but had luminal irregularities at its middle portion; there was a tight stenosis at the middle right coronary artery immediately distal to a right ventricle branch. Distally, the right coronary artery divided into a moderate-sized posterior descending artery and posterolateral branches. A 50% stenosis was noted at the proximal posterior descending artery. Septal collaterals filled the distal obtuse marginal branch from the right coronary artery. In this patient, despite the presence of severe resting wall motion abnormalities and severe multivessel coronary artery disease, the thallium-201 (Fig. 1), sestamibi (Fig. 1), and contrast echocardiogram (Figs. 2–4) showed the presence of myocardial perfusion in most regions of the left ventricle, and therefore, presumably, the presence of viability. The patient underwent CABG to the left anterior descending, left circumflex, and posterior

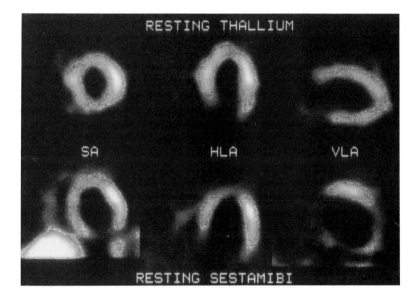

Figure 1 Example of the visual assessment of myocardial viability by thallium-201 SPECT (upper row) and by sestamibi SPECT (lower row) in a patient with severe resting wall motion abnormalities. From left to right, the views shown are: the short axis view (left), the horizontal long axis view (center), and the vertical long axis view (right). In this particular example, the thallium images show no perfusion defect, whereas the sestamibi shows a perfusion defect in the posterior wall (5:30–6:30 o'clock) in the short axis, and in the bottom part of the vertical long axis figure.

PRE   POST
Parasternal Long Axis

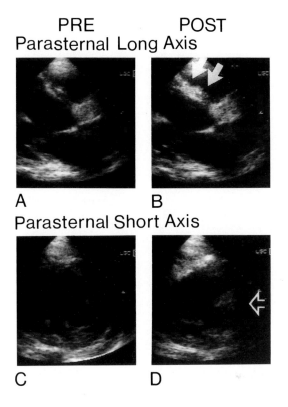

A   B
Parasternal Short Axis

C   D

Figure 2 Parasternal long axis (A and B) and short axis (C and D) views of patient MN. The images to the left are pre-echo contrast administration and the images to the right are post-echo contrast administration. In this example, the contrast is administered into the left main coronary artery. An increase in brightness, or contrast effect, is noted in the septum (solid arrow). The lateral wall (open arrow) shows dropout of the image and therefore cannot be evaluated in this view.

descending arteries, and as early as 10 min after CABG, an improvement in global ventricular function could already be appreciated (Fig. 5).

III. METHODS USED TO ASSESS MYOCARDIAL VIABILITY

Several methods have been used to assess the presence or absence of myocardial viability. Generally speaking, these methods depend on the demonstration of myocardial perfusion, myocardial metabolism, or an inotropic

PRE   POST
Apical 4 Chamber

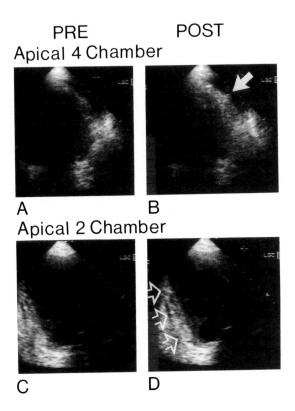

A   B
Apical 2 Chamber

C   D

Figure 3 Apical four-chamber (A and B) and two-chamber (C and D) views of patient MN. In this example, the lateral wall (solid arrow) shows a contrast effect, but the apex and septal walls are not well visualized and therefore cannot be evaluated well in this view. The inferior wall (open arrows) does not show any significant contrast effect.

response to a stimulus. The methods that use the demonstration of perfusion as the basis for the presence of viability include positron emission tomography (PET), thallium-201 imaging, sestamibi imaging, and myocardial contrast echocardiography. The first of these techniques, PET, uses, in addition to the assessment of perfusion, indices of metabolism to demonstrate viability. Methods that use the inotropic response to a stimulus include dobutamine-echocardiography, postextrasystolic potentiation, and nitroglycerin administration.

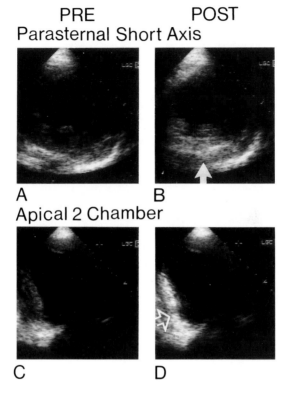

PRE   POST
Parasternal Short Axis

A   B
Apical 2 Chamber

C   D

Figure 4   Parasternal short axis (A and B) and two-chamber (C and D) views before and after echo-contrast administration in the right coronary artery in patient MN. The posterior wall (solid arrows) and the inferior wall (open arrow) show a contrast effect.

A. Positron Emission Tomography

Positron emission tomography has been successfully used to assess myocardial viability (6–8,30–33). This technique has the distinct advantage of allowing for the assessment of both myocardial perfusion and metabolism. This is particularly important since severely ischemic but viable myocardium might show almost no flow, despite the presence of myocardial metabolism. Under normal circumstances, the myocardium uses fatty acids for its metabolism. However, when blood flow and oxygen supply decrease, anaerobic metabolism ensues, and consequently, the myocardium begins using glucose

Pre CABG   Post CABG

| DIASTOLE | SYSTOLE | DIASTOLE | SYSTOLE |

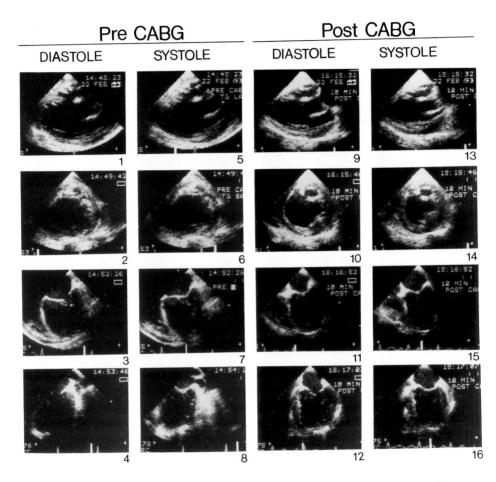

Figure 5 Left ventricular function assessment by echocardiographic views before and after CABG in patient MN, including long axis (first row), short axis (second row), the apical four-chamber (third row), apical two-chamber (fourth row) views, in both end-diastole and in end-systole. An improvement in global function is seen post-CABG in all views.

instead of fatty acids as a source of energy (34). A high ratio of regional glucose utilization to myocardial flow has been found to be a reliable sign of severely ischemic but viable muscle (6).

Tillisch et al. (6) studied 17 consecutive patients with resting wall motion abnormalities with PET. Sixteen of these patients had a history of myocardial infarction. Wall motion was graded on a 0 (normal) to 4 (dyskinetic) scale. Positron emission tomography was performed with $^{13}NH_3$ and ^{18}FDG, normalizing all counts to the maximum counts obtained in all planes. All patients were then revascularized by CABG. Seventy-three regions were found to have abnormal resting wall motion, 37 (51%) of which improved postoperatively (43% with mild hypokinesis, 57% with severe hypokinesis, and 43% with akinesis). Resting wall motion abnormalities were predicted preoperatively to be reversible if ^{18}FDG uptake (tracer of metabolism) was normal or increased and if $^{13}NH_3$ uptake (tracer of flow) was normal (pattern A) or decreased (pattern B); wall motion abnormalities were predicted to be irreversible if both $^{13}NH_3$ and ^{18}FDG uptake were depressed (pattern C). Twenty-two of the revascularized regions with preoperative pattern A (88%), 13 of 16 regions with pattern B (81%), and only 2 of 26 regions with pattern C (7.6%) showed a postoperative improvement in wall motion. Of interest, 28 of 73 regions with baseline wall motion abnormalities (39%) had pathological Q waves on ECG; of these, 15 regions improved postoperatively. On the other hand, the remaining 13 regions showed no viability by PET, and only one of the 12 revascularized regions improved postoperatively.

Several studies have demonstrated that PET is a better predictor of myocardial viability than thallium-201 scintigraphy (8,30,32). This probably relates to the improved imaging resolution of PET and to its added benefit of also assessing metabolism. The advantage of PET over thallium is apparently lost when sophisticated quantitative analysis of perfusion by thallium is undertaken (31). The disadvantages of PET relate to its high cost, nonportability, and need of an in situ cyclotron to produce the ^{18}F-deoxyglucose.

B. Thallium-201 Imaging

Thallium-201 imaging (Fig. 1) has been used successfully by various groups to detect myocardial viability (8,30–32,35–48). In essence, thallium-201 is a potassium analog and, as such, is extracted from the blood by the cells of the myocardium in proportion to blood flow. In routine clinical practice, the thallium is injected intravenously at the peak of stress (i.e., treadmill, dipyridamole, adenosine, etc.) and the myocardium is then imaged within a few minutes. If the myocardium shows a relative perfusion defect, this then demonstrates a disparity of myocardial blood flow between one or more regions in the heart. Once this occurs, one is left to decide what the underlying abnormality of flow is. This abnormality can be due to ischemia during stress, to a previous myocardial infarction, or to myocardial hibernation. To distinguish among these three possibilities, one must resort to redistribution imaging 4 h after stress imaging. The presence of redistribution, or a filling-in of the perfusion defect at 4 h, documents viable but "ischemic" myocardium, whereas the lack of redistribution indicates either a scar or hibernating myocardium. Since the decision to revascularize a certain area of the heart might depend on the proof of viability, the distinction between scar and hibernation is self-evident.

Dilsizian et al. (40) studied 100 patients with known coronary artery disease (CAD). All patients had a 2-mCi injection of thallium-201 at peak exercise followed by single photon emission computed tomography (SPECT) with a gamma camera immediately after exercise, and 3–4 h later. A second injection (1 mCi) of thallium was performed then and reinjection imaging was done 10–125 min later. Both qualitative and quantitative thallium analysis were performed on all images. All patients underwent coronary arteriography and gated blood-pool cardiac scintigraphy as well. Of 100 patients, 20 patients underwent PTCA, followed 3–6 months later by repeat thallium exercise SPECT, radionuclide, and coronary angiography. Ninety-two of the patients showed perfusion defects during exercise for a total of 260 abnormal regions (qualitative analysis) and 259 regions (quantitative analysis). Of these 260 regions, 172 regions (66%) showed persistent defects at redistribution (87 showed partial reversibility and 85 showed no reversibility). After reinjection of thallium, 42 of 85 regions (49%) with no reversibility showed increased thallium uptake. Similarly, the quantitative analysis showed an improved thallium uptake in 40% of "fixed" defects. In the 20 patients undergoing PTCA, 15 of 23 regions (65%) with persistent defects on redistribution imaging showed enhanced thallium uptake during reinjection imaging. On repeat imaging 3–6 months post-PTCA, 13 of 15 regions (87%) were found to have normal stress and redistribution thallium uptake and improved regional wall motion. These data suggest that the routine 4-h redistribution imaging underestimates the presence of viable myocardium (36–38). This may relate in part to the slow nature of thallium redistribution and in part to the low levels of thallium present in the blood hours after the initial administration. To deal with the slow redistribution, some investigators have advocated waiting up to 24 h to reassess redistribution when a fixed defect is present at 4 h (38). However, in many cases this is impractical, and in others, the myocardial counts can be so low as to make the interpretation of images difficult. To deal with the low levels of thallium during redistribution, early or late reinjection of thallium poststress can be done (40–45). Whereas these strategies do indeed seem to reduce the overestimation of scar by thallium, they also add to the cost and radiation involved in this procedure.

Among the advantages of thallium imaging are the facts that it is widely used in this country and that the parameters of viability are, though mostly subjective, well known and accepted.

C. Technetium-99m-Methoxyisobutyl Isonitrile (Sestamibi)

Recently, technetium-99m-methoxyisobutyl isonitrile (Fig. 1), better known as sestamibi, has been used to identify dysfunctional but viable myocardium

(45,46). This agent does not redistribute in the myocardium and has a much shorter half-life than thallium. Several studies using sestamibi have shown that its sensitivity and specificity for diagnosing coronary artery disease are comparable to that of thallium scintigraphy (47–49). However, in comparative studies, it appears to be less reliable than thallium in detecting myocardial viability (45–46).

Marzullo et al. (46) studied 14 patients with resting regional wall motion abnormalities due to a previous myocardial infarction. All patients underwent a resting thallium injection with early (10 min) and late (16 h) imaging, a resting sestamibi, and a dobutamine-echocardiogram. Fifty segments (group 1) had normal wall motion and < 50% coronary stenosis. Fifty-seven (group 2) segments showed normal wall motion and > 50% stenosis; and 75 segments (group 3) showed abnormal wall motion abnormalities and > 50% stenosis. Early thallium-201, delayed thallium-201, sestamibi, and dobutamine echocardiography correctly identified 79%, 86%, 75%, and 82%, respectively, of the postoperative viable segments and 92% of the postoperative nonviable segments.

D. Myocardial Contrast Echocardiography

Myocardial contrast echocardiography (MCE) (Figs. 2–4) is a relatively new technique for assessing myocardial perfusion (50). In this technique, minuscule ($< 10\ \mu$m) microbubbles of air are produced by a process called sonication (51) and are then injected into the coronary arteries or into the aortic root while the heart is imaged with two-dimensional echocardiography. As the microbubbles pass through the myocardium, a "contrast" effect is observed in the myocardium; this contrast effect occurs because the microbubbles act as potent reflectors of sound waves (52). With this technique, myocardial regions without blood flow appear as absolute (i.e., dark) perfusion defects, whereas regions with reduced blood flow appear as regions with "relative" perfusion defects (i.e., less bright than normally perfused areas) (53–55).

This technique has been used to demonstrate areas at risk both experimentally and clinically (56–58). It has been used to demonstrate the improvement in myocardial perfusion that follows PTCA (58,59) and CABG (60,61). Myocardial contrast echocardiography has also been used to assess collateral blood flow (62–64); this is particularly important to our present discussion since in the presence of critical lesions and/or total occlusions the viability of the muscle previously perfused by a patent artery will totally depend on the flow provided by collaterals for its survival. The concept is clearly demonstrated in a recent study by Sabia et al. (65). In this study, 33 patients with recent myocardial infarctions (12 ± 7 days) underwent an MCE study during catheterization. All of these patients had totally occluded infarct-related arteries, and thus flow to the infarcted areas, if present, would have to come retrogradely via collaterals. A significant correlation ($r = 0.67$, $p < 0.01$) was observed between peak creatine kinase levels and the percentage of myocardium not perfused by either antegrade or collateral flow. Likewise, a significant negative correlation ($r = -0.57$, $p < 0.01$) was observed between MCE-defined spatial extent of collateral flow and regional function. Along these lines, we have recently demonstrated in an animal model of thrombosis-thrombolysis that, as assessed by MCE, the degree of collateral flow observed during thrombosis can predict the eventual recovery of function post-thrombolysis (66).

Two recent papers (67,68) have addressed the ability of MCE to predict the recovery of regional function in patients after previous myocardial infarctions who were subjected to revascularization or thrombolysis to improve flow to the region demonstrating resting wall motion abnormalities. Ito et al. (67) studied 39 patients presenting with acute anterior myocardial infarction who demonstrated total occlusions of the left anterior descending coronary artery during angiography. At the time of angiography, MCE was performed before and after thrombolysis ($n = 10$) or PTCA ($n = 29$) of the culprit vessel. All patients had angiographically successful reperfusion. A significant perfusion defect was noted before thrombolysis or PTCA in all patients, but only in nine patients postreperfusion. The patients showing "perfusion" after thrombolysis had significant improvements of regional function and ejection fraction at 4 weeks. On the other hand, the patients showing persistent perfusion defects had no improvements in function at follow-up. This study demonstrates two important findings. First, it shows that a patient can have an angiographically open epicardial artery after thrombolysis and still have low microcirculatory blood flow. The microcirculation is, in fact, more important than the patency status for recovery of function. Second, the study highlights the value of MCE to assess the degree of the microcirculation after reperfusion.

The second study (68) examined 43 patients undergoing PTCA post-MI. Myocardial contrast echocardiography was performed before and after successful PTCA. Regional wall motion was scored using a 1 to 5 scale, where 1 = normal function and 5 = dyskinesis. An angiographically successful PTCA was observed in 34 patients, and an unsuccessful PTCA in 9 patients. As assessed by MCE (i.e., evidence of perfusion in the region with abnormal resting wall motion), the percentage of the infarct bed supplied by collateral flow was similar in patients in whom PTCA was successful and in patients in whom it was not ($73 \pm 5\%$ vs. $67 \pm 14\%$, p = NS). The 32 patients with abnormal wall motion at baseline showed significant inverse correlations between the percentage of the infarct bed supplied by collateral flow at baseline and the wall motion 1 month later. Furthermore, a significant improvement in wall motion score was seen. At follow-up, the patients showing extensive collateral flow at baseline and successful PTCA had significant improvements in wall motion ($p < 0.001$), whereas the patients with poor collateral flow at baseline despite successful PTCA did not show any improvements in wall motion. In this study, MCE was again more predictive of functional recovery than angiography was.

E. Dobutamine Echocardiography

The use of dobutamine echocardiography to assess myocardial viability has recently been recognized (33,46). Briefly, if a resting regional contractile abnormality is secondary to stunning, the addition of low-dose intravenous dobutamine (5 to 10 μg/kg/min) will result in an improvement in contractile function. While several explanations have been proposed to explain this finding, it is probably the result of an improvement in the metabolism-contractile coupling. The dobutamine echocardiography test has been found to be safe and effective in predicting viability (33,46), and, in at least one small study, comparable to PET scanning (33).

Pierard et al. (33) studied 17 patients treated with intravenous thrombolysis within 3 h of a first acute anterior myocardial infarction. Dobutamine echocardiography was performed 7 ± 4 days after thrombolysis at doses of 5 and 10 mg/kg/min for 5 min. Positron emission tomography was performed at rest with N_{13} ammonia (flow tracer) and with ^{18}F-deoxyglucose (metabolism tracer). Based on the presence or absence of viability as assessed by PET (described earlier), the patients were divided into three groups: group 1A (five patients with normal perfusion in the area at risk); group 1B (six patients with decreased flow but abnormally high glucose to perfusion ratios); and group 2 (six patients with parallel decreases in perfusion and glucose uptake). Systolic wall thickening improved with dobutamine in all group 1A patients, in three of six group 1B patients, and in none of the group 2 patients. Concordance between dobutamine echocardiography and PET was observed in 79% of the segments examined. Though these results are encouraging, more studies are necessary to establish the value of this technique in a larger number of patients.

One potential disadvantage of the technique, at least theoretically, relates to the presence of myocardial hibernation, rather than stunning, as the underlying mechanism of regional contractile dysfunction. In this instance, a resting wall motion abnormality would not be expected to improve during dobutamine administration, since the abnormality relates more to a state of chronically depressed myocardial blood flow, which in the presence of critical coronary stenosis or occlusions would not be expected to improve during dobutamine administration. A recent study (69) suggests that hibernation occurs in a sizable number of patients with resting wall motion abnormalities, implying that the number of patients with potentially falsely negative dobutamine-echocardiograms could be significant. The use of inducing a premature ventricular beat to detect viable muscle in the presence of a regional contractile abnormality is similar to a dobutamine echocardiogram (i.e., if the contractility improves, the region is viable) (70,71). Though this method appears to be able to detect the presence of viable muscle, it is unclear what the underlying mechanism of the dysfunction could have been in those studies; again, hibernation would not, at least in theory, be expected to show an improvement with a premature beat, while stunning would.

F. Nitroglycerin

The use of nitroglycerin to uncover viable but dysfunctional muscle (72, 73) is probably based on the fact that a reduction of preload results in an improved myocardial oxygen supply/demand ratio by decreasing the intracavitary pressure effect on the subendocardium.

IV. LIMITATIONS TO THE CLINICAL ASSESSMENT OF MYOCARDIAL VIABILITY

As explained earlier, the demonstration of viable myocardium in the presence of resting wall motion abnormalities requires the demonstration of myocardial perfusion and/or metabolism, or an improvement of the resting wall motion abnormality in response to some intervention [i.e., dobutamine,

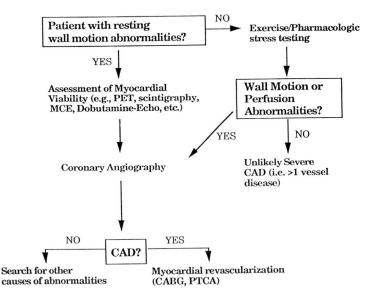

Figure 6 Proposed algorithm of myocardial viability assessment and treatment. CAD = coronary artery disease; CABG = coronary artery bypass grafting; MCE = myocardial contrast echocardiography; PTCA = percutaneous transluminal coronary angioplasty.

premature ventricular contraction (PVC), revascularization] (Fig. 6). If one thus decides that a region of myocardium showing hypokinesis or akinesis is indeed viable (though temporarily dysfunctional) but in need of revascularization to regain function, a potential problem might arise if the revascularization procedure is unsuccessful. In this instance, the regional function would not improve after the unsuccessful revascularization; however, the preoperative assessment would have "incorrectly" identified the tissue as viable. This problem has recently been demonstrated by Ragosta et al. (74). These investigators found that thallium-201 SPECT predicted regional myocardial viability before revascularization with a good sensitivity, specificity, and predictive accuracy. However, when these investigators examined the predictive accuracy of cases only with successful revascularization, they found a significantly higher accuracy for the technique to detect viability.

V. TREATMENT OF MYOCARDIAL HIBERNATION AND STUNNING

As described above, the primary underlying abnormality in myocardial hibernation is the chronically depressed myocardial blood flow (27). It follows then that an improvement in myocardial blood flow after successful thrombolysis, PTCA, or CABG will result in an improvement in contractile function. Though several studies would tend to support this (19–25), the concept of hibernation has recently been challenged, and an alternative explanation to the regional contractile dysfunction (i.e., that it is due to repetitive episodes of severe ischemia) has been suggested (69).

On the other hand, the primary abnormality in myocardial stunning is a defect in the energy-contractility coupling mechanism, a result of a severe but relatively short (< 15 min) period of ischemia mediated by the release of oxygen-free radicals. In this instance, the treatment can be directed toward improving the contractile function with catecholamines (75–78), with calcium (79), or by preventing the disruption of the primary abnormality by the use of oxygen-free radical scavengers (15). Several clinical studies are underway to explore the relative value of each of these strategies.

VI. SUMMARY

This chapter is an attempt to provide the reader with an up-to-date summary regarding the existing evidence that resting wall motion abnormalities do not equate to irreversibly damaged myocardium, and thus stress the importance of determining whether myocardial viability is present in patients exhibiting resting wall motion abnormalities. As explained earlier in this chapter, these abnormalities in contractility can be due to myocardial "stunning," myocardial "hibernation," or scar; the first two represent viable but temporarily dysfunctional myocardium that, under the appropriate conditions, can regain its normal function. Myocardial "stunning" represents a prolonged myocardial dysfunction state that follows a severe ischemic event; by definition, in this entity, the regional dysfunction persists despite the reestablishment of adequate blood flow. On the other hand, hibernation relates to a more chronic state in which a persistent decrease in regional flow leads (perhaps as an adaptive response) to prolonged myocardial dysfunction. Thus, the diagnosis of these two entities relies on the simultaneous assessment of regional myocardial perfusion and function. The concept of hibernation has recently been challenged and an alternative explanation to the regional contractile dysfunction (i.e., due to repetitive episodes of severe ischemia) has been suggested. Methods of assessment of myocardial viability include thallium-201 and sestamibi scintigraphy, PET scanning, myocardial contrast echocardiography, dobutamine echocardiography, and post-PVC and post-nitroglycerin improvement in regional function. Each of these techniques has advantages and disadvantages. While thallium-201 imaging is the most known and used method of assessing viability, the slow redistribution of thallium and the need for reinjection render it a time-consuming and costly process. Sestamibi, which takes less time because of its shorter half-life, has proven less reliable in detecting viability than its more popular counterpart. Though PET provides more sophisticated imaging resolution and information than the other methods (e.g., by assessment of metabolism), its cost and need for a cyclotron on site have limited its widespread use. In addition, some of the newer technological methods (i.e., MCE and dobutamine echocardiography) appear to be useful in detecting viability; however, these are "new" technologies, and their value will need to be tested in a larger number of patients.

ACKNOWLEDGMENT

This chapter was written during the tenure of Clinician-Scientist Award No. 92004390 of the American Heart Association.

REFERENCES

1. Takaro T, Hultgren HN, Lipton MJ, Detre KM. The VA Cooperative randomized study of surgery for coronary arterial occlusive disease. II. Subgroup with significant left main lesions. Circulation 1976;54(suppl III):III-107–III-117.
2. Alderman EL, Fisher LD, Litwin P, et al. Results of coronary artery bypass surgery in patients with poor left ventricular function (CASS). Circulation 1983;68: 785–795.

3. Passamani E,Davis BD, Gillespie MJ, Killip T, and the CASS principal investigators and their associates. A randomized trial of coronary artery bypass surgery: Survival of patients with low ejection fraction. N Engl J Med 1985;312: 1665-1671.

4. European Coronary Surgery Study Group. Long-term results of prospective randomised study of coronary artery bypass surgery in stable angina pectoris. Lancet 1982;1173-1180.

5. Flameng W, Wouters L, Sergeant P, et al. Multivariate analysis of angiographic, histologic and electrocardiographic data in patients with coronary artery disease. Circulation 1984;70:7-17.

6. Tillisch J, Brunken R, Marshall R, et al. Reversibility of cardiac wall motion abnormalities predicted by positron tomography. N Engl J Med 1986;314:884-888.

7. Brunken R, Rillisch J, Schwaiger M, et al. Regional perfusion, glucose metabolism, and wall motion in patients with chronic electrocardiographic Q wave infarctions: Evidence for persistence of viable tissue in some infarct regions by positron emission tomography. Circulation 1986;73:951-963.

8. Tamaki N, Yonekura Y, Yamashita K, et al. Relation of left ventricular perfusion and wall motion with metabolic activity in persistent defects on thallium-201 tomography in healed myocardial infarction. Am J Cardiol 1988;62:202-208.

9. Kolibask AJ, Goodenow JS, Busk CA, Teltalman MR, Lewis RP. Improvement of myocardial perfusion and left ventricular function after coronary artery bypass grafting in patients with unstable angina. Circulation 1979;59:66-74.

10. Chatterjee K, Swan JHC, Parmley WW, Sustaita H, Marcus HS, Matloff J. Influence of direct myocardial revascularization of left ventricular asynergy and function in patients with coronary heart disease. Circulation 1973;47:276-286.

11. Priest MF, Curry GC, Smith LR, et al. Changes in left ventricular segmental wall motion following randomization to medicine or surgery in patients with unstable angina. Circulation 1978;58(suppl I):I-62-I-68.

12. DeFeyter PJ, Suryapranata H, Surruys PW, Beatt K, Van Den Brand M, Hugenholtz PG. Effects of successful percutaneous transluminal coronary angioplasty on global and regional left ventricular function in unstable angina pectoris. Am J Cardiol 1987;60:993-997.

13. Renkin J, Wijns W, Ladha Z, Col J. Reversal of segmental hypokinesis by coronary angioplasty in patients with unstable angina, persistent T wave inversion, and left anterior descending coronary artery stenosis. Additional evidence for myocardial stunning in humans. Circulation 1990;82:913-921.

14. de Zwaan C, Cheriex EC, Braat SHJG, Stappers JLM, Wellens HJJ. Improvement of systolic and diastolic left ventricular wall motion by serial echocardiograms in selected patients treated for unstable angina. Am Heart J 1991;121: 789-797.

15. Bolli R. Mechanism of myocardial "stunning." Circulation 1990;82:723-738.

16. Kloner RA, Przyklenk K, Patel B. Altered myocardial states: The stunned and hibernating myocardium. Am J Med 1989;86(suppl 1A):14-22.

17. Fournier C, Boujon B, Hebert JL, et al. Stunned myocardium following coronary spasm. Am Heart J 1991;121:593–595.
18. Mathias P, Kerin NZ, Blevins RD, Cascade P, Rubinfire M. Coronary vasospasm as a cause of stunned myocardium. Am Heart J 1987;113:383–385.
19. Topol EJ, Weiss JL, Brinker JA, et al. Regional wall motion improvement after coronary thrombolysis with recombinant tissue plasminogen activator: Importance of coronary angioplasty. J Am Coll Cardiol 1985;6:426–433.
20. Schmidt WG, Sheehan FH, von Essen R, Uebis R, Effert S. Evolution of left ventricular function after intracoronary thrombolysis for acute myocardial infarction. Am J Cardiol 1989;63:497–502.
21. Bourdillon PDV, Broderick TM, Williams ES, et al. Early recovery of regional left ventricular function after reperfusion in acute myocardial infarction assessed by serial two-dimensional echocardiography. Am J Cardiol 1989;63:641–646.
22. Stewart JR, Blackwell WH, Crute SL, Loughlin V, Greenfield LJ, Hess ML. Inhibition of surgically induced ischemia/reperfusion injury by oxygen free radical scavengers. J Thorac Cardiovasc Surg 1983;86:262–272.
23. Johnson DL, Horneffer PJ, Dinatale JM, Gott VL, Gardner TJ. Free radical scavengers improve functional recovery of stunned myocardium in a model of surgical coronary revascularization. Surgery 1987;102:334–340.
24. Ballantyne CM, Verani MS, Short HD, Hyatt C, Noon GP. Delayed recovery of severely "stunned" myocardium with the support of a left ventricular assist device after coronary artery bypass graft surgery. J Am Coll Cardiol 1987;10: 710–712.
25. Breisblatt WM, Stein KL, Wolfe CJ, et al. Acute myocardial dysfunction and recovery: A common occurrence after coronary bypass surgery. J Am Coll Cardiol 1990;15:1261–1269.
26. Rahimtoola SH. A perspective on the three large multicenter randomized clinical trials of coronary bypass surgery for chronic stable angina. Circulation 1985; 75(suppl V):V-123–V-135.
27. Rahimtoola SH. The hibernating myocardium. Am Heart J 1989;117:211–221.
28. Gradman A, Deedwania P, Cody R, et al. Predictors of total mortality and sudden death in mild to moderate heart failure. J Am Coll Cardiol 1989;14: 564–570.
29. Cohn JN, Rector TS. Prognosis of congestive heart failure and predictors of mortality. Am J Cardiol 1988;62:25A.
30. Brunken R, Schwaiger M, Grover-McKay MG, Phelps ME, Tillisch J, Schelbert HR. Positron emission tomography detects tissue metabolic activity in myocardial segments with persistent thallium perfusion defects. J Am Coll Cardiol 1987;10:557–567.
31. Bonow RO, Dilsizian V, Cuocolo A, Bacharach SL. Identification of viable myocardium in patients with chronic coronary artery disease and left ventricular dysfunction. Comparison of thallium scintigraphy with reinjection and PET imaging with ^{18}F-fluorodeoxyglucose. Circulation 1991;83:26–37.
32. Tamaki N, Ohtani H, Yamashita K, et al. Metabolic activity in the areas of new fill-in after thallium-201 reinjection: Comparison with positron emission tomography using fluorine-18-deoxyglucose. J Nucl Med 1991;32:673–678.

33. Pierard LA, De Landsheere CM, Berthe C, Rigo P, Kulbertus HE. Identification of viable myocardium by echocardiography during dobutamine infusion in patients with myocardial infarction after thrombolytic therapy: Comparison with positron emission tomography. J Am Coll Cardiol 1990;15:1021–1031.
34. Camici P, Araujo L, Spinks T, Lammertsma AA, Jones T, Maseri A. Myocardial glucose utilization in ischemic heart disease: Preliminary results with ^{18}F-fluorodeoxyglucose and positron emission tomography. Eur Heart J 1986;7 (suppl C):19–23.
35. Berger BC, Watson DD, Burwell LR, et al. Redistribution of thallium at rest in patients with stable and unstable angina and the effect of coronary artery bypass surgery. Circulation 1979;60:1114–1125.
36. Gibson RS, Watson DD, Taylor GJ, et al. Prospective assessment of regional myocardial perfusion before and after coronary revascularization surgery by quantitative thallium-201 scintigraphy. J Am Coll Cardiol 1983;1:804–815.
37. L,iu P, Kiess MC, Okada RD, et al. The persistent defect on exercise thallium imaging and its fate after revascularization: Does it represent scar or ischemia? Am Heart J 1985;110:996–1001.
38. Kiat H, Berman DS, Maddahi J, et al. Late reversibility of tomographic myocardial thallium-201 defects: An accurate marker of myocardial viability. J Am Coll Cardiol 1988;12:1456–1463.
39. Patel TC, Gibbons RJ, Mullany CJ. Resting thallium-201 scintigraphy for identifying viable myocardium in a patient with severe left ventricular dysfunction. Mayo Clin Proc 1993;68:63–67.
40. Dilsizian V, Rocco TP, Freedman NM, Leon MB, Bonow RO. Enhanced detection of ischemic but viable myocardium by the reinjection of thallium after stress-redistribution imaging. N Engl J Med 1990;323:141–146.
41. Rocco TP, Dilsizian V, McKusick KA, Fischman AJ, Boucher CA, Strauss HW. Comparison of thallium redistribution with rest "reinjection" imaging for the detection of viable myocardium. Am J Cardiol 1990;66:158–163.
42. Ohtani H, Tamki N, Yonekura Y, et al. Value of thallium-201 reinjection after delayed SPECT imaging for predicting reversible ischemia after coronary artery bypass grafting. Am J Cardiol 1990;66:394–399.
43. Mori T, Minamiji K, Kurogane H, Ogawa K, Yoshida Y. Rest-injected thallium-201 imaging for assessing viability of severe asynergic regions. J Nucl Med 1991;32:1718–1724.
44. Dilsizian V, Smeltzer WR, Freedman NM, Dextras R, Bonow RO. Thallium reinjection after stress-redistribution imaging. Does 24-hour delayed imaging after reinjection enhance detection of viable myocardium? Circulation 1991;83:1247–1255.
45. Cuocolo A, Pace L, Ricciardelli B, Chiariello M, Trimarco B, Salvatore M. Identification of viable myocardium in patients with chronic coronary artery disease: Comparison of thallium-201 scintigraphy with reinjection and technetium-99m methoxyisobutyl isonitrile. J Nucl Med 1992;33:505–511.
46. Marzullo P, Parodi O, Reisenhofer B, et al. Value of rest thallium-201/technetium-99m sestamibi scans and dobutamine echocardiography for detecting myocardial viability. Am J Cardiol 1993;71:166–172.

47. Kiat H, Maddashi J, Roy LT, et al. Comparison of Tc-99m methoxy isobutyl isonitrile with thallium-201 evaluation of coronary artery disease by planar and tomographic methods. Am Heart J 1989;117:1-11.
48. Sinusas AJ, Beller GA, Smith WH, Vinson EL, Brookeman V, Watson DD. Quantitative planar imaging with technetium-99m methoxyisobutyl isonitrile: Comparison of uptake patterns with thallium-201. J Nucl Med 1989;30:1456-1463.
49. Wackers FJTH, Berman DS, et al. Technetium-99m hexakis 2-methoxyisobutyl isonitrile: Human biodistribution, dosimetry, safety and preliminary comparison to thallium-201 for myocardial perfusion imaging. J Nucl Med 1989;30: 301-311.
50. Klicpera M, Glogar D, Mayr H, Mohl W, Losert U, Kaindl F. Myocardial perfusion evaluated by contrast echocardiography: A preliminary report. Chest 1982;82:751-756.
51. Feinstein SB, Ten Cate F, Zwehl W, et al. Two dimensional contrast echocardiography: I. In vitro development and quantitative analysis of echo contrast agents. J Am Coll Cardiol 1984;3:14-20.
52. Meltzer RS, Tickner EG, Sahines TP, Popp RL. The source of ultrasound contrast effect. J Clin Ultrasound 1980;8:121-127.
53. Kemper AJ, O'Boyle JE, Sharma S, et al. Hydrogen peroxide contrast-enhanced two-dimensional echocardiography: Real-time in vivo delineation of regional myocardial perfusion. Circulation 1983;68:603-611.
54. Armstrong WF, West SR, Mueller TM, Dillon JC, Feigenbaum H. Assessment of location and size of myocardial infarction with contrast enhanced echocardiography. J Am Coll Cardiol 1983;2:63-69.
55. Tei C, Sakamaki T, Shah PM, et al. Myocardial contrast echocardiography: A reproducible technique of myocardial opacification for identifying regional perfusion deficits. Circulation 1983;67:585-593.
56. Kaul S, Pandian NG, Okada RD, Pohost GM, Weyman AE. Contrast echocardiography in acute myocardial ischemia. I. In vivo determination of total left ventricular "area at risk." J Am Coll Cardiol 1984;4:1;272-1282.
57. Cheirif B, Zoghbi WA, Bolli R, O'Neill PG, Hoyt BD, Quinones MA. Assessment of regional myocardial perfusion by contrast echocardiography. II. Detection of changes in transmural and subendocardial perfusion during dipyridamole-induced hyperemia in a model of critical coronary stenosis. J Am Coll Cardiol 1989;14:1555-1565.
58. Lang RM, Feinstein SB, Feldman T, Neumann A, Chua KG, Borow KM. Contrast echocardiography for evaluation of myocardial perfusion: Effects of coronary angioplasty. J Am Coll Cardiol 1986;8:232-235.
59. Cheirif J, Zoghbi WA, Raizner AE, et al. Assessment of myocardial perfusion in humans by contrast echocardiography. I. Evaluation of regional coronary reserve by peak contrast intensity. J Am Coll Cardiol 1988;11:735-743.
60. Spotnitz WD, Keller MW, Watson DD, et al. Success of internal mammary bypass grafting can be assessed intraoperatively using myocardial contrast echocardiography. J Am Coll Cardiol 1988;12:196-201.

61. Mudra H, Zwehl W, Klauss V, et al. Intraoperative myocardial contrast echocardiography for assessment of regional bypass perfusion. Am J Cardiol 1990; 66:1077–1081.
62. Widimsky P, Cornel JH, Ten Cate FJ. Evaluation of collateral blood flow by myocardial contrast enhanced echocardiography. Br Heart J 1988;59:20–22.
63. Spotnitz WD, Matthew TL, Keller MW, Powers ER, Kaul S. Intraoperative demonstration of coronary collateral flow using myocardial contrast two-dimensional echocardiography. Am J Cardiol 1990;65:1259–1261.
64. Lim Y-J, Nanto S, Masuyama T, et al. Coronary collaterals assessed with myocardial contrast echocardiography in healed myocardial infarction. Am J Cardiol 1990;66:556–561.
65. Sabia PJ, Powers ER, Jayaweera, Ragosta M, Kaul S. Functional significance of collateral blood flow in patients with recent acute myocardial infarction. A study using myocardial contrast echocardiography. Circulation 1992;85:2080–2089.
66. Cheirif BJ, Wray RA, Bravenec J, Brown D, Quiñones MA, Mickelson JK. Contrast echo assessment of collateral flow in a model of coronary thrombosis and delayed reperfusion: Relation to regional function. Circulation 1991;84(suppl II):II-358.
67. Ito H, Tomooka T, Sakai N, et al. Lack of myocardial perfusion immediately after successful thrombolysis. A predictor of poor recovery of left ventricular function in anterior myocardial infarction. Circulation 1992;85:1699–1705.
68. Sabia PJ, Powers ER, Ragosta M, Sarembock IJ, Burwell LR, Kaul S. An association between collateral blood flow and myocardial viability in patients with recent myocardial infarction. N Engl J Med 1992;327:1825–1831.
69. Vanoverschelde J-LJ, Wijns, W, Depre C, et al. Mechanisms of chronic regional postischemic dysfunction in humans. New insights from the study of non-infarcted collateral-dependent myocardium. Circulation 1993;87:1513–1523.
70. Popio KA, Gorlin R, Bechtel DJ, Levine JA. Postextrasystolic potentiation as a predictor of potential myocardial viability: Preoperative analyses compared with studies after coronary bypass surgery. Am J Cardiol 1977;39:944–953.
71. Hamby RI, Aintablian A, Wisoff BG, Hartstein ML. Response of the left ventricle in coronary artery disease to postextrasystolic potentiation. Circulation 1975;51:428–435.
72. Helfant RH, Pine R, Meister SG, Feldman MS, Trout RG, Banka VS. Nitroglycerin to unmask reversible asynergy. Correlation with postcoronary bypass ventriculography. Circulation 1974;50:108–113.
73. Chesebro JH, Ritman EL, Frye RL, et al. Regional myocardial wall thickening response to nitroglycerin. A predictor of myocardial response to aortocoronary bypass surgery. Circulation 1978;57:952–957.
74. Ragosta M, Beller GA, Watson DD, Kaul S, Gimple LW. Quantitative planar rest-redistribution ^{201}Tl imaging in detection of myocardial viability and prediction of improvement in left ventricular function after coronary bypass surgery in patients with severely depressed left ventricular function. Circulation 1993; 87:1630–1641.

75. Mercier JC, Lando U, Kanmatsus K, et al. Divergent effects of inotropic stimulation on the ischemic and severely depressed reperfused myocardium. Circulation 1982;66:397–400.
76. Ellis SE, Wynne J, Braunwald E, Henschke CI, Sandor T, Kloner RA. Response of reperfusion-salvaged, stunned myocardium to inotropic stimulation. Am Heart J 1984;107:9–13.
77. Arnold JMO, Braunwald E, Sandor T, Kloner RA. Inotropic stimulation of reperfused myocardium with dopamine: Effects on infarct size and myocardial function. J Am Coll Cardiol 1985;6:1026–1034.
78. Becker LC, Levine JH, DiPaula AF, Guarnieri T, Aversano TR. Reversal of dysfunction in postischemic stunned myocardium by epinephrine and postextrasystolic potentiation. J Am Coll Cardiol 1986;7:580–589.
79. Ito BR, Tate H, Kobayashi M, Schaper W. Reversibly injured, postischemic canine myocardium retains normal contractile reserve. Circ Res 1987;61:834–846.

6

Coronary Laser Angioplasty

Lawrence Deckelbaum
West Haven Veterans Affairs Medical Center and
Yale University School of Medicine, New Haven, Connecticut

I. INTRODUCTION

A. Potential of Laser Angioplasty

With the widespread growth and success of percutaneous transluminal coronary angioplasty (PTCA), the realization of several constraints and limitations of balloon angioplasty stimulated the development of alternative revascularization approaches such as laser angioplasty. Despite success rates exceeding 90% in the treatment of isolated stenotic lesions, coronary angioplasty is much less successful in treating total occlusions, with success rates falling below 70% (1,2). Angioplasty is best suited for the treatment of discrete atherosclerotic stenoses, with lower success rates and more difficult application in patients with diffuse atherosclerotic disease (3). As a result, there are a large number of patients with coronary artery disease who are candidates for neither bypass surgery nor balloon angioplasty because of the diffuse nature of their atherosclerotic coronary disease. Moreover, despite an initially high primary success rate, coronary angioplasty is still plagued by a restenosis rate as high as 57% (4).

The potential advantages of laser angioplasty address the limitations of balloon angioplasty. Laser is an acronym for a phrase that describes the etiology of laser radiation: Light Amplification by Stimulated Emission of

Radiation. There are unique laser qualities that arise from the manner in which laser light is generated. Laser light is very uniform and can therefore be emitted as a very narrow beam of energy that can be focused into and transmitted by flexible silica fibers.

The appeal of laser technology for revascularization lies in the fact that intense energy can be delivered in a precisely controlled manner to any site, such as intravascular lesions, that is accessible to an optical fiber.

Because laser energy can vaporize atherosclerotic plaque, there may be no requirement for a preexisting channel, and therefore laser angioplasty may have a high success rate for the treatment of chronic coronary occlusions. In its best embodiment, laser angioplasty offers the potential of passing a fiberoptic catheter through the entire length of the coronary circulation while vaporizing all atherosclerotic plaque along the arterial wall. This applicability for the treatment of diffuse atherosclerotic disease would offer treatment opportunities currently unavailable with conventional bypass surgery or angioplasty. Finally, in contrast to balloon angioplasty where the plaque material is fractured, compressed, or displaced, laser angioplasty will vaporize the plaque material and convert it to gaseous products and microscopic particulate matter (5). It is hoped that this bulk removal of plaque material could improve acute procedural success rates, decrease complication rates, treat "untreatable" lesions or lesions not amenable to conventional techniques, and decrease restenosis rates.

B. History of Laser Angioplasty

1. Continuous Wave Lasers

The ability of laser energy to vaporize atherosclerotic plaque was first demonstrated in 1963 by McGuff and colleagues (6), only 3 years after the first laser was developed by Maiman. The first intravascular recanalization using lasers was reported by Choy who used argon laser radiation for thrombolysis in animals. In 1983, Choy performed the first clinical laser angioplasty using an argon laser and bare fiber intraoperatively (7). The high incidence of complications (perforation and occlusion) was in part due to the rigid catheter, the small amount of tissue ablated, and the laser-induced thermal damage.

In an attempt to minimize the risk of arterial perforation due to laser ablation and mechanical trauma from the optical fiber, several approaches were persued. Olive-shaped metal tips were placed on the terminal ends of the silica fibers used for laser angioplasty. These hollow tips converted the laser light energy into heat energy to achieve recanalization by tissue vaporization and mechanical compression of plaque material in a process referred to as laser thermal angioplasty. Percutaneous coronary procedures were performed in 1987. Despite success of the system in the peripheral circulation, coronary laser thermal angioplasty was a disappointment. Of the 15 patients reported in the literature (3 intraoperative, 12 percutaneous) (8–10), only 60% (9 patients) had a successful procedure. There were one perforation, three acute occlusions, and four abrupt closures or myocardial infarctions postprocedure.

Another approach to enhancing safety was to use a multifiber coronary laser catheter consisting of an array of fibers circumferentially arranged around a guidewire lumen. The use of multiple smaller fibers enhanced catheter flexibility over that using single larger fibers, and the passage over a guidewire decreased the likelihood of perforation from irradiation of the vessel wall. Cote (11) reported percutaneous multifiber coronary laser angioplasty in 23 patients using a four-fiber catheter coupled to an argon laser. He reported a 100% success rate with reduction in the mean stenosis from 97% to 14% following adjunctive balloon angioplasty. The continuous-wave argon laser was operated in a chopped or intermittent manner to deliver brief pulses of argon laser irradiation to minimize thermal damage.

2. Pulsed Lasers

Concerns regarding laser thermal damage as witnessed with laser thermal angioplasty resulted in the development of pulsed laser angioplasty systems. Laser radiation at a variety of wavelengths from the ultraviolet to the infrared can vaporize atherosclerotic plaque. However, the choice of wavelength and energy parameters determines the efficiency of plaque ablation and the extent of thermal damage to the surrounding tissue. Continuous-wave lasers have power output that is constant over time. Continuous-wave laser radiation, such as that emitted by the argon (Nd:YAG) or CO_2 lasers, will vaporize tissue with thermal damage to the adjacent tissue. Consistent pathological findings at the perimeter of the laser crater are a superficial zone of coagulation necrosis and a subjacent zone of polymorphous lacunae. Pulsed lasers delivery energy in brief pulses, each of which is separated by an emission-free interval. Pulsed lasers can have very high peak powers that exceed the average power by several orders of magnitude. As a result, delivery of laser energy in the pulsed mode eliminates gross and microscopic evidence of thermal injury (12). Isner and Grundfest have each reported the ability of the excimer laser at 308 nm to ablate vascular tissue with minimal thermal damage (13–15). Deckelbaum (12) described tissue ablation with minimal thermal damage that could be achieved using a variety of pulsed lasers at ultraviolet, visible, and infrared wavelengths if appropriate parameters of pulse duration and fluence, or energy density (mJ/cm^2) were chosen. Whether minimization of thermal damage with pulsed laser ablation results from nonthermal mechanisms of tissue ablation is a matter of controversy

(16). Nonthermal mechanisms include tissue removal by direct bond breaking of the peptide bonds of organic molecules (photoablation), or by tissue fragmentation by shock waves generated by high-peak power laser pulses (photodisruption). The large photon energy at the excimer wavelength of 308 nm suggests the possibility of a photoablative mechanism of excimer laser ablation. Alternatively, "clean" ablation could result from a thermal mechanism with optimization of the laser parameters. A short laser pulse duration to minimize thermal diffusion from the irradiated tissue, a low repetition rate to enable tissue cooling during the relatively long interpulse interval, and a large pulse fluence to completely vaporize the irradiated tissue volume (dispelling hot gases and particulate matter and leaving little heat to be conducted to adjacent tissue) may remove tissue by a thermal process in which heat dissipation has been optimized and no surrounding thermal damage occurs (12,17). Excimer laser parameters employed for laser angioplasty are consistent with these requirements, and analysis of the products of excimer laser ablation (18) is consistent with a thermal ablation process.

In 1988, Litvack et al. reported the first percutaneous coronary angioplasty performed with a pulsed excimer laser coupled to a multifiber catheter (19). In 1990, the first percutaneous pulsed holmium laser angioplasty (infrared wavelength 2.1 μm) was performed also with a multifiber catheter (20). In 1992 and 1993, the FDA approved marketing of the LAIS Dymer 200+ (Advanced Interventional Systems, Irvine, CA) and Spectranetics CVX-300 (Spectranetics, Colorado Springs, CO) coronary laser angioplasty systems, respectively. In Europe, a Technolas MAX-10 (Fa. Technolas, Graefelfing, Germany) excimer laser coronary angioplasty system has also been used clinically. In announcing the first coronary excimer laser angioplasty (ELCA) system approval in January 1992, the FDA Commissioner David A. Kessler said, "This device will help save lives. It will definitely provide a benefit to heart patients who would not do well with balloon angioplasty." It is estimated that by mid-1993 5000 ELCAs had been performed worldwide. Fewer holmium laser angioplasties have been performed (approximately 600) since this system (Eclipse 2100, Eclipse Surgical Technologies, Palo Alto, CA) is limited to investigational use pending FDA approval.

II. METHODS

A. System Parameters

Excimer lasers are gas lasers that emit pulsed laser radiation in the ultraviolet. The specific wavelength is determined by the composition of the gases in the laser cavity. Lasing is induced by transmitting a high-voltage electrical discharge through the gas mixture. Current clinical excimer lasers contain a mixture of xenon and chloride (XeCl) and lase at 308 nm. Higher excimer wavelengths (e.g., 351 nm) are less capable of ablation without thermal damage, and lower wavelengths (e.g., 248 nm) are more difficult to transmit through conventional silica optical fibers. The word "excimer" is a contraction of the words "excited dimer," with the dimer being a molecule made up of two atoms, in this case xenon and chloride. To facilitate fiberoptic coupling and transmission of excimer laser radiation, the pulse duration of clinical excimer lasers has been "stretched" from values used for industrial applications. Parameters employed for laser angioplasty using the LAIS (21) or Spectranetics (22) systems are pulse durations of 185 ns or 135 ns, respectively, repetition rates of 25 Hz or 20 Hz, respectively, and fluences (pulse energy density) of 30–60 mJ/mm². The Technolas system operates at a shorter pulse duration of 55 ns, a repetition rate of 2–40 Hz, and a fluence of 42–51 mJ/mm² (23).

Holmium lasers are solid-state lasers that emit pulsed radiation in the mid-infrared portion of the spectrum. Lasing is induced by a flashlamp discharge that excites holmium atoms embedded in a crystal laser rod. The emitted wavelength is 2–2.1 μm at a pulse energy up to 4 J, a pulse duration of 250 μs, and a repetition rate of 5 Hz (24). The major differences in laser tissue interaction between holmium and excimer lasers arises from the fact that ultraviolet wavelengths are predominantly absorbed by tissue proteins and nucleic acids, whereas infrared wavelengths are absorbed by tissue water. Tissue has a higher absorption coefficient at 308 nm than at 2.1 μm (characteristic absorption depths of 50 μm and 286 μm, respectively) (25). As a result of the shorter pulse duration and stronger tissue absorption, lower pulse energies are used for excimer than for holmium laser ablation (approximately 100-fold difference).

Both excimer and holmium laser angioplasty systems are coupled to multifibers over the guidewire catheters. Figure 1 shows a multifiber coronary laser catheter consisting of an array of 61-μm diameter fibers circumferentially arranged around a guidewire lumen. The laser radiation is emitted from the catheter in a ring or halo shape and, as a result, cores out the obstructive plaque in the coronary artery resulting in a neolumen approximating the catheter diameter. The active area (area occupied by optical fiber) of these catheters is approximately 20–30% of the total surface area at the tip excluding the guidewire lumen. Laser catheters range in external diameter from 1.3–2.0 mm with common sizes being 1.3, 1.6, and 2.0 mm for AIS catheters, 1.4, 1.7, and 2.0 mm for Spectranetics, and 1.4, 1.5, 1.7, and 2.0 mm for Eclipse catheters. Catheters are available in standard over-the-wire or monorail formats, as well as in concentric and, recently, eccentric fiber configurations. The latter eccentric catheters are suitable for eccentric le-

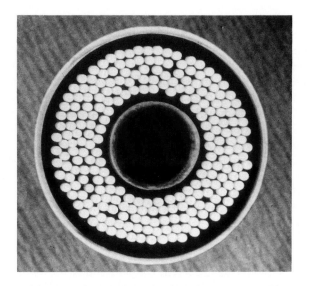

Figure 1 A multifiber coronary laser angioplasty catheter (Spectranetics 1.7-mm diameter concentric) is shown above. The catheter consists of approximately 245 61-μm fibers arranged concentrically around a guidewire lumen. The laser irradiation is emitted in a ring or halo shape.

sions and may be capable of achieving greater debulking by multiple passes through the lesion at varying orientations.

B. Procedural Parameters

The procedural similarities between excimer laser angioplasty and balloon angioplasty are greater than their differences. Patients receive heparin, aspirin, and vasodilators (e.g., calcium channel blockers and nitrates) prior to, during, and following the procedure as part of standard PTCA treatment. Conventional coronary angioplasty large lumen guide catheters are employed, with 8-French catheters for 1.3–1.7-mm diameter laser catheters, and 9-French catheters for 2.0-mm laser catheters. The left Judkins curve may be chosen slightly oversized to avoid an acute angle in the secondary bend. An appropriate size laser catheter is usually ≈ 1 mm smaller than the target vessel diameter. Similar to balloon angioplasty, laser angioplasty requires the crossing of the lesion with a 0.014- to 0.018-in. guidewire over which the concentric multifiber catheter is then advanced. An extra support guidewire may be used to enhance laser catheter support. After placement of the guidewire through the lesion, the laser catheter is advanced and positioned proximal to the lesion. Eccentric catheters are oriented for maximal lesion contact. Laser parameters are chosen: excimer repetition rate of 20–25 Hz and fluence of 40–50 mJ/mm² (lower range for saphenous vein graft or restenotic lesions, higher rate for native coronary lesions or calcified restenotic lesions); holmium repetition rate of 5 Hz and pulse energy of 250–700 mJ/pulse. Lasing is then started with catheter advancement through the lesion at a rate of 0.5–1.0 mm/s. The guidewire is maintained taut to support the laser catheter and maintain its intraluminal orientation. Several laser trains (e.g., 3–5 s each) may be performed before the lesion is crossed by the laser catheter (a "pass"). On occasion, several passes may be performed with the same size or larger catheters in an attempt to maximize debulking of the lesion. Following laser ablation, adjunctive balloon angioplasty is performed in most cases. The undersizing of the laser catheter with respect to the vessel enhances safety at the expense of neolumen size, and therefore requires a secondary procedure, usually PTCA. Additional procedural details and nursing considerations are well described in Reference 26. Typical angiographic results from laser angioplasty are shown in Figure 2.

Coronary arterial perforation is a rare complication of laser angioplasty that is almost never seen with conventional balloon angioplasty. Management of perforation involves reversal of anticoagulation (e.g., with protamine), prolonged balloon inflation (e.g., with an autoperfusion balloon if necessary), and percutaneous pericardial drainage if cardiac tamponade develops. Because laser angioplasty is performed over a guidewire, a balloon catheter can usually be advanced over the same guidewire and inflated at the site of perforation to prevent further extravasation of blood. Perforation is best avoided by selecting a catheter >1 mm smaller than the target vessel and by avoiding bifurcation lesions or acutely angled lesions (>45°). If the laser catheter cannot be advanced through a lesion, forceful advancement may result in loss of guidewire support and direct the laser catheter at the vessel wall instead of the lumen. To avoid this possibility, the operator should consider increasing the fluence, using a smaller laser catheter, or abandoning the procedure if 10–15 s of laser time fails to result in laser catheter advancement through the stenosis (22).

Specimens retrieved by directional atherectomy immediately after laser angioplasty have documented acute pathological alterations resulting from in vivo laser angioplasty similar to that predicted by experimental studies in vitro (27). Fine edge disruption with infrequent foci of vacuolar injury was seen following excimer laser irradiation, whereas frequent vacuolar injury with rare thermal damage was seen following holmium laser irradiation. The absence of thermal damage following excimer laser angioplasty has also been confirmed angioscopically (28).

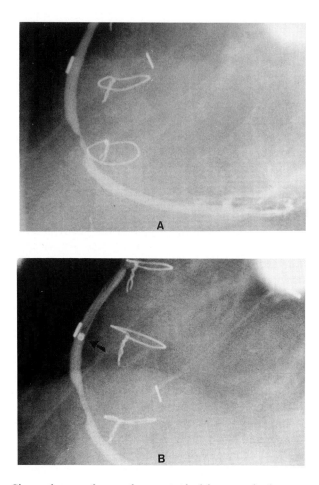

Figure 2 Cineangiogram frames from a typical laser angioplasty procedure are shown above. (A) The initial angiogram revealed a long stenotic lesion in a saphenous vein graft to the right coronary artery. A guidewire was passed through the vessel across the stenosis. (B) A 2.0-mm diameter concentric multifiber catheter coupled to an excimer laser was then passed over the guidewire through the stenosis. Following laser angioplasty, a neolumen was created approximating the diameter of the catheter. The radiopaque distal marker of the laser catheter is seen in the proximal vessel (arrow). (C) The final result following adjunctive balloon dilatation shows minimal residual stenosis at the site of the prior lesion.

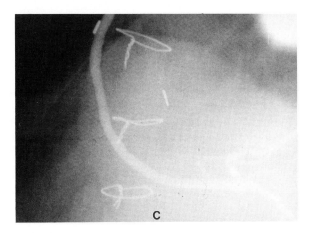

Figure 2 Continued

It is difficult to quantitate the magnitude of tissue ablation following a laser catheter pass. Torre (29), Margolis (30), and Bittl (31) reported that postlaser minimal luminal diameters were comparable to the size of the catheter used (0–0.2 mm). This observation is consistent with laser ablation of arterial tissue as opposed to catheter-induced mechanical dilation of the artery. The later mechanism would be expected to be associated with elastic recoil as seen with PTCA where the final minimal lumen diameter ranges from 30–60% less than the balloon's inflated diameter (32–34). Intracoronary ultrasonography (35) has also suggested that there is less residual plaque and less vessel stretch following laser as compared to balloon angioplasty alone.

Table 1 The Effect of Laser Debulking on Subsequent Balloon Dilatation (mean values shown)

Catheter diameter	1.4 mm	1.7 mm	2.0 mm
	$n = 6$	$n = 57$	$n = 12$
Diameters (mm)			
Reference vessel	3.04	3.08	3.02
Lesion site			
prelaser	0.49	0.49	0.44
postlaser	1.40	1.62	2.04
PTCA balloon size	2.90	3.00	2.92
Post-PTCA	2.04	2.22	2.88

Updated from Reference 42.

Torre et al. (29) reported an observation supporting the benefit of plaque debulking prior to balloon angioplasty (Table 1). When comparably sized vessels were treated with ELCA followed by adjunctive balloon angioplasty, the degree of laser debulking correlated with the final lumen diameter. Seventy-five 3.0-mm diameter vessels with 85% stenosis were treated with 1.4-, 1.7-, or 2.0-mm diameter laser catheters prior to 3.0-mm diameter balloon catheter dilatation. The final vessel diameters were 2.0, 2.2, and 2.9 mm, respectively, demonstrating less elastic recoil in the vessels treated with the larger diameter laser catheters with presumably greater plaque ablation.

III. RESULTS

A. Clinical Success

Since only excimer laser coronary angioplasty systems have been FDA approved, and since the majority of clinical cases and publications report on results of excimer laser angioplasty, the details of the subsequent discussion will focus predominantly on these systems. Data on holmium laser angioplasty results are rather similar to those of the excimer laser angioplasty, and most issues apply to both systems. The holmium laser angioplasty experience will be referred where data differ substantially.

For the analysis of laser angioplasty results, clinical success was defined as a reduction by ⩾20% of the narrowing of the vessel diameter to a ⩽50% residual stenosis in the absence of a major in-hospital complication (i.e., myocardial infarction, emergency coronary artery bypass grafting, or death). Laser success was defined as a reduction by ⩾20% of the narrowing of the vessel diameter. Lesions were graded according to the A, B, or C classification of the ACC/AHA Task Force as modified by Ellis et al. (3) to include types B1 and B2, depending on whether one or more complex features were present.

The reported results using either the Spectranetics or LAIS excimer laser angioplasty systems are rather comparable. Overall, laser angioplasty has a procedural success rate of 86–94% with a major complication rate of 5–7% (30,31,36–38). Laser success occurred in 82–85%. Failure of laser angioplasty occurred more often due to inability to advance the catheter to the site of the lesion due to prestenotic vessel tortuosity than to inability to pass the laser catheter through the lesion (39). Based on quantitative angiographic data from the AIS (30,36) and Spectranetics (31) registries, the mean lesion percent stenosis of 80–87% is reduced to 43–50% following laser angioplasty, and to a final residual stenosis of 21–29% following adjunctive balloon angioplasty. Adjunctive balloon angioplasty was performed more frequently in later series with incidences ranging from 47% (36) to 88% (31). These data are consistent with the smaller series of patients undergoing ELCA using the Technolas system who experienced a mean stenosis reduction from 90–52% following laser angioplasty, and to 25% after adjunctive balloon dilatations (23). Laser alone produced a residual stenosis ≤50% in only 55% of treated lesions (31).

The reported results using Eclipse holmium laser angioplasty are similar, with a procedural success rate of 94–95%, a laser success rate of 79–83%, and a major complication rate of approximately 5% (40,41). Mean percent stenosis decreased from 89–57% following laser angioplasty, and to a final residual stenosis of 22% after balloon angioplasty. Most patients had adjunctive PTCA. Comparable success rates with both holmium and excimer laser angioplasty have also been reported from the experience of a single center (42).

Excimer laser coronary angioplasty has been successful in cases of PTCA failure (21,37,43). In these instances, ELCA debulking was effective in facilitating balloon crossing of a long rigid stenosis that could not be crossed after guidewire passage through the lesion, and/or in overcoming prominent elastic recoil of the stenosis after PTCA, and/or in dilating hard lesions that resisted balloon dilatation even at high pressure.

The results of excimer laser angioplasty appear to be somewhat insensitive to lesion complexity. Equivalent ELCA success rates have been reported for simple and complex lesions (31): 91% for type A, 91% for type B1, 89% for type B2, and 95% for type C lesions. Major complication rates were also not higher in complex lesions: 6% for type A, 6% for B1, 9% for B2, and 3% for type C lesions. Similar insensitivity of success and complication rates to AHA/ACC Task Force classification was also found in the other series that addressed this question (21,39).

Multivariate analysis (31,37) identified that bifurcation lesions (odds ratio = 0.16) and tortuous vessels (odds ratio = 0.48) reduced the likelihood of clinical success of ELCA. On the other hand, restenosis lesions, ostial lesions, and saphenous vein graft lesions were associated with a greater likelihood of clinical success. However, the multivariate model could account for only 23% of the variability in clinical success, suggesting that it is still difficult to predict the clinical outcome in a specific patient. In another series (36), multivariate analysis showed lesion eccentricity to be the only independent predictor for the occurrence of a major procedural complication (odds ratio = 3.32) or expressed inversely for clinical success (odds ratio = 0.30). However, in this series, eccentric catheters were not utilized, and 20% of the lesions with no complications had a high eccentricity index. Although angiographic evidence of thrombus was an uncommon occurrence in ELCA-treated lesions (9% of lesions), when present it decreased the clinical success rate to 58% and was associated with a 25% incidence of embolization, a

33% incidence of myocardial infarction, and a 17% incidence of abrupt closure (44). The presence of intracoronary thrombus was the most important (negative) predictor of clinical success in this analysis. In contrast to this observation with excimer laser ablation, holmium laser angioplasty has been used successfully for recanalization in patients with acute myocardial infarction (45), where the presence of thrombus is a near universal occurrence.

B. Complications

Risk of myocardial infarction during the ELCA procedure or during hospitalization was 3-4% (30,31,36,38,46). The risk of abrupt closure was 5-7% with two-thirds occurring in the catheterization laboratory and one-third occurring later in-hospital. Abrupt closure was treated with balloon angioplasty with success in more than half the cases. Bypass surgery was required at some time during hospitalization in 3-4% (30,31). Coronary spasm was reported in 2-4% (30,47), although another study (48) suggested a much higher incidence of persistent mild vasospasm. This vasospasm was demonstrated angiographically 1 day following ELCA by a 0.2-mm increase in vessel diameter following intracoronary nitroglycerin. This same study also reported a 38% incidence of vasospasm during the ELCA procedure (in 38 patients) which is a higher incidence than that reported in other series, and may have resulted from longer lasing times. Complication rates were relatively independent of AHA/ACC Task Force classification (21,31). Predictors of major complications were bifurcation lesions and eccentric stenoses (36,37). A decreased risk of complications was seen in the "alpha" lesion group consisting of calcified stenoses, saphenous vein graft lesions, total occlusions, lesions >10 mm long, ostial lesions, and unsuccessful balloon dilatations (37). The risk of death from ELCA was 0.6% (46). The reported complications of holmium laser angioplasty are similar (40) to those of ELCA with an incidence of myocardial infarction of 2%, perforation, 2%, emergency bypass surgery, 3%, dissection, 5%, and death, 0.3%.

In one series (31), 5.5% of patients undergoing ELCA showed evidence of significant dissection that impaired flow, resulted in myocardial infarction, or required bypass surgery. Overall incidence of excimer laser-induced dissections has been reported to be 16% angiographically (36). Angioscopy following excimer laser angioplasty (28) has documented irregular recanalized channels with intraluminal flaps and plaque fractures. Intracoronary ultrasound also suggests that the incidence of dissections following laser and adjunctive balloon angioplasty may be higher than appreciated angiographically (35). The presence of a dissection correlated with the occurrence of an important complication (odds ratio = 3.9). A lower dissection rate following holmium than excimer laser angioplasty was reported in the small experience of a single center (42). In vitro data (49), however, demonstrated larger dissections following holmium irradiation of aorta than following excimer irradiation.

The etiology of these dissections appears to be due to the pulsed laser energy delivery. Mechanical trauma to the arterial wall due to passage of the laser catheter might contribute to the incidence of dissection, but this was probably more a factor in the first generation of laser catheters that used larger diameter fibers and were much stiffer than current catheters. Adjunctive balloon angioplasty probably does play a major role in arterial wall dissections; however, many of the dissections are noted after laser angioplasty alone. In vitro studies (50,51) have shown that pulsed excimer or holmium laser ablation is associated with photoacoustic effects such as rapidly expanding and collapsing cavitation bubbles and acoustic shock waves that may play an important role in causing these arterial dissections. Time-resolved photography revealed forceful vapor bubble formation during excimer or holmium laser ablation that resulted in tissue elevation up to 2.5 mm. Irradiation and vaporization of blood probably contributes to cavitation bubble formation and acoustomechanical trauma without any procedural benefit. In blood, each excimer laser pulse generated a fast-expanding and imploding vapor bubble whose size was proportional to the pulse energy. In vivo, excimer laser irradiation coaxially in a rabbit artery produced an intraluminal bubble that resulted in microsecond dilatation (to a 50% increase in vessel diameter) and invagination of the arterial segment (50). This was associated with histological dissections and extensive wall damage far beyond the penetration depth of the 308-nm laser light. It is possible that this mechanical distention of the vessel is a potent stimulus for smooth muscle cell proliferation and an increase in vasomotor tone contributing to restenosis and vasospasm, respectively (51). Abela (52) postulated that multiple layers of dissection could cause the artery to puff up similar to a "mille-feuilles" pastry. This swelling in the arterial wall as a result of multilayered dissection planes could be the etiology of angiographic "spasm" or acute occlusion following laser angioplasty. Balloon dilatation is often effective in compressing these layers back together and restoring the vessel lumen.

Vessel perforation has been reported to occur in 1–3% of cases (22,30,36). Of the patients with perforation, 39–50% had a major complication resulting directly from perforation (e.g., cardiac tamponade, myocardial infarction, or need for emergency bypass surgery) and the other 50–61% had no clinical complications after successful sealing of the puncture site. No patient with perforation died. A large catheter-to-vessel ratio was an important risk factor as vessel perforation occurred in 8.3% of lesions in which the laser catheter was ≤0.5 mm smaller than the diameter of the target vessel, but occurred only in 1.5% of lesions in which the laser catheter was >1 mm smaller than

than the target vessel. Multivariate analysis revealed that bifurcation lesions, target vessel diameter <2.25, diabetes mellitus, and female gender were associated with increased risk of vessel perforation. Long lesions and calcified lesions were not at increased risk. Follow-up angiography in 12 patients whose perforation was sealed with balloon angioplasty revealed an aneurysm in one patient (8% incidence). The incidence of perforation has declined by avoiding higher risk lesions and by careful catheter sizing such that the incidence of perforation has been decreasing to 0.4% in the last 1000 patients treated in the AIS registry (46).

Coronary artery aneurysm formation has been rarely reported following excimer laser angioplasty: once following balloon sealing of a laser-induced perforation (22), and once following an uncomplicated stand-alone excimer laser angioplasty (53). The authors speculated that ablation into the media may have been responsible for aneurysm formation in the latter case.

Regarding potential long-term effects, experimental and epidemiological studies have demonstrated the carcinogenic potential of UV-B (280–320 nm) at fluences comparable to those used during laser angioplasty. Cytotoxic and mutagenic effects of 308-nm irradiation are due to error-prone repair mechanisms. However, it is not known if there is any risk of a single intravascular exposure to 308-nm irradiation, or if vascular tissue is susceptible to UV carcinogenesis (54).

C. Restenosis

It was hypothesized that by ablating atherosclerotic plaque laser angioplasty could decrease the restenosis rate by decreasing the plaque mass, diminishing elastic recoil that contributes to restenosis, and by decreasing vessel injury-induced smooth muscle cell proliferation. Unfortunately, there is no evidence that laser angioplasty has a lower overall restenosis rate than balloon angioplasty (55). In a subgroup of 95 ELCA patients undergoing quantitative angiography, Bittl (31) reported the mean minimal lumen diameter had increased from 2.3 ± 0.5 to 1.2 ± 1.0 mm, and the mean percent stenosis had decreased from $21 \pm 14\%$ to $56 \pm 32\%$ at restudy an average of 5.2 months postprocedure. Lumen diameter at follow-up did not correlate with the post-laser lumen diameter but did correlate with the postprocedural lumen diameter after adjunctive balloon angioplasty. Overall restenosis rate was 48%. However, only 31% had clinical evidence of restenosis with recurrence of angina, positive exercise treadmill test, myocardial infarction, or need for revascularization.

In contrast to balloon angioplasty, ELCA had a trend toward a lower restenosis rate in saphenous vein grafts than in native coronary arteries (31, 37). Relative risk analysis revealed that lesion length was a predictor of restenosis, whereas adjunctive PTCA and vessel diameter >3.0 mm were predictors of freedom from restenosis (37). As reported for other interventional modalities, the risk of restenosis following excimer laser angioplasty is related to the vessel diameter immediately postprocedure. The minimal lumen diameter at 3- to 6-month follow-up was directly related to reference vessel diameter and to minimal lumen diameter after laser and balloon treatment. The lowest likelihood of restenosis occurred when laser ablation and balloon dilatation were used in large vessels to produce a lumen that approached the reference diameter of the vessel (56).

D. Niche Applications

The absence of any randomized clinical trial comparing PTCA and ELCA makes it difficult to determine which lesions are best treated by laser angioplasty. However, comparison with historical controls suggests certain niche applications. ELCA success >90% has been reported (21,30,31,57) in certain lesions that have responded poorly to balloon angioplasty. These include diffuse disease (lesion length >10 mm), lesions in saphenous vein grafts older than 3 years, ostial lesions, chronic total occlusions, and type B and C lesions. PTCA results in these lesions range from 61–84% (3). On the other hand, some investigators perceive no advantage of excimer laser over balloon angioplasty for the treatment of discrete uncomplicated lesions (21). These comparisons must be interpreted cautiously as historical PTCA controls may differ in patient selection and do not represent what is achievable using current techniques and equipment. It will be important for the greater acceptance and growth of laser angioplasty to confirm these benefits in randomized clinical trials.

The currently approved indications for excimer laser angioplasty are listed in Table 2. Laser angioplasty appears to be safe and effective for the treatment of saphenous vein graft lesions, aorto-ostial lesions, long lesions, moderately calcified lesions, total occlusions that can be crossed with a guidewire, and balloon dilatation failures. These niches have been proposed for laser angioplasty because the success rate for ELCA treatment of these lesions appears to be higher than that with balloon angioplasty when compared

Table 2 Indications for Coronary Laser Angioplasty

Long lesions (> 10–20 mm long)
Saphenous vein graft lesions
Moderately calcified lesions
Aorto-ostial lesions
Total occlusions that can be crossed with a guidewire
Lesions that cannot be crossed or dilated with a balloon catheter

with historical controls. Restenosis lesions may also be appropriate for laser angioplasty as both laser success and procedural success (37,38,58) were higher in restenosis lesions than in de novo lesions.

With the current catheter technology, optimal lesions for laser angioplasty are probably those causing very high-grade stenoses or total occlusions in large vessels; in these cases, a large multifiber catheter can be safely used, and the large plaque cross-sectional area maximizes the percent of contact of the catheter face with the atheroma resulting in the greatest amount of plaque debulking.

IV. DISCUSSION

The development of the current laser angioplasty systems based on pulsed lasers coupled to concentric multifiber over-the-wire catheters has reflected a compromise between efficacy and safety. As a result, laser angioplasty is still limited by guidewire dependency, inadequate plaque ablation, laser-induced arterial injury, and restenosis. The future growth and acceptance of laser angioplasty will depend on how effectively these problems are addressed.

Passing the laser catheter over a guidewire adds safety; however, it limits the application of the procedure to lesions that can be crossed with a guidewire. Chronic total occlusions that cannot be crossed by a guidewire still cannot be treated by laser angioplasty. The recent introduction of fiberoptic laser guidewires for primary recanalization of chronic total occlusions by direct plaque ablation may effectively expand the application of the current laser angioplasty systems.

Choosing the diameter of the laser catheter to be approximately 1 mm less than the normal vessel diameter affords a margin of safety and minimizes the risk of complications but results in less plaque ablation. As a result, the laser created neolumen diameter is usually inadequate, and requires adjunctive balloon angioplasty to achieve an optimal result. Newer catheters may be capable of achieving more complete plaque ablation. Directional or eccentric multifiber catheters may be able to achieve larger neolumens (59, 60). Both Spectranetics and LAIS have developed 1.7- to 1.8-mm diameter over-the-wire catheters with eccentric placement of the optical fibers. Preliminary experience suggests that these catheters may be effective for highly eccentric lesions and bifurcation lesions. It might be possible to achieve a neolumen larger than the catheter diameter with multiple catheter passes at different orientations throughout the stenotic artery.

Feedback systems based on fluorescence spectroscopy (61,62) or intravascular ultrasound (35) may also be capable of safely guiding greater plaque ablation. Fluorescence spectroscopy is capable in vitro of discriminating normal and atherosclerotic artery, and of guiding recanalization of total occlusions (61). Preliminary in vivo trials have begun to evaluate the efficacy of fluorescence spectroscopy to determine catheter tissue contact, to guide eccentric catheter orientation, and to confirm the adequacy of saline infusion in clearing blood from the catheter–tissue interspace (62).

Pulsed laser angioplasty results in arterial wall injury reflected by an incidence of coronary dissection approximating 20% during clinical procedures. Although this dissection rate may be lower than that reported with balloon angioplasty, laser-induced dissections occur unpredictably, and are associated with the major complications of the procedure. Minimizing the number of laser passes, minimizing irradiation of blood, and/or decreasing laser pulse energy may decrease the incidence of laser-induced dissections.

The use of saline infusion into the coronary artery during laser angioplasty is being investigated to displace blood and minimize acoustomechanical injury (63,64). In vitro experiments documented that excimer laser ablation in blood resulted in a bubble diameter of 1.2 mm and an acoustic pressure of 15 kbar as compared to no acoustic signal or bubble formation in saline (63). A four-fold dilution of blood reduced the bubble diameter to 0.48 mm and the pressure to 0.25 kbar. In another experiment (64), the magnitude of the pressure pulse was reduced 60% in a 10% blood solution, and 95% in saline, as compared to that in whole blood. The difference is due to the strong absorption of 308-nm radiation by blood as compared to saline. The transmission through 1 mm of saline was 100% but only 59% through a 10% blood/saline solution (64).

Another approach to reduce arterial wall injury is the use of multiplexing, or sequential firing of the laser into sections of the multifiber catheter to decrease the pulse energy and thereby reduce acoustomechanical damage. An 11-fold reduction in shock wave and acoustic pressure, reduction of histological acoustic injury, and decreased neointimal proliferation in an animal model were reported following multiplexing (65,66).

The major problem that laser angioplasty has yet failed to resolve is that of restenosis. The hypothesis driving laser angioplasty has been that plaque ablation by laser radiation, as opposed to plaque displacement by a balloon catheter, would result in a lower restenosis rate. This hypothesis has still to be proven. The unaltered restenosis rate following laser angioplasty may be due to the inadequate plaque ablation and/or the neointimal proliferation in response to the mechanical injury induced by laser dissections or adjunctive balloon angioplasty. Efforts aimed at increasing plaque ablation or reducing arterial wall injury, described above, may therefore be effective in lowering the restenosis rate.

V. CONCLUSIONS

Laser angioplasty is fighting for a niche in the cardiac interventionalist's therapeutic armamentarium. Several niche applications of laser angioplasty have been approved, but increasing acceptance by physicians and patients will depend on successfully addressing the problems outlined above. For any new interventional technology such as laser angioplasty, one must consider whether the new technology can do something that conventional approaches cannot or whether the new technology can do something less expensive than the conventional approaches. If developments in laser angioplasty enable recanalization of total occlusions and treatment of coronary stenoses with a low incidence of complications and a low rate of restenosis, then the answer to both of these questions for laser angioplasty will be "yes." Of all the new coronary interventional approaches, laser angioplasty is probably the least "mature" in that it has the greatest potential for ongoing refinement and improvement. Hopefully, as this development occurs, the full potential of laser angioplasty will be realized.

REFERENCES

1. DiSciascio G, Vetrovec GW, Cowly MJ, et al. Early and late outcome of percutaneous transluminal angioplasty for subacute and chronic total coronary occlusion. Am Heart J 1986;111:833–839.
2. Holmes DR, Vlietstra RE, Reeder GS, et al. Angioplasty in total coronary artery occlusion. J Am Coll Cardiol 1984;3:845–849.
3. Ellis SG, Vandeormael MG, Cowley MJ, et al. Coronary morphologic and clinical determinants of procedural outcome with angioplasty for patient selection. Circulation 1990;82:1193–1202.
4. Topol EJ, Leya F, Pinkerton CA, et al. A comparison of directional atherectomy with coronary angioplasty in patients with coronary artery disease. The CAVEAT study group. N Engl J Med 1993;329:221–227.
5. Isner JM, Clarke RH, Donaldson RF, et al. Identification of photoproducts liberated by in-vitro argon laser irradiation of atherosclerotic plaque, calcified cardiac valves and myocardium. Am J Cardiol 1985;55:1192–1196.
6. McGuff PE, Bushnell D, Soroff HS, et al. Studies of the surgical applications of laser (light amplification by stimulated emission of radiation). Surgical Forum 1963;14:143–145.
7. Choy DSJ, Stertzer RH, Myler RK, et al. Human coronary laser recanalization. Clin Cardiol 1984;7:377–381.
8. Cumberland DC, Oakley GDG, Smith GH, et al. Percutaneous laser assisted coronary angioplasty (letter). Lancet 1986;II:214.
9. Cumberland DC, Taylor DI, Welsh CL, et al. Percutaneous laser thermal angioplasty: Initial clinical results with a laser probe in total peripheral artery occlusions. Lancet 1986;I:1457–1459.

10. Sanborn TA, Faxon DP, Kellett MA, et al. Percutaneous coronary laser thermal angioplasty with a metallic capped fiber. J Am Coll Cardiol 1987;9(suppl A): 104A.

11. Cote G, Smith A, Andrus S, et al. Immediate results of percutaneous argon laser coronary angioplasty. Circulation 1989;80(suppl II):II-477.

12. Deckelbaum LI, Isner JM, Donaldson RF, et al. Reduction of laser-induced pathologic tissue injury using pulsed energy delivery. Am J Cardiol 1985;56: 662-666.

13. Grundfest WS, Litvack IF, Goldenberg T, et al. Pulsed ultraviolet lasers and the potential for safe laser angioplasty. Am J Surg 1985;150:220-226.

14. Grundfest WS, Litvack F, Forrester JS, et al. Laser ablation of human atherosclerotic plaque without adjacent tissue injury. J Am Coll Cardiol 1985;5:929-933.

15. Isner JM, Donaldson RF, Deckelbaum LI, et al. The excimer laser: gross, light microscopic and ultrastructural analysis of potential advantages for use in laser therapy of cardiovascular disease. J Am Coll Cardiol 1985;6:1102-1109.

16. Isner JM, Steg PG, Clarke RH. Current status of cardiovascular laser therapy. IEEE J Quantum Electron 1987;QE-23:1756-1771.

17. Deckelbaum LI, Isner JM, Donaldson RF, et al. Use of pulsed energy delivery to minimize tissue injury resulting from carbon dioxide laser irradiation of cardiovascular tissues. J Am Coll Cardiol 1986;7:898-908.

18. Clarke RH, Isner JM, Donaldson RF, et al. Gas chromatographic-light microscopic correlative analysis of excimer laser photoablation of cardiovascular tissues: Evidence of a thermal mechanism. Circ Res 1987;60:429-437.

19. Litvack F, Grundfest WS, Goldenberg T, et al. Percutaneous excimer laser angioplasty of aortocoronary saphenous vein grafts. J Am Coll Cardiol 1989;14: 803-808.

20. Geschwind HJ, Dubois-Rande JL, Zelinsky R, et al. Percutaneous coronary mid-infra-red laser angioplasty. Am Heart J 1991;122:552-558.

21. Cook SL, Eigler NL, Shefer A, et al. Percutaneous excimer laser coronary angioplasty of lesions not ideal for balloon angioplasty. Circulation 1991;84:632-643.

22. Bittl JA, Ryan TJ, Keaney JF, et al. Coronary artery perforation during excimer laser coronary angioplasty. J Am Coll Cardiol 1993;21:1158-1165.

23. Werner G, Buchwald A, Unterberg C, et al. Excimer laser angioplasty in coronary artery disease. Eur Heart J 1991;12:24-29.

24. Eclipse 2100 specification sheet. Eclipse Surgical Technologies, Palo Alto, CA.

25. Deckelbaum LI. System design considerations for laser angioplasty. Tex Heart Inst J 1989;16:150-157.

26. Goodking J, Coombs V, Golobic R. Excimer laser angioplasty. J Heart Lung 1993;22:26-35.

27. Isner JM, Rosenfield K, White CJ, et al. In vivo assessment of vascular pathology resulting from laser irradiation. Circulation 1992;85:2185-2196.

28. Nakamura F, Kvasnicka J, Uchida Y, et al. Percutaneous angioscopic evaluation of luminal changes induced by excimer laser angioplasty. Am Heart J 1992; 124:1467-1472.

29. Torre SR, Sanborn TA, Sharma SK, et al. Percutaneous coronary excimer laser angioplasty quantitative angiographic analysis demonstrates improved angioplasty results with larger laser catheters. Circulation 1990;82(suppl III):III-671.
30. Margolis JR, Mehta S. Excimer laser coronary angioplasty. Am J Cardiol 1992; 69:3F-11F.
31. Bittl JA, Sanborn TA. Excimer laser-facilitated coronary angioplasty. Circulation 1992;86:71-80.
32. Hanet C, Wijns W, Michel X, et al. Influence of balloon size and stenosis morphology on immediate and delayed elastic recoil after percutaneous transluminal coronary angioplasty. J Am Coll Cardiol 1991;18(2):506-511.
33. Isner JM, Rosenfield K, Losordo DW, et al. Combination balloon ultrasound imaging catheter for percutaneous transluminal angioplasty. Circulation 1991; 84(2):739-754.
34. Rensing BJ, Hermans WR, Beatt KJ, et al. Quantitative angiographic assessment of elastic recoil after percutaneous transluminal coronary angioplasty. Am J Cardiol 1990;66:1039-1044.
35. Tenaglia AN, Tcheng JE, Kisslo KB, et al. Intracoronary ultrasound evaluation of excimer laser angioplasty (abstr). Circulation 1992;86(suppl I):I-516.
36. Ghazzal ZM, Hearn JA, Litvack F, et al. Morphological predictors of acute complications after percutaneous excimer laser coronary angioplasty. Circulation 1992;86:820-827.
37. Bittl JA, Sanborn TA, Tcheng JE, et al. Clinical success, complications and restenosis rates with excimer laser coronary angioplasty. Am J Cardiol 1992; 70:1533-1539.
38. Litvack F, Margolis J, Cummins F, et al. Excimer laser coronary registry: Report of the first consecutive 2080 patients (abstr). J Am Coll Cardiol 1992;19 (suppl A):276A.
39. Baumbach A, Haase K, Karsch KR. Usefulness of morphologic parameters in predicting the outcome of coronary excimer laser angioplasty. Am J Cardiol 1991;68:1310-1315.
40. Knopf WD, Parr KL, Moses JW, et al. Multicenter registry report. Circulation 1992;86(suppl I):I-511.
41. Knopf W, Parr K, Moses J, et al. Holmium laser angioplasty in coronary arteries (abstr). J Am Coll Cardiol 1992;19(suppl A):352A.
42. Geschwind HJ, Nakamura F, Kvasnicka J, et al. Excimer and holmium yttrium aluminum garnet laser coronary angioplasty. Am Heart J 1993;125:510-522.
43. Watson LE, Gantt S. Excimer laser coronary angioplasty for failed PTCA. Cathet Cardiovasc Diagn 1992;26:285-290.
44. Estella P, Ryan TJ, Landzberg JS, et al. Excimer laser-assisted coronary angioplasty for lesions containing thrombus. J Am Coll Cardiol 1993;21:1550-1556.
45. de Marchena E, Mallon S, Posada JD, et al. Direct holmium laser assisted balloon angioplasty in acute myocardial infarction. Am J Cardiol 1993;71:1223-1225.
46. Litvack F, Eigler NL, Forrester JS. In search of the optimized excimer laser angioplasty system. Circulation 1993;87:1421-1422.

47. Sanborn TA, Torre SR, Sharma SK, et al. Percutaneous coronary excimer laser-assisted balloon angioplasty. J Am Coll Cardiol 1991;17:94–99.
48. Baumbach A, Haase KK, Voelker W, et al. Effects of intracoronary nitroglycerin on luman diameter during early follow-up angiography after coronary excimer laser atherectomy. Eur Heart J 1991;12:726–731.
49. van Leeuwen TG, van Erven L, Meertens JH, et al. Origin of arterial wall dissections induced by pulsed excimer and mid-infrared laser ablation in the pig. J Am Coll Cardiol 1992;19:1610–1618.
50. van Leeuwen TG, Meertens JH, Velema E, et al. Intraluminal vapor bubble induced by excimer laser pulse causes microsecond arterial dilation and invagination leading to extensive wall damage in the rabbit. Circulation 1993;87:1258–1263.
51. Isner JM, Pickering JG, Mosseri M. Laser-induced dissections. J Am Coll Cardiol 1992;19:1619–1621.
52. Abela GS. Abrupt closure after pulsed laser angioplasty. J Interventional Cardiol 1992;5:259–262.
53. Preisack MB, Voelker W, Haase KK, et al. Case Report: Formation of vessel aneurysm after stand alone coronary excimer laser angioplasty. Cathet Cardiovasc Diagn 1992;27:122–124.
54. Feld MS, Kramer JR. Mutagenicity and the XeCl excimer laser. Am Heart J 1991;6:1803–1806.
55. Buchwald AB, Werner GS, Unterberg C, et al. Restenosis after excimer laser angioplasty of coronary stenoses and chronic total occlusions. Am Heart J 1992;123:878–885.
56. Bittl JA, Kuntz RE, Ahmed WH, et al. The effect of acute procedural results on restenosis after excimer laser-facilitated angioplasty. Circulation 1992;86 (suppl I):I-532.
57. Holmes DR, Forrester JS, Litvack F, et al. Chronic total obstruction and short-term outcome: The excimer laser coronary angioplasty registry experience. Mayo Clin Proc 1993;68:5–10.
58. Reeder GS, Bresnahan JF, Holmer DR, et al. Excimer laser coronary angioplasty. Cathet Cardiovasc Diagn 1992;25:195–199.
59. Henson KD, Leon MB, Pichard AD, et al. Successful directional excimer laser coronary angioplasty in unfavorable lesion morphologies. J Am Coll Cardiol 1993;21:385A.
60. Ghazzal ZM, Leon MB, Shefer A, et al. The novel directional laser catheter. J Am Coll Cardiol 1993;21:288A.
61. Garrand TJ, Stetz ML, O'Brien KM, et al. Design and evaluation of a fiberoptic fluorescence guided laser recanalization system. Lasers Surg Med 1991;11:106–116.
62. Scott JJ, Desai SP, Deckelbaum LI. Optimization of laser angioplasty catheter position using arterial fluorescence feedback. Lasers Surg Med 1993;13(suppl 5):12.
63. Grunkemeier JM, Gregory KW. Acoustic measurements of cavitation bubbles in blood, contrast and saline using an excimer laser. Circulation 1992;86(suppl IV):16.

64. Tcheng JE, Phillips HR, Wells LD, et al. A new technique for reducing pressure pulse phenomena during coronary excimer laser angioplasty (abstr). J Am Coll Cardiol 1993;21(suppl A):386A.

65. Xie DY, Hassenstein S, Oberhoff M, et al. Preliminary evaluation of smooth excimer laser coronary angioplasty (SELCA) in vitro. Circulation 1992;86(suppl I):I-653.

66. Oberhoff M, Hassenstein S, Hanke H, et al. Smooth excimer laser coronary angioplasty (SELCA). Circulation 1992;86(suppl I):I-800.

7

Coronary and Saphenous Vein Graft Stents

Christopher J. White
Health Care International Medical Center, Glasgow, Scotland

Stephen R. Ramee
Ochsner Medical Institutions, New Orleans, Louisiana

I. INTRODUCTION

Placement of noncoronary intravascular stents was first described in 1969 by Charles Dotter who experimented with metal and plastic tubes and coils in canine iliac vessels as an adjunct to angioplasty (1). Over the past 25 years there have been myriad stent designs developed and tested for both peripheral and coronary vascular applications. Current iterations of vascular stents have married the advanced technology of balloon angioplasty catheters and both metal and polymeric stents. Polymeric stents have the special properties of being biodegradable and of undergoing phase changes from liquid to solid. This allows a liquid applied or "poured" onto the vessel surface to be hardened in place. The term "arterial paving" was coined to describe this process (2).

Metal stents, be they self-expanding or balloon-expandable designs, may be configured as either wire coils or a tubular mesh. Self-expanding stents are designed with an external constraining membrane that holds the compressed stent on the delivery catheter. When the membrane is withdrawn, the stent is released from the catheter to expand against the arterial wall. Balloon-expandable stents are tightly crimped on angioplasty balloons and are deployed by inflating the balloon.

There are two broad clinical indications for stent implantation. The first is to prevent recurrent stenosis or restenosis after angioplasty, and the second is to salvage a failed angioplasty. Current data suggest that there is a direct relationship between maximizing the luminal area after angioplasty and lowering the incidence of restenosis (3). It has also been shown that the more aggressively the artery is dilated, the more prolific will be the healing response contributing to restenosis (4). The efficacy of stents for restenosis reduction will depend on their ability to create a vascular lumen large enough to compensate for the intimal proliferative response after arterial injury.

Abrupt occlusion is the major cause of morbidity and mortality associated with failed angioplasty procedures. Conventional methods of restoring arterial patency, such as long balloon inflations, the use of slightly larger balloons, and thrombolytic infusions, may often be successful; but too often emergency coronary bypass surgery is necessary. The inability to routinely maintain coronary perfusion in the face of an abrupt occlusion necessitates on-site surgical back-up for those patients in whom conventional "salvage" angioplasty fails. The ability of stents to reliably restore vessel patency during salvage angioplasty procedures is expected to have a positive impact on reducing the morbidity and mortality of the procedure, and reduce costs as well by making routine surgery stand-by unnecessary.

For stents to be accepted as a viable therapeutic option, the potential benefits must outweigh the potential complications. The major risks of stent placement include thrombosis and hemorrhagic complications. All of the current stent designs are thrombogenic and pose a risk of "subacute" thrombosis, the sudden thrombotic occlusion of a stent vessel 24 h to several weeks after implantation. While there are a growing number of coronary stent and saphenous vein graft stents for the clinician to choose from, our laboratory experience has been with the Wiktor® coronary stent and the Palmaz-Schatz® biliary stent. This chapter will review the methods, clinical results, and complications experienced with each of these stents, and conclude with an analysis based on our experience.

II. CORONARY STENTS

The Wiltor® stent (Medtronic, Inc., San Diego, CA) is a unique balloon-expandable tantalum coil stent currently undergoing clinical trials to determine the efficacy and safety of the device for reducing restenosis, and for salvaging a failed angioplasty (bailout). The stent is 17 mm in length, composed of a single strand of tantalum wire, 0.005-in. in diameter, wound in a semihelical coil, and tightly crimped on a 2.0-cm-long conventional angioplasty balloon (Prime™, Medtronic, Inc., San Diego, CA) (Fig. 1). This configuration allows the stent to be placed on a balloon catheter with minimal

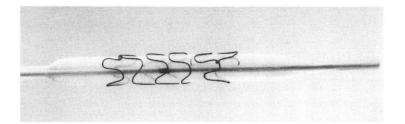

Figure 1 Wiktor® stent.

increase in the balloon profile. The coil design confers flexibility to the balloon-mounted stent and this flexibility allows the stent to easily pass through the tight bends in standard coronary guiding catheter configurations as well as to negotiate the tortuosity of the native coronary arteries.

Tantalum was chosen as the metal for this stent for several reasons. Most importantly, tantalum is much more radiopaque than stainless steel wire of this dimension. Tantalum, a long-standing component of intracardiac pacemaker leads, is known to be biologically inert. An inelastic metal, tantalum displays very little elastic recoil and tends not to "spring back" to its original configuration as stainless steel does. Finally, presumably because of the repulsion of negatively charged blood elements, particularly platelets, electronegative metals such as tantalum have been associated with relative "thromboresistance" when compared with electropositive metals such as stainless steel (5).

The Wiktor® stent may be placed using standard 8-French guiding catheters. All commercially available guiding catheter configurations are compatible with delivery of this stent. When using the Wiktor® stent, every attempt should be made to obtain optimal guiding catheter seating to aid delivery of the balloon-mounted stent to the target lesion. The stent should be sized 10–15% larger than the reference vessel diameter, and all lesions should be predilated before stent placement. In elective restenosis lesions, predilation can be performed with a balloon 0.5 mm smaller than the estimated final stent diameter. In patients who receive stents as a consequence of a suboptimal angioplasty result, the investigator should determine whether the stent should be the same size as the initial balloon used or 0.5 mm larger.

The stent was delivered on 3.0-, 3.5-, 4.0- and 4.5-mm balloons. Due to the redundant coils in this design, the stent does not shorten when the balloon is inflated. The inelasticity of tantalum results in very little recoil of the stent once it has been expanded. The in vivo recoil of the Wiktor® stent has been quantitatively measured at 3% (6). This allows stent deployment with a balloon sized to the desired stent diameter (i.e., a 3.0-mm balloon is used to deploy a 3.0-mm stent). In contrast, stent deployment with a stainless steel coil stent (Gianturco-Roubin, Cook Inc., Bloomington, IN) requires 0.5-mm oversized balloons (i.e., a 3.5-mm balloon is used to deploy a 3.0-mm stent) (7). There is a theoretical concern that using oversized balloons to deliver stents may cause coronary artery dissections at the proximal or distal portion of the balloon which would not be covered by the stent.

A. Wiktor® Stent Procedure

1. Wiktor® Stent Placement

The tantalum wire is wound directly onto the balloon delivery catheter and packaged for use. Negative pressure is applied to the balloon to check for "pin-hole" leaks that would cause balloon failure during deployment. The stent delivery catheter is advanced over an 0.018-in. or 0.014-in. angioplasty guidewire. Care must be taken not to snag any of the coils of the stent during introduction through the Tuoy-Borst adapter. Because this stent has no covering sheath, it is very difficult to retrieve once it has exited the guiding catheter. For this reason, during balloon predilation, the adequacy of guiding catheter support must be determined. If the guiding catheter initially chosen does not provide excellent support, it should be changed for a more supportive guiding catheter before introducing the stent.

The excellent radiopacity of tantalum leaves no doubt about the location of the proximal and distal coils of the stent. It is quite easy, using contrast injections to visualize sidebranches, to precisely place the stent either proximal to or distal to a sidebranch, or to place the stent in the proximal left anterior descending or left circumflex coronary artery without having any portion of the stent in the left main coronary artery.

Once the stent has been positioned, the balloon catheter is inflated to 4 atm pressure (balloon nominal inflation pressure) for 15–30 s. The balloon is deflated and contrast injections are performed to confirm patency. The balloon catheter is then withdrawn into the guiding catheter, and angiography is performed. In our experience, the radiopacity of the tantalum wire does not interfere with our ability to assess the angiographic results of stent placement. At this time, additional inflations with the same balloon at the same or higher pressures or with a larger balloon can be performed if necessary to optimize the lumen diameter. Occasionally, with larger delivery balloons ⩾4.0 mm, it is necessary to advance the balloon catheter before withdrawal to minimize the risk of the "wings" of the deflated balloon to snag the coils of the stent. As mentioned above, with the guidewire remaining across the lesion, multiple options are available to increase the final stent diameter. The compliant stent delivery balloon can be inflated to slightly higher pressures (6–8 atm), or a larger balloon may be used.

Recrossing the deployed stent with a guidewire carries the risk of the guidewire traveling outside the stent, i.e., between the stent wire and the vessel wall. This external location may be very difficult to determine with fluoroscopy, and can result in significant distortion of the stent geometry when attempting to advance a balloon over the misplaced guidewire. To avoid this, we use a very tight "J" curve (almost a loop) on the guidewire when recrossing the stent.

In the event that it is necessary for a second stent to be placed distal to the initially placed stent, this can usually be accomplished without difficulty. The need for a second distal stent arises when attempting to "tack up" dissection flaps, if the initial stent does not satisfactorily cover the distal portion of the dissection. When at all possible, the most distal extent of the dissection should be stented first to avoid having to cross a deployed stent with an undeployed stent due to the risk of catching or snagging a coil of the deployed stent with a coil of the undeployed stent. When placing multiple stents, the radiopacity of the tantalum coils allows great precision when positioning the second stent.

2. Stent Retrieval

If the balloon-mounted stent is unable to reach the target lesion, generally due to inadequate guiding catheter support, the operator has two options. The first is to deploy the stent proximal to the lesion. The second option is to attempt to withdraw the undeployed balloon-mounted stent back into the guiding catheter, and remove it from the body. Great care must be taken to align the lumen of the guiding catheter and the balloon catheter to avoid scraping the stent off of the balloon during withdrawal into the guiding catheter. The radiopacity of the stents allows the operator to clearly visualize the stent coils catching on the lip of the guiding catheter. If the undeployed stent is unable to be withdrawn into the guiding catheter, the position of the balloon catheter and the guiding catheter should be fixed by tightening the O-ring of the Tuoy-Borst adapter, and the guiding catheter and the stent delivery catheter are withdrawn as a unit to the femoral arterial sheath. Under fluoroscopic guidance, the stent should be gently withdrawn into the femoral sheath and removed from the body.

If the stent becomes dislodged from the balloon catheter but remains on the guidewire, it may be retrieved using a loop snare. The snare is loaded onto the guidewire and advanced to the stent. The loop of the snare is then tightened and the single strand of tantalum wire can be removed by withdrawing the snare. This procedure of snaring the stent may also be used to retrieve a stent that has embolized to a peripheral vessel. The radiopacity of the stent facilitates locating the embolized stent and guiding its removal.

B. Wiktor® Stent Clinical Experience

Patient selection for coronary Wiktor® stent implantation is based upon meeting the entry criteria of two trials aimed at either (1) reducing the incidence of restenosis after angioplasty or (2) reestablishing coronary patency after failed angioplasty (bailout). For the restenosis reduction trials, the inclusion criteria require that the patient be at increased risk for restenosis after angioplasty. Patients were enrolled in the "bailout trial" if they demonstrated acute or threatened closure of the vessel undergoing angioplasty or if they demonstrated a suboptimal angioplasty result (i.e., if they had a critical reduction in coronary flow after angioplasty or if we were unable to reduce the residual stenosis to less than 50% of the reference diameter).

All patients were required to be potential candidates for surgical revascularization. Objective evidence of coronary ischemia, a positive treadmill stress test, a clinical history of angina pectoris, or evidence of ischemia on their electrocardiogram was required. For elective implantation of stents in the restenosis trial, patients had to have a left ventricular ejection fraction ⩾30%. Patients at increased risk of bleeding complications were excluded. For example, patients with recent or active gastrointestinal bleeding, any prior history of bleeding problems, the inability to safely take oral anticoagulants, an intolerance to aspirin, or chronic liver disease were excluded.

Vessel selection criteria included both native coronary arteries and saphenous vein bypass grafts. The target vessel was required to be at least 3.0 mm in diameter up to a maximum of 4.5 mm in diameter at the lesion site. Left main coronary artery lesions were excluded. For elective stent implantation in the restenosis trial, vessels that contained angiographically visible thrombus were excluded.

All lesion types (ACC/AHA criteria A, B, and C) (8) 15 mm or less in length were considered acceptable for stent implantation. In patients with acute or threatened occlusion (bailout trial), multiple stent implantation was permitted to cover extensive dissections.

1. Wiktor® Multicenter Restenosis Trial

Elective implantation of the Wiktor® balloon expandable tantalum coil stent was attempted in 198 patients (139 native coronary arteries and 59 saphenous vein grafts). Patients were preteated with 325 mg of aspirin, dipyridamole 75 mg t.i.d., and a calcium antagonist. Low molecular weight dextran was given intravenously beginning at least 2 h before the procedure at 100 ml/h.

Restenosis lesions were predilated with 0.5-mm undersized balloons, while suboptimal result patients usually had their dilating balloon matched to the reference artery size. Additional heparin (5000–10,000 IU) was administered as needed to maintain the activated clotting time ⩾300 s and "optimal" guiding catheter seating was obtained before stent placement. We commonly used left Amplatz catheters for right coronary artery and left circumflex artery stent placement, and left Judkins catheters for left anterior descending coronary artery stent placement.

Successful stent delivery was accomplished in 190 of 198 (96%) patients (Fig. 2). In the successfully implanted patients, multiple stents were placed in 23 (12%) patients and single stents were placed in 167 (89%) patients. Eight patients failed to have the stent successfully implanted, three due to excessive proximal vessel tortuosity, two due to inadequate guiding catheter support, one due to stent embolization, one due to balloon catheter damage of a deployed stent, and one due to inability to cross a predilated lesion with the balloon-mounted stent. The mean hospital stay was 6 ± 3 days.

The arterial sheath was removed 4–24 h after the procedure. Patients received intravenous dextran (50–100 cc/h) until therapeutic anticoagulation with intravenous heparin was obtained with a partial thromboplastin time between 70 and 90 s. Heparin was continued until the patient's protime was 18–22 s. The heparin was then gradually tapered and discontinued over 12 h ensuring that the protime remained above 18 s. At discharge, patients were taking aspirin, dipyridamole, a calcium antagonist, and warfarin. Oral anti-

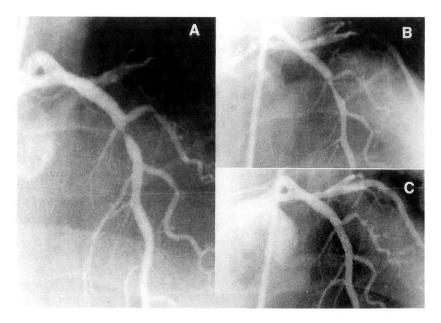

Figure 2   (A) Baseline angiogram of mid-LAD lesion. (B) Post-angioplasty result with residual stenosis > 50% due to elastic recoil. (C) Post-Wiktor® stent placement.

coagulation with warfarin was continued for 3 months and titrated to pro-long the protime to 18–20 s.

Follow-up data were available in 166 of 190 (87%) patients at a minimum of 5 months after stent implantation with clinical restenosis present in 51 (31%) patients. Follow-up angiography was obtained in 101 (51%) patients. Angiographic restenosis ($\geq$50% diameter narrowing) was present in 26 (26%) of the 101 patients. Complications associated with elective stent implantation are shown in Table 1.

The European experience with elective implantation of the Wiktor® stent for reducing restenosis reflects a high rate of implantation success ranging from 98% in a multicenter trial of 50 consecutive patients with one or more prior episodes of restenosis (6) to 100% in eight elective patients with restenosis (9). The European Multicenter Wiktor® Stent Trial (6) for preventing restenosis reported no procedural or stent-related deaths. There were no instances of acute stent thrombosis; however, subacute thrombosis with myocardial infarction occurred in five (10%) patients. Of the five patients with subacute thrombosis, however, four were not adequately anticoagulated at the time of stent thrombosis. Significant bleeding complications occurred in 11 (22%) patients, including 6 patients who required blood transfusion for femoral access complications, 3 patients who had gastrointestinal bleeding, and 2 patients who had hematuria. The angiographic restenosis rate in this study was 29%.

We are encouraged by the high success rate of implantation of this device. However, we are concerned that the early complications of elective stent implantation may exceed any future benefit obtained in reducing restenosis. Since the majority of these complications are related to stent thrombosis or to the aggressive anticoagulation regimen employed to prevent thrombosis, it would seem appropriate to focus on reducing the thrombogenicity of

Table 1 Complications of Wiktor® Stent Placement

Complications	Restenosis trial ($n = 198$)		Bailout trial ($n = 152$)	
	(n)	(%)	(n)	(%)
Stent death	2	1.0	1	0.7
All death	9	4.5	14	9.2
Myocardial infarction	14	7.1	17	11.1
Stroke	1	0.5	0	0
Transfusion	17	8.6	8	5.3
Emergency bypass	7	3.5	12	7.9
Stent thrombosis	11	5.5	12	7.9

these devices with the development of antithrombogenic materials, or coatings, to improve the risk-to-benefit ratio for the elective indication of restenosis reduction.

2. Wiktor® "Bailout" Trial

The U.S. Multicenter Wiktor® Stent Trial for acute or threatened closure, or "bailout," is currently in progress. To be considered eligible, patients are required to have either acute or threatened closure of the dilated vessel after balloon angioplasty or a suboptimal angioplasty result with a residual stenosis $> 50\%$.

Success was defined as reduction of the diameter stenosis to $< 50\%$ with resolution of the acute coronary ischemia. Placement of the Wiktor® stents was attempted in 152 patients (180 lesions)—25 with acute closure, 75 with threatened occlusion, and 52 with a suboptimal result with $> 50\%$ residual stenosis. Stent placement in native coronary arteries ($n = 97$) or vein grafts ($n = 55$) between 3.0 and 4.5 mm was attempted in patients with failed angioplasty and no contraindication to anticoagulation. Stents were placed with conventional angioplasty equipment including 8-French guiding catheters and 0.014-in. or 0.018-in. guidewires. Successful placement of 204 of 215 (95%) attempted stents was obtained in 147 of 152 (97%) patients, and 175 of 180 (97%) lesions (Fig. 3).

There were 11 failed attempts at placing stents in nine patients, including four patients who were successfully stented on the second attempt and five patients who received no stent, because of an inability to reach the target lesion ($n = 3$), failure to cross the lesion ($n = 2$), dislodgement of the stent from the balloon ($n = 1$), stent placement in a false lumen ($n = 1$), stent embolization ($n = 1$), inadequate guide catheter support ($n = 1$), and stent damage ($n = 2$). Complications both in-hospital and during follow-up are shown in Table 1.

There have been two published series of patients from Europe who have received the Wiktor® stent for acute or subacute closure after angioplasty. Buchwald and coworkers (10) reported on 11 patients with otherwise unmanageable occlusion after angioplasty. Successful "bailout" was accomplished in every case. In a more recent report, Burger and colleagues (9) described their experience with the Wiktor® stent in 20 patients with threatened or acute closure after angioplasty. Successful implantation was accomplished in 19 of 20 (95%) patients. The single failure occurred in a left circumflex coronary artery due to inadequate guiding catheter support and successful coronary bypass surgery was performed. At 6 months follow-up, 12 (60%) of the patients with failed balloon angioplasty had patent arteries. Reasons for failure to maintain stent patency included the single patient with failure to deliver the stent, two patients with acute thrombosis, two patients with subacute thrombosis, one patient with restenosis, and two patients who died.

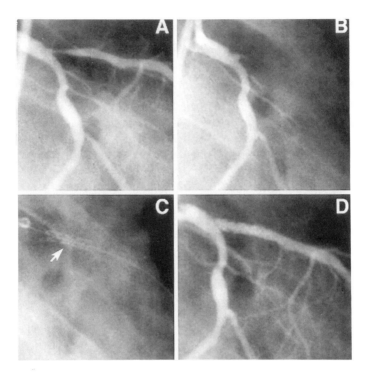

Figure 3 (A) Baseline angiogram with proximal LAD stenosis. (B) Abrupt occlusion following angioplasty. (C) Placement of a Wiktor® stent as a "bailout" device. (D) Final angiogram with restored patency of the LAD. LAD = left anterior descending.

The European investigators stressed the stent's radiographic opacity and flexibility as the key to their high rate of implantation success. And although they still acknowledged the significant bleeding complications that can occur with aggressive anticoagulation regimens, they emphasized that the stent's failures during this trial were often related to suboptimal anticoagulation regimens.

C. Complications

As summarized in the individual trials above, the major risks related to the Wiktor® stent include stent thrombosis and the risk of hemorrhage complications related to the vigorous anticoagulation regime used to prevent possible stent thrombosis. It appears that the risk of stent thrombosis is lower in elective settings than in the more urgent abrupt occlusion environment.

III. BILIARY STENTS FOR SAPHENOUS VEIN GRAFT STENOSES

Percutaneous angioplasty in stenotic or occluded saphenous vein coronary bypass grafts has been associated with less favorable results, including a lower primary success rate, a higher procedural complication rate, and a higher restenosis rate than in native coronary arteries (11–14). These suboptimal results and the significant clinical need for a percutaneous therapy for failed saphenous vein bypass grafts have stimulated investigation into the application of newer technologies, such as atherectomy, laser-assisted angioplasty, and the use of endovascular stents.

The placement of stents into saphenous vein grafts has several potential advantages based upon the ability of stents to maximize the acute gain after angioplasty, which has been associated with a lower restenosis rate (13,15), and to minimize the risk of angiographic dissection (16) after angioplasty in native coronary arteries.

Early reports describing the placement of the Palmaz-Schatz® coronary stent (Johnson and Johnson Interventional Systems, Warren, NJ) in aortocoronary saphenous vein grafts have been encouraging both for acute success and long-term patency. Data from a multicenter trial revealed procedural success in 220 of 224 (98%) vein grafts attempted with a restenosis rate of 26% (17). Strumpf et al. (18) reported their single center experience with this Palmaz-Schatz® device in 26 patients with saphenous vein graft disease. They achieved successful stent implantation in all lesions with a restenosis rate of 13%. Complications included stent embolism in 2 (8%) patients, stent thrombosis in 1 (4%) patient, and bleeding complications in 5 (19%) patients. We and others have hypothesized that many of these complications may be overcome by using the Palmaz biliary stent. First, the biliary stent is not articulated and is also available in 10-, 15-, and 20-mm lengths, which allows more uniform coverage of the lesion. Others (19) have suggested that because the coronary device distorts when its diameter is expanded ≥5.0 mm, the larger biliary stent is more suitable for use in these saphenous vein grafts.

A. Biliary Stent Procedure

We placed 57 stents (Palmaz, Johnson and Johnson Interventional Systems, Warren, NJ) in 37 patients with 40 stenotic or occlusive lesions in coronary saphenous vein bypass grafts that measured ≥3.5 mm in diameter. Patients were pretreated at least 1 day before stent placement with 325 mg of aspirin per day, dipyridamole 75 mg t.i.d., and a calcium channel blocker. Before stent implantation, patients were started on low molecular weight dextran at 100 ml/h, which was continued until adequate heparinization had been achieved after sheath removal. Percutaneous femoral access was obtained with an 8-French hemostatic sheath. Ten thousand units of heparin were administered and an 8-French Hockey Stick or multipurpose angioplasty guiding catheter (Sherpa®, Medtronic, Inc., San Diego, CA) was advanced to the ostium of the target vein graft. The lesion was crossed with an 0.018-in. (High Torque Floppy®, ACS, Santa Clara, CA) or 0.016-in. (Flex®, U.S.C.I., Billerica, MA) guidewire. Predilation of the lesion was performed with a 0.5-mm undersized balloon, based upon visual estimation of the reference diameter of the graft.

The nonarticulated stainless steel stent, Palmaz 104 (10-mm length, 4- to 9-mm expansion range), or Palmaz 154 (15-mm length, 4- to 9-mm expansion range) (Fig. 4) was then hand-crimped onto the delivery balloon. We took great care not to "cigarette roll" the stent while hand-crimping the device on the balloon to avoid scratching or tearing the delivery balloon. Negative pressure was then applied to confirm that there were no leaks in the balloon. While holding the crimped stent tightly with forefinger and thumb to prevent expansion, the balloon was partially inflated with 1 atm pressure to create a "dumbbell" effect to prevent migration of the stent during delivery. The inflation device was then returned to a neutral position and the stent advanced over the guidewire to the predilated target lesion.

Before stent placement, the patient's activated clotting time was determined and, if <300 s, additional heparin was administered. It was occasionally necessary to adjust the position of the guiding catheter minimizing acute bends in the guiding catheter to allow this nonarticulated stent to pass freely to the graft. After positioning the stent at the site of the lesion, negative

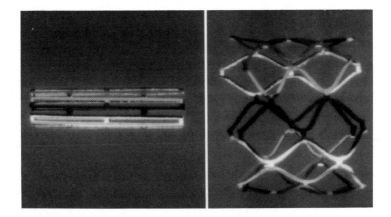

Figure 4 Balloon-expandable biliary stent (JJIS 104).

pressure was again applied to the balloon to confirm the integrity of the balloon. The balloon was then inflated to 6 atm for 15–30 s. Stents were placed in tandem when necessary without overlap, a technique that was facilitated by the relative radiopacity of this stainless steel stent. After stent deployment, the balloon was withdrawn, and angiography was performed. Further balloon inflations with higher pressures or with larger balloons were performed in an attempt to minimize the residual stenosis at the lesion site, and to slightly overdilate the stent if possible.

After stent placement, the activated clotting time was allowed to decline to between 160 and 180 s at which time the arterial sheath was removed and hemostasis was obtained with hand pressure. Intravenous heparin was then given, without a bolus, to maintain the partial thromboplastin time between 70 and 90 s. The dextran-40 infusion was continued until adequate heparinization was achieved. Warfarin (10 mg) was administered orally for 3 days and titrated to achieve a protime of 18–20 s. Patients were kept at bed rest for 36–48 h to minimize the risk of access site complications. At discharge, patients were taking aspirin 325 mg per day, dipyridamole 75 mg t.i.d., warfarin, and a calcium channel blocker. Oral anticoagulation with warfarin was continued for at least 3 months.

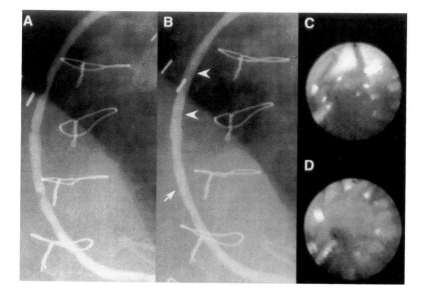

Figure 5   (A) Baseline angiogram of a right saphenous vein bypass graft. (B) Angiogram following placement of three JJIS 104 stents (arrowheads). (C) and (D) Angioscopy of the stented segments.

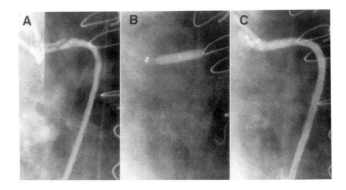

Figure 6   Placement of a biliary stent at the site of a dissection in a saphenous vein graft stent.

B. Biliary Stent Clinical Experience

Successful stent placement was accomplished in all patients and all lesions without stent embolism or abrupt occlusion (Figs. 5 and 6). Seven stents were placed at sites of prior restenosis, 5 stents were placed in de novo lesions, and 28 stents were placed after a suboptimal angioplasty result in a vein graft. Single stents were placed in 28 vein grafts, and multiple (2–4) stents were placed in 12 grafts.

The percent diameter stenosis was reduced from a baseline of $75.6 \pm 1.0\%$ to $4.4 \pm 6.6\%$ ($p < 0.001$). The baseline minimal lumen diameter of the lesion was measured to be 0.7 ± 0.7 mm and increased to 3.9 ± 0.5 mm ($p < 0.001$) after stent placement.

C. Complications

There was one aborted stent delivery due to a tear in the balloon. This was discovered before attempting to deploy the stent, when negative pressure was applied to the balloon and blood returned from the inflation lumen. The stent was uneventfully withdrawn into the guiding catheter and removed while still mounted on the balloon. A second stent and balloon were then reinserted and successfully deployed.

In-hospital complications included subacute stent thrombosis in 2 (5%) patients, acute myocardial infarction in 2 (5%) patients, death in 1 (3%) patient, bleeding complications in 2 (5%) patients, and access site-related problems in 5 (14%) patients. No patient required emergency bypass surgery.

IV. CONCLUSIONS

The Wiktor® stent offers several advantages as an adjunctive device for potential use in reducing the incidence of restenosis after angioplasty and as a "bailout" device for failed angioplasty. Its most outstanding attribute is its excellent radiopacity, a result of its tantalum composition. The ability to positively identify the margins of the stent with routine fluoroscopy allows the stent to be placed with precision and confidence. The flexibility conferred by the coil configuration of the stent allows the use of all commercially available configurations of guiding catheters, placement in tortuous and distal vessels, and an encouragingly high rate of procedural successes both in elective and emergent situations. The coil configuration also avoids the problem of "stent jail" encountered with wire mesh stents or tubular slotted steel designs. The coil design allows guidewire and balloon access to diseased sidebranches arising from the stented segment of an artery. Finally, the Wiktor® stent is balloon expandable without a covering sheath. This greatly simplifies deployment of the stent and is identical to inflating a balloon on the target lesion. There is no requirement for the operator to perform extra tasks, such as withdrawing a covering sheath before deployment, and no uncertainty regarding the stent's final location in the artery associated with self-expanding devices.

The disadvantages of the Wiktor® stent are linked to its advantages. For example, the radiopacity of the tantalum wire poses some difficulty for automated edge-detection programs used for quantitative angiography; however, this has not been a problem for the clinical assessment of angiographic results after stent placement. The flexibility of the coil design has raised concerns about the mechanical strength of the stent and its ability to scaffold the endolumenal surface of the dilated artery. Quantitative assessment of the stent immediately after deployment and at 6-month angiographic follow-up has failed to demonstrate significant recoil or compression of the stent due to elastic forces exerted by the dilated artery (6). Finally, the fact that the stent delivery is not encumbered by a covering safety sheath also means that, once the stent has exited the guiding catheter, the risk of stent embolization or deployment of the stent proximal to the target lesion is markedly increased if the stent cannot be advanced to the stenosis.

We have demonstrated the feasibility and safety of placing nonarticulated stainless steel biliary stents into stenotic or occluded saphenous vein grafts. Our purpose in exploring this application for nonarticulated stents was to improve the immediate and long-term results of percutaneous treatment of stenotic coronary saphenous vein grafts. Current approaches, including laser-assisted angioplasty, directional atherectomy, or balloon angioplasty, are associated with less favorable results in vein grafts than in native coronary arteries. Consequently, affected patients and their physicians are searching for a better alternative to repeat coronary bypass surgery for failed saphenous vein grafts.

The benefits of using these stents in this study included the use availability of 10-mm-long stents, which are sufficient to completely cover the majority of lesions and minimize the amount of metal placed in the vessel. In addition, the absence of the articulation allowed uniform coverage of these discrete lesions without a gap. The biliary stent has slightly thicker stainless steel struts than the articulated coronary stent, which markedly improves the fluoroscopic visibility of the stent and aids in the precision with which they can be placed. We found that we could easily juxtapose stents without overlap, leaving a smaller gap between tandem stents than the 1.0-mm space inherent in the articulated coronary stent (Palmaz-Schatz®) design.

However, while the stents used in this study had many advantages over articulated designs, they also presented some limitations. The stent is delivered without a covering sheath which presents more risk than a stent delivered with a covering sheath (i.e., the Palmaz-Schatz® coronary device). The retrieval of the undeployed stent back into the guiding catheter is a difficult procedure. When using stents without covering sheaths, care must be taken when withdrawing the undeployed stent into the guiding catheter so that the tip of the guiding catheter does not scrape the stent off of the balloon and therefore cause either systemic or coronary stent embolization. In addition, because the lack of an articulation in the stent limits its length to 15 mm so that bends and curves in the guiding catheters and vein grafts can be negotiated, longer, nonarticulated stents are limited to the straighter right coronary saphenous vein grafts that can be cannulated with "multipurpose" shaped guiding catheters.

To minimize failure of the stent delivery, we advocate the following precautions: (1) predilate lesions to ensure that the lesion is expandable and minimize the stenosis that the high-profile balloon-mounted stent must cross; (2) carefully select the target lesions so as to avoid angulated ($>90°$) segments; (3) ensure **optimal** guiding catheter position during balloon predilation; (4) use firm guidewires to provide a more solid "rail" over which to advance the stent; and (5) use non-PET delivery balloons to avoid scratching or tearing the balloon with the stent which can result in failure to deploy the stent.

The risk-to-benefit analysis of placing coronary stents for reducing restenosis remains to be determined in randomized trials. The risk of subacute thrombosis and bleeding complications is a significant concern when electively placing these devices in patients in whom the balloon angioplasty procedure was initially successful. The immediate benefit of stent placement in patients with failed angioplasty is more apparent, although a comparison with alternative strategies such as prolonged inflation with perfusion balloons and temporary stents is warranted.

Although the ability of a stent to salvage a failed angioplasty will be of great benefit, this indication will apply to only a minority of patients undergoing angioplasty. The larger potential application of stents lies in their ability to possibly reduce the incidence of restenosis, thereby sustaining vessel patency after percutaneous angioplasty. However, the placement of stents adds significantly to the cost and morbidity of an elective angioplasty procedure. The use of multiple balloons to predilate and deploy the stent, the cost of the stent itself, and the prolonged hospitalization necessary to ensure adequate anticoagulation contribute to this increased cost. The morbid events of subacute stent thrombosis and bleeding complications are more frequent than with angioplasty alone. We must ask ourselves, "What magnitude of reduction in the incidence of restenosis justifies these risks?" A randomized trial will be necessary to objectively assess the risk-to-benefit ratio of elective stenting to prevent restenosis.

REFERENCES

1. Dotter CT. Transluminally-placed coilspring endarterial tube grafts: long-term patency in canine popliteal artery. Invest Radiol 1969;4:329–332.
2. Slepian MJ, Schmidler A. Polymeric endoluminal paving/sealing: A bio-degradable alternative to intracoronary stenting (abstr). Circulation 1988;78(II):409A.
3. Kuntz RE, Safian RD, Carrozza JP, Fishman RF, Mansour M, Baim DS. The importance of acute luminal diameter in determining restenosis after coronary atherectomy or stenting. Circulation 1992;86:1827–1835.
4. Strauss BH, Serruys PW, de Scheerder IK, et al. Relative risk analysis of angiographic predictors of restenosis within the coronary Wallstent. Circulation 1991; 84:1636–1643.
5. Sawyer PN, Srinivasan S. Studies on the biophysics of intravascular thrombosis. Am J Surg 1967;114:42–60.
6. de Jaegere PP, Serruys PW, Bertrand M, et al. Wiktor stent implantation in patients with restenosis following balloon angioplasty of a native coronary artery. Am J Cardiol 1992;69:598–602.
7. Roubin GS, Cannon AD, Agrawal SK, et al. Intracoronary stenting for acute and threatened closure complicating percutaneous transluminal coronary angioplasty. Circulation 1992;85:916–927.
8. Ryan TJ, Faxon DP, Gunnar RM, et al. Guidelines for percutaneous transluminal coronary angioplasty: A report of the American College of Cardiology/American Heart Association Task Force on Assessment of Diagnostic and Therapeutic Cardiovascular Procedures (Subcommittee on Percutaneous Transluminal Coronary Angioplasty). J Am Coll Cardiol 1988;12:529–545.
9. Burger W, Sievert H, Steinmann J, et al. Acute and mid-term experiences with the Wiktor stent in acute complications and restenosis after coronary angioplasty. J Intervent Cardiol 1992;5:147–157.

10. Buchwald A, Unterberg C, Werner G, Voth E, Kreuzer H, Wiegand V. Initial clinical results with the Wiktor stent: A new balloon-expandable coronary stent. Clin Cardiol 1991;14:374–379.

11. Reeves F, Bonan R, Cote G, et al. Long-term angiographic follow-up after angioplasty of venous coronary bypass grafts. Am Heart J 1991;122:620–627.

12. Platko WP, Hollman J, Whitlow PL, Franco I. Percutaneous transluminal angioplasty of saphenous vein graft stenosis: Long-term follow-up. J Am Coll Cardiol 1989;14:1645–1650.

13. Reeder GS, Bresnahan JF, Holmes DR Jr, et al. Angioplasty for aortocoronary bypass graft stenosis. Mayo Clin Proc 1986;61:14–19.

14. Ernst SM, van der Feltz TA, Ascoop CA, et al. Percutaneous transluminal coronary angioplasty in patients with prior coronary artery bypass grafting: Long-term results. J Thorac Cardiovasc Surg 1987;93:268–275.

15. Kuntz RE, Safian RD, Levine MJ, Reis GJ, Diver DJ, Baim DS. Novel approach to the analysis of restenosis after the use of three new coronary devices. J Am Coll Cardiol 1992;19:1493–1499.

16. Fischman DL, Savage MP, Leon MB, et al. Effect of intracoronary stenting on intimal dissection after balloon angioplasty: Results of quantitative and qualitative coronary analysis. J Am Coll Cardiol 1991;18:1445–1451.

17. Leon MB, Ellis SG, Pichard AD, Baim DS, Heuser RR, Schatz RA. Stents may be the preferred treatment for focal aortocoronary vein graft disease (abstr). Circulation 1991;84:II-249.

18. Strumpf RK, Mehta SS, Ponder R, Heuser RR. Palmaz-Schatz stent implantation in stenosed saphenous vein grafts: Clinical and angiographic follow-up. Am Heart J 1992;123:1329–1336.

19. Freidrich SP, Davis SF, Kuntz RE, Carrozza JP, Baim DS. Investigational use of the Palmaz-Schatz biliary stent in large saphenous vein grafts. Am J Cardiol 1993;71:439–441.

8

Coronary Atherectomy: Directional, Rotational, and Extraction Catheters

Alaa E. Abdelmeguid
Brooklyn Veterans Affairs Medical Center, Brooklyn, New York

Patrick L. Whitlow
The Cleveland Clinic Foundation, Cleveland, Ohio

I. INTRODUCTION

Despite advanced technology, percutaneous transluminal coronary angioplasty (PTCA) continues to be plagued by the limitations of abrupt closure and restenosis. In addition, decreased success and increased complications are observed in the treatment of complex lesions (e.g., ulcerated, calcified, vein graft, long lesions, etc.). New modalities for plaque removal, ablation, and scaffolding have been developed to improve success, reduce residual stenosis, minimize dissection and abrupt closure, expand the treatment of lesions currently unfavorable for PTCA, and potentially reduce the incidence of restenosis.

In this chapter, the roles of directional, rotational, and extraction atherectomy devices will be examined. The discussion will focus on the indications for these new devices and the niches that each of them may fill in the field of interventional cardiology. A description of the device and its method of use will be only briefly mentioned, since this has been discussed elsewhere. Several technical approaches that have been found helpful in using these devices will be discussed.

II. DIRECTIONAL CORONARY ATHERECTOMY (DCA)

A. Methods

1. Description and Technique

Directional coronary atherectomy involves the selective excision and removal of obstructive atheromatous or abnormally proliferating lesions from the vessel wall. The directional coronary atherectomy catheter (Devices for Vascular Intervention, Inc., Redwood City, CA) (Fig. 1) consists of a metal housing with an affixed balloon and a flexible nose cone collection chamber at the distal end of a hollow rigid tube. Within the housing, there is a retractable cup-shaped cutter that is activated by an external hand-held motor driven unit connected by a torque cable.

After placing a routine PTCA guidewire distal to the target stenosis, the atherectomy catheter is advanced into the lesion and oriented so that the cutting window faces the bulk of the atheroma. The balloon is inflated to 5–10 psi, buttressing the housing in place and pushing the atheroma into the cutting window. When the cutter is retracted, the balloon pressure is increased to 10–80 psi. The motor driven unit is then activated, and a lever allows the operator to slowly advance the cutter through the lesion as it rotates at 2000 rpm. The balloon is then deflated, the catheter reoriented, and the procedure repeated until the desired result is achieved. The excised atheroma is stored in the distal nose cone, which is emptied at the end of the procedure or whenever it becomes full and prevents free movement of the guide-

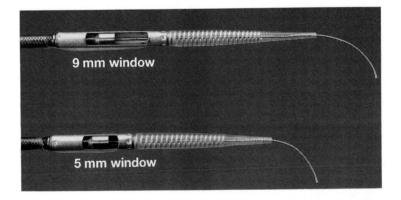

Figure 1   Directional atherectomy catheters: the SCA-EX Atherocath has a 9-mm cutting window, and the modified "short-cutter" can negotiate tortuosity with a tighter radius of curvature. (Courtesy of Devices for Vascular Intervention, Inc., Redwood City, CA.)

wire. Alternatively, an exchange length wire may be used and the device removed and emptied every 8–12 cuts. Appropriate sizing of the device, sufficient number of cuts, and adequate balloon inflation pressure are necessary for optimal tissue removal.

2. Technical Considerations

Guiding Catheters. The guide catheter is not as deeply seated as with PTCA to avoid guide-induced trauma or undue stress to the artery as the rigid Atherocath exits at an angle from the guide tip. It is important to ensure coaxial alignment of the atherectomy guide and the target artery under fluoroscopy. An 11-French guide can provide better support in the unusual circumstance when a 9.5- or 10-French guide fails to provide the necessary support. Typically, pulling back on the guide, turning clockwise (or occasionally counterclockwise) orients the guiding catheter and Atherocath shaft in the proper plance, and is much more successful than power positioning (1).

Guidewire. The guidewire should be positioned in the major target vessel distally avoiding entrapment of the wire in a side branch and eliminating the possibility of tip fracture if the wire should spin with the torque cable. The position of the wire should be checked before activation of the cutter, since retracting the cutter may cause proximal guidewire migration. If the guidewire is not freely mobile, the cutter should not be activated; instead, the entire system should be pulled out as a unit, the collection chamber cleared of atheroma, and the process repeated. We have found the ACS (Advanced Cardiovascular Systems, Santa Clara, CA) extrasupport guidewire, and the nitenol Microvena wire (Medtronic, Inc., Minneapolis, MN) to be particularly useful in providing support when advancing the Atherocath.

Atherocath. A final residual stenosis of 0–10% is the goal (2). This result is achieved by using an Atherocath that is one size larger than the original manufacturer's FDA approved guidelines for directional atherectomy (Table 1). We currently use a 6-French Atherocath for a 2.5- to 2.8-mm artery,

Table 1 Atherocath Sizing

Reference vessel segment (mm)	Size recommendation (F)	
	Manufacturer's	New
2.5–2.9	5	6
3.0–3.4	6	7-EX
3.25–3.4	6	7-Surlyn
3.5–3.9	7	7-Graft
≥4.0	7-Graft	7-Graft

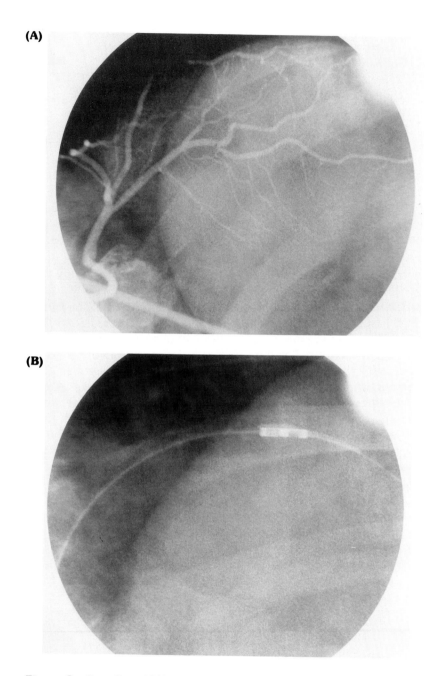

Figure 2 Complicated bifurcation lesion in the left anterior descending located in a major curve. (A) Preintervention arteriogram, RAO cranial view. (B) 7-French Short Cutter Atherocath across the lesion. (C) Postatherectomy result confirming minimal residual stenosis. (Courtesy of Charles A. Simonton, M.D., Charlotte, NC.)

(C)

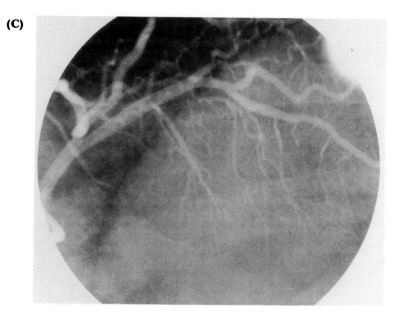

Figure 2 Continued

7-French EX device for a 2.8- to 3.2-mm vessel, a 7-French Surlyn device for 3.0- to 3.5-mm vessel, and 7-French graft device for vessels ≥3.5 mm. Higher inflation pressures (45–80 psi) usually yield more atheroma with the same size device after standard inflation pressures (10–45 psi) cease to yield tissue. The 5-French device is rarely used since atherectomy is seldom utilized in vessels <2.4 mm in diameter (*vide infra*). The modified EX device, while frequently easier to advance and cross the stenosis without nose cone trauma, extracts less tissue in large vessels than the original Surlyn device, which results in a smaller minimal luminal diameter. For this reason, Surlyn devices are almost always used in vessels ≥3.25 mm unless there is another lesion or major curve that raises concern for nose cone trauma to the distal artery. If a residual stenosis of ≥10% remains, the balloon inflation pressure is first increased to 30–40 psi and finally to 40–80 psi before upsizing the device. If ≥10% residual stenosis still exists, adjunctive PTCA or a larger Atherocath is used to optimize the angiographic result. The new short cutter device (with cutting window length of 6 mm, instead of the usual 10-mm length) sometimes allows passage to the target stenosis when proximal vessel tortuosity or calcification could prevent a normal length cutter from reaching the target (Fig. 2).

Adjunctive PTCA. Predilatation with conventional balloon angioplasty is performed only when difficulty in crossing the lesion is anticipated, or when the atherectomy catheter cannot be advanced across the stenosis. Both situations have been rare in our experience. Post-DCA angioplasty is performed if a significant stenosis remains after the atherectomy, with a target residual stenosis of 0–10% (2,3).

B. Clinical Outcome

1. Acute Results

The extent of luminal improvement after DCA appears to be due to a combination of Dotter effect, PTCA effect, and tissue removal (4). Compared to conventional balloon angioplasty, DCA results in a larger lumen with less incidence of dissection (5,6). Recent studies reviewing the procedural outcome of DCA have shown success and complication rates comparable to those associated with PTCA (7–10) (Table 2). The incidence of acute closure with DCA is comparable to that of PTCA (~ 4%), with most of these abrupt closures occurring in the lab (6). Similar to PTCA, directional atherectomy is very effective in treating focal, noncalcified lesions, but is less effective in treating lesions associated with diffuse disease, calcification, proximal vessel tortuosity, or degenerated saphenous vein grafts (SVG) (7,8). It should be noted, however, the DCA has been shown to be well suited for lesions with irregular complex contour which traditionally had a high complication rate when treated with PTCA (7) (vide infra), and in treating selected lesions that failed attempted PTCA (11). Side branch closure is unusual postatherectomy; however, if indicated, a side branch can be wired and protected by a nitenol Microvena wire (Medtronic, Inc., Minneapolis, MN) that cannot be cut by the Atherocath (12).

The Coronary Angioplasty Versus Excisional Atherectomy Trial (CAVEAT) was the first prospective randomized comparison of DCA versus PTCA. The recently published results showed that DCA has a higher success rate: 89% versus 80%, $p < 0.001$; at the expense of a higher rate of early complications: 11% versus 5%, $p < 0.001$ [death: 0% versus 0.4%; clinically detected myocardial infarction (MI): 6% versus 3%; emergency coronary artery bypass grafting (CABG): 3% versus 2%; abrupt closure 7% versus 3%] (10).

Table 2 Directional Atherectomy: Acute Procedural Results

	N	Success (%)	MI (%)	CABG (%)	Death (%)
Hinohara 1991 (8)	382	94	5.0	4.6	0.3
Ellis 1991 (7)	378	88	1.8	5.5	1.0
Fishman 1992 (9)	190	98	0.0	0.5	0.0
CAVEAT 1993 (10)	1012	89	6.0[a]	3.0	0.0

[a]Detected clinically by site.

2. Restenosis

Despite a better acute angiographic result compared with PTCA, the incidence of restenosis has only been mildly reduced by the use of DCA. The recently completed CAVEAT study demonstrated an acute luminal gain of 1.04 mm for DCA compared to 0.85 mm for PTCA ($p < 0.0001$). However, late loss was also more prominent in the DCA group (-0.54 mm vs -0.41 for PTCA; $p = 0.003$), resulting in a similar final net gain (0.47 mm for DCA vs 0.40 mm for PTCA; $p = 0.30$) (10).

Fishman et al. analyzed 225 atherectomies and reported an angiographic restenosis rate of 32% (9). They showed that a lower restenosis rate was associated with a postprocedure lumen diameter > 3 mm, a serum cholesterol level $\leqslant 200$ mg/dl, and recent myocardial infarction. Hinohara et al. showed that a higher restenosis rate was associated with DCA of saphenous vein grafts, hypertension, a long lesion ($\geqslant 10$ mm), a small vessel diameter (< 3 mm), a noncalcified lesion, and the use of a smaller device (6 F) (13).

The only restenosis data that directly compare DCA to PTCA came from the CAVEAT study and showed a 6-month angiographic restenosis rate of 50% for DCA versus 57% for PTCA ($p = 0.06$) (10). It is possible that the restenosis rate for DCA in CAVEAT could have been even more favorable if a more aggressive strategy including adjunctive PTCA had been utilized to obtain a more optimal postprocedure diameter (3).

When performing a DCA, the approach should be to strive for 0–10% residual stenosis (with or without adjunct PTCA). This rationale is based on a growing body of evidence that suggests that the best predictor of 6-month residual stenosis is the immediate postprocedural lumen diameter (9).

C. Specific Lesion Selection

1. Saphenous Vein Graft (SVG) Lesions

Acute success rates of directional atherectomy of nondegenerated SVGs are comparable to those with conventional angioplasty of native vessels ($> 90\%$) (14). The procedural success is similar to that for DCA in native coronary vessels. The recently completed CAVEAT II trial, which randomized 305 patients with de novo focal SVG stenoses to DCA or PTCA, found a low incidence of major procedural complications (death: 1.6% for DCA versus 1.5% for PTCA; Q-wave MI: 1.6% for DCA versus 1.5% for PTCA; CABG: 0% for DCA versus 1.5% for PTCA), and procedural success was more common for DCA (89%) than PTCA (79%). Target vessel revascularization by 6 months was improved for DCA compared to PTCA (24% versus 35%, $p < 0.05$) (15).

Notably, unlike PTCA, the age of saphenous vein graft, per se, does not appear to adversely affect the results of directional atherectomy. Pomerantz et al. reported a 93% success rate for directional atherectomy of SVGs in a group where 86% of the patients had SVGs that were > 3 years old (14). Abdelmeguid et al. found no difference in acute or short-term complication rates of DCA when comparing young (≤ 36 months old) versus old (> 36 months) SVGs (16). These results are in marked contrast with the significantly worse results of PTCA in >36-month SVGs (17). It is important to note, however, that severely degenerated SVGs are usually excluded from DCA series, and therefore these results cannot be extrapolated to degenerated SVGs with obvious friable grumous material.

As previously discussed, a high incidence of restenosis after atherectomy of SVGs (>50%) has been reported by Hinohara et al. (13). However, a more recent study in which the investigators attempted to obtain the largest possible acute lumen diameter showed a 26% restenosis rate, thus raising the possibility that the previously reported high restenosis rates in SVGs might have been related, in part, to suboptimal final procedural results (14). A 0–10% residual stenosis with DCA is the goal, regardless of the target vessel, in an attempt to reduce restenosis.

2. Proximal LAD

PTCA of the proximal LAD has been associated with a restenosis rate exceeding 50%. The recently completed CAVEAT trial has shown that DCA of the proximal LAD has a higher success rate (93% versus 85%) and a lower restenosis rate (42% versus 58%) compared with PTCA (10). However, the smaller cohort presented in the Canadian Coronary Atherectomy Trial (18) did not confirm these results. DCA has become the first choice at Cleveland Clinic in treating a discrete, de novo, less than heavily calcified stenosis of the proximal LAD in a vessel ≥3 mm in diameter.

3. Complex and Thrombus-Associated Lesions

Large thrombi are a contraindication for DCA. However, the presence of a small amount of clot with underlying complex, eccentric morphology does not adversely affect the results of DCA (6). Indeed, in this situation, the Atherocath is the device of choice in our practice. Ellis et al. reported on a subgroup of 30 patients with complex, probably thrombus-associated stenoses, who were treated with DCA, and found 100% success rate and 0% complication rate (7). Traditionally, these patients had a higher than usual risk of procedural complications when treated with PTCA (19,20). The relatively soft nature of the stenosis and the removal of the nidus from thrombus formation by the atherotome make such lesions particularly well suited for treatment with DCA.

The excision of complex, ulcerated plaque by DCA could theoretically improve the risk of intervention in patients with unstable angina to the level of those with stable angina. This hypothesis was tested in a recent study from the Cleveland Clinic (21). In that study, Abdelmeguid et al. studied 287 consecutive patients who underwent directional atherectomy for a single de novo stenosis (21). Seventy-seven patients had stable angina (group I), 110 patients had progressively worsening angina in the absence of rest or postinfarction angina (group II), and 100 patients had rest and/or post-infarction angina (group III). The results of the study showed that major ischemic complications (death, Q-wave infarction, emergency bypass surgery) occurred more frequently in group III (7% versus 1.3% for group I and 0.9% for group II; $p = 0.03$). There was no difference in death or Q-wave infarction among the three groups, but emergency surgery was more frequent in group III (5% versus 1.3% for group I and 0% for group II; $p = 0.05$). Clinical follow-up was obtained in 98.5% of successful procedures for a mean follow-up period of 22 months (range 9–52 months) and revealed a higher incidence of hospitalization for angina in group III ($p = 0.05$), and a trend toward more bypass surgery and myocardial infarction in the same group ($p = 0.09$ and 0.16, respectively). There was no difference in repeat percutaneous interventions among the three groups (19–24%, $p = 0.75$).

These results show that, like angioplasty, the definition of unstable angina is important in determining the acute outcome of directional atherectomy. In the absence of rest or post-MI angina, the acute results of DCA in patients with progressive angina are not significantly different from those obtained in stable angina. The results also suggest that both the acute and short-term outcome in unstable angina are not greatly affected by atherectomy, but more so by the pathophysiology of unstable angina itself, which imparts a worse outcome with atherectomy (or angioplasty) than the same intervention with stable angina. Therefore, in the setting of rest or post-MI angina, especially in the presence of intracoronary thrombus or complex morphology, it is felt that the atherectomy procedure should be postponed whenever possible, and that the patient should be anticoagulated in an attempt to "cool off" the unstable plaque. However, in many instances this is not clinically feasible, and the ischemic time during the procedure should be minimized using more frequent but brief device insertions. Meticulous attention should be paid to systemic anticoagulation, and the ACT should not be allowed to drop below 350 s throughout the DCA procedure. The patient is kept on heparin overnight after a successful procedure in the setting of unstable angina. New antiplatelet drugs (e.g., 7E3) and specific thrombin inhibitors (e.g., Hirudin) may improve the results of DCA in this setting, and their role is under investigation.

4. Bifurcation Lesions

The major limitation of PTCA in bifurcation lesions is side branch occlusion. The incidence of this complication increases from 1% for type I bifurcation lesions (where a normal branch vessel originates near the lesion of the parent vessel), to 4% for type II bifurcation lesions (where the side branch has no or minimal disease, but originates from the stenosis of the parent vessel), to 13–34% for type III lesions (where the parent vessel and side branch are involved in a single severe stenosis) (22). The most common etiology of side branch occlusion with PTCA is the "snow plow" effect resulting from shifting plaque during balloon inflation in the parent vessel. Side branch occlusion may also occur by extension of balloon-induced dissections of the parent vessel.

In contrast to PTCA, the mechanism of DCA involves tissue removal, which reduces the incidence of shifting plaques as well as dissection, and may potentially improve the results of percutaneous revascularization of bifurcation lesions.

The technical approach to DCA of bifurcation lesions is different from that of PTCA (22). The stenosis of the parent vessel is crossed first with the guidewire, followed by atherectomy. Then the guidewire is redirected across the stenosis in the side branch to allow PTCA or DCA of the side branch. Because of the potential for guidewire entrapment or fracture, it is our approach at the Cleveland Clinic to treat the parent vessel and the branch sequentially. The modified kissing atherectomy approach, described by Leya et al. in one patient using two Nitinol wires to protect the side branch during atherectomy, needs to be substantiated in further studies, since the risk and safety of the Nitinol double-wire technique remain unclear, and especially that branch protection during DCA is generally unnecessary because branches can almost always be cannulated from within the smooth lumen of the atherectomized parent vessel (12).

The CAVEAT investigators have recently reported their results comparing DCA versus PTCA for the treatment of bifurcation lesions (23). Lesions treated with DCA had a higher postprocedural diameter: 1.9 versus 1.6 mm, $p = 0.001$ and a higher angiographic success rate: 88% versus 74%, $p = 0.001$. However, this occurred at the expense of a higher incidence of acute ischemic complications (death, MI, and CABG): 9.5% versus 3.7%, $p = 0.006$). At 6 months follow-up, the minimal luminal diameter was higher: 1.4 versus 1.1 mm, $p = 0.001$, and the restenosis rate lower: 50% versus 61%, $p = 0.02$, for DCA-treated lesions.

Side branch occlusion occurs in 3–4% of bifurcation lesions treated with DCA (9). Important predictors of side branch occlusion after DCA include ostial branch stenosis >50% and the presence of dissection, and they can be managed by PTCA or DCA (24).

In summary, bifurcation lesions in vessels >2.5 mm in diameter seem to be well suited for DCA using conventional 6- or 7-French devices. However, significant calcification within or near a bifurcation remains a strong predictor of procedural failure due to inability to cross the lesion with the Atherocath. Improvement in the design of the Atherocath (e.g., short cutter devices) may ultimately expand its use for bifurcation lesions.

5. Rescue Atherectomy for Failed PTCA

DCA has been proposed as a rescue technique for failed or suboptimal PTCA in an attempt to avoid myocardial infarction, or emergency bypass surgery. McCluskey et al. from the Cleveland Clinic recently reported the largest series of patients treated with rescue DCA for failed PTCA (100 patients with 103 treated lesions) (11). The etiology of failed PTCA in that study was primarily from dissections (50.5%), recoil (41.8%), and recurrent thrombosis in 7.8%. Complete vessel closure was present in 22.3% of the lesions. The average percent stenosis was 79% before PTCA, 56% after PTCA, and 24% after rescue DCA. Rescue DCA was successful in 94 of 103 lesions (91.3%). In the subgroup of patients with failed PTCA (TIMI grade 0–2 flow or acute closure after PTCA), TIMI grade 3 flow was restored in 30 of 33 patients (90.9%). Complications included 1 perforation, 2 deaths within 24 h, and 6 patients requiring bypass surgery.

The technique of rescue atherectomy allows rapid reestablishment of flow in acutely closed vessels or vessels with unstable morphology. However, to avoid perforation, care needs to be taken by using appropriately sized devices at low inflation pressures. Moreover, long spiral dissections are not appropriate for salvage DCA.

Prospective randomized trials will be required to determine the ultimate utility and cost effectiveness of rescue atherectomy compared to other methods such as perfusion balloons, permanent and temporary stents. Until these studies are completed, however, rescue DCA appears to be a safe and effective technique for treating potentially unstable and serious complications of failed PTCA (11).

6. Ostial Lesions

PTCA of ostial lesions has been traditionally associated with a lower success rate, a higher complication rate, and a higher restenosis rate (25). Theoretically, DCA may be useful in limiting the elastic recoil associated with these lesions. However, adequate backup has been a problem with aorto-ostial lesions, and has resulted in low success rates in this subset of ostial stenoses. Rotational atherectomy may be better suited for such lesions (especially in the presence of calcification) because the Rotablator device does not require substantial guide backup, thus making the procedure less technically challenging. However, non-aorto-ostial bifurcation lesions are well suited for DCA with high success and low residual stenosis (22).

7. Restenotic Lesions

Recent evidence shows that the incidence of restenosis after DCA is higher for restenotic lesions compared with de novo lesions (13). Hinohara et al.

Table 3 Directional Coronary Atherectomy

Indications
  Stenosis in proximal or midsegments of large-size vessel in
    the absence of contraindications /
  Saphenous vein graft lesions
  Bifurcation lesions
  Lesions failing angioplasty

Contraindications
  Large thrombi
  Excessive proximal tortuosity
  Diffuse disease (>20 mm)
  Small vessel (<2.5 mm)
  Degenerated SVGs
  Moderate to heavy calcification
  Extensive or spiral dissections

reported a restenosis rate in native coronary arteries of 31% for primary lesions, and 28% and 49% for lesions treated with one and two previous angioplasty procedures (13). The restenosis rate for saphenous vein grafts was 53% for primary lesions, and 58% and 82% for lesions treated with one and two previous angioplasty procedures. For these reasons, DCA is avoided in lesions that have restenosed more than once, unless it is felt that the final minimal luminal diameter achieved can be improved by DCA compared to previous procedures and other techniques. Table 3 summarizes our current indications and contraindications for directional atherectomy.

III. ROTATIONAL ATHERECTOMY

A.   Methods

1.   Description and Technique

The Rotablator® consists of an elliptically shaped brass burr coated with 5- to 10-μm diamond chips bonded to a flexible drive shaft (Fig. 3). The drive shaft and the burr rotate at 150,000 to 200,000 rpm as they are advanced over an 0.009-in. stainless steel guidewire. After wiring the stenosis, the Rotablator® is tracked just proximal to the lesion and subsequently activated. The operator uses a control knob to slowly advance the rotating burr over the guidewire and through the lesion, resulting in micro abrasion of the obstructing atheroma. If adjunctive intervention is required, which is frequently the case, the Rotablator® can be exchanged over the guidewire for a larger burr or another definitive device (usually a PTCA or DCA catheter).

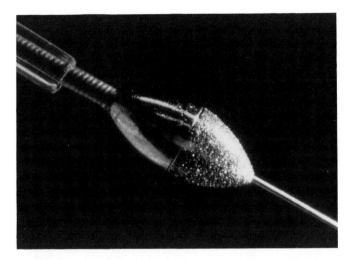

Figure 3 Magnified view of the Rotablator® burr, sheath, and drive shaft over an 0.009-in. guidewire. (Courtesy of Heart Technology, Redmond, WA.)

Because of its high rotational speed, the Rotablator® preferentially ablates inelastic, noncompliant, atheromatous tissue. Plaque-free wall segments are spared from mechanical trauma because their viscoelastic properties make them deflect around the rotating burr. Intravascular ultrasound has provided insight into the mechanism of action of the Rotablator® (26). After rotablation atherectomy, the intima–lumen interface was unusually distinct and circular (Fig. 4). Intravascular ultrasound also showed an increase in lumen size, a decrease in plaque-plus-media area, and in the arc of target lesion calcification, and no change in target lesion external elastic membrane cross-sectional area.

2. Technical Considerations

Temporary Pacing. Transient bradyarrhythmias and heart block are not uncommon with the Rotablator® and may be related to transient ischemia of the atrioventricular node caused by increased viscosity in the microcirculation secondary to micro particles generated during the procedure, micro cavitation resulting from the high-speed rotation or vibration of the guidewire (27). Bradyarrhythmias are especially common with rotablation of the RCA, but they can occur during rotablation of the circumflex or the LAD. A temporary pacemaker is inserted when performing rotablation of the RCA, a dominant circumflex, or when rotablating the LAD or circumflex if the RCA is occluded and receives collateral blood flow from the left coronary system.

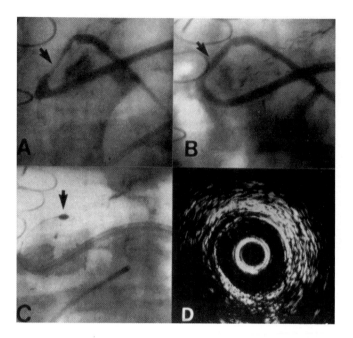

Figure 4 The Robablator. (A) Angiogram of a patient with a long saphenous vein graft lesion (black arrow) that failed PTCA with balloon pressures up to 20 atm. (B) Angiogram after Rotablator procedure with up to a 2.5-mm burr. (C) Rotablator burr passing through the lesion. (D) Intravascular ultrasound image of the final lumen after Rotablator and adjunctive PTCA (3.5-mm balloon). Note round, sharp edge of the lumen–intima interface and the absence of intimal fracture. (Courtesy Ref. 26.)

Systemic vasodilation is common during and just after each Rotablator® run, especially in right coronary artery procedures. Special attention to adequate fluid administration prior to Rotablator® runs (pulmonary wedge pressure of 15–20 mm Hg) minimizes hypotension. Venous filling pressure is extremely important when spasm occurs with the Rotablator® pass, because while spasm may be relieved with nitrates or verapamil administration, these agents exacerbate systemic vasodilatation and hypotension. Alpha-adrenergic agents should be readily available and liberally used if hypotension, not responsive to fluid challenge, persists.

Guiding Catheters.   The diameter of the guiding catheter is dictated by the size of the burr used; 8-French guides can accommodate burrs with diameters up to 1.75 mm; 9-French guides accommodate burrs with diameters up to 2.25 mm. Burrs of 2.5 mm currently require a 10-French guide. All customary guide catheter shapes can be utilized with the Rotablator®.

Guidewire. The 0.009-in. Rotablator® guidewire is not as maneuverable as usual PTCA wires and may be difficult to position across a tight stenosis in a tortuous vessel. The type C Rotablator wire is extremely flexible and safe, but not as easily steered as the stiffer type A wire. If a Rotablator wire cannot be positioned distally across a stenosis, a traditional PTCA wire [bare wire or preloaded into a flexible sheath (Probing Sheath, USCI, Billerica, MA; or Tracker catheter, Target Therapeutics, Fremont, CA)] is steered into position. The 0.009-in. Rotablator wire will frequently track along the path of the PTCA guidewire, and the extra wire may be removed. Alternatively, a sheath may be tracked over the wire beyond the lesion, and the PTCA wire exchanged for the noncoated Rotablator wire.

Rotablator Burrs/Adjunctive PTCA. Burr diameters vary from 1.25–2.5 mm for coronary arteries. In diffusely diseased vessels or in vessels with moderate lesion length (7–20 mm) or severe stenoses (i.e., stenoses with large plaque burden compared to the size of the run-off bed), a small burr size (i.e., 1.5 or 1.75 mm) is used and gradually upsized in an attempt to minimize the load of micro particle embolization during burr passage. Passing the burr slowly with only minimal forward pressure against the stenosis, in runs ≤45 s may reduce slow flow and spasm. Intracoronary and systemic nitroglycerin as well as 30–50 cc saline flushes after each Rotablator run may also help minimize ischemia. The rotablation procedure is currently stopped at a burr/artery ratio of ~ 0.80 or when a residual stenosis of <20% is achieved. The largest, safest residual lumen is frequently obtained with adjunctive PTCA. A trial is planned to determine whether attempting to achieve the largest safest residual lumen with rotablation (Rotablator alone) or to utilize the Rotablator® followed by adjunctive PTCA is the best strategy to minimize restenosis, presumably by decreasing the residual plaque burden without deeply injuring the arterial wall (*vide infra*). The burr is gradually upsized (in 0.25- to 0.5-mm increments) without skipping to the final burr size early in the procedure in de novo lesions longer than 5 mm. Using a single large burr as proposed by Zacca et al. may cause more complications in de novo stenoses, though this strategy works well with restenotic lesions (28). The sequential utilization of smaller to larger burrs decreases plaque burden over time and may lower the risk of dissection, micro embolism, and slow flow. Indeed, when Stertzer et al. analyzed 23 lesions in which there was either a severe dissection, occlusion, or perforation, they showed that in 61% of these cases, burr sizes were skipped and that in 26% of these cases a relatively large burr was used as the first device (29). The device is continuously rotated during advancement of the burr, and the speed is not allowed to drop below 90% of the free-running speed, which is an indication of excessive load being placed on the burr due to rapid advancement. Rotablation is stopped if a dissection has been identified to avoid its extension. If slow flow is observed, intracoronary nitroglycerin or verapamil are utilized to normalize flow prior to each Rotablator® pass. If slow flow or severe spasm persist, then PTCA generally restores normal flow quickly.

B. Clinical Outcome

1. Acute Results

In reviewing the results of rotational atherectomy, it should be noted that most Rotablator® patients have complex morphology (Type B_2 or C lesions) that is known to convey an adverse effect on the results of PTCA. Despite that, the angiographic success, complication profile, and restenosis associated with rotational atherectomy appear to compare favorably with PTCA (Table 4) (29–32). Whitlow et al. reported on 874 lesions in 745 patients treated with the Rotablator and found that lesion calcification, eccentricity, lesion length > 10 mm, and vessel tortuosity did not have an adverse effect on angiographic success (33). Moreover, unlike PTCA, cumulative effects of angiographic risk factors on success were not apparent; in fact, type A, B_1, B_2, and C lesions had comparable angiographic success rates (97%, 94%, 95%, and 95%, respectively). However, major complications (i.e., death, MI, and bypass surgery) were increased with more complex lesion morphology: 0% for type A lesions, 7% for type B_1, 8% for type B_2, and 15% for type C lesions. Popma et al. found that angulation $\geqslant 45°$ was the only risk factor for procedural failure (i.e., angiographic failure or death or Q-wave MI or emergency CABG) ($p < 0.005$; odds ratio 3.67) and that minor complications (recurrent ischemia, abrupt closure, repeat PTCA) were related to proximal tortuosity ($p < 0.05$; odds ratio 3.36), bifurcation lesions ($p < 0.05$; odds 2.31), and de novo lesions ($p < 0.001$; odds ratio 5.68) (34). Whitlow et al. analyzed 1153 patients who underwent rotational ablation, and showed that bifurcation lesions carry an increased risk of side branch compromise (1.5% versus 0.3%; $p = 0.06$) and acute occlusion (6.2% versus 2.8%; $p = 0.009$) (35). There was also a trend toward more major complications (death, Q-wave MI, E-CABG) in bifurcation lesions (4.8% versus 2.9%; $p = 0.15$). Cowley et al. also

Table 4 Rotational Atherectomy: Acute Results

	N	Success (%)	Q-wave MI (%)	non-Q-wave MI (%)	CABG (%)	Death (%)
Buchbinder 1991 (30)	745	94	0.8	4.6	1.4	0.0
Bertrand 1992 (32)	129	86	2.3	5.5	1.6	0.0
Stertzer 1993 (29)	302	95	3.3	11.0	1.2	0.0
Cowley 1993 (31)	1362	95	0.9	4.6	2.1	0.8

MI = myocardial infarction; CABG = coronary artery bypass grafting.

showed that bifurcation lesions are associated with a higher rate of Q-wave MI (2.2 versus 0.6%; $p < 0.05$). On the other hand, the overall angiographic success rate was not significantly different compared with lesions that were not at a bifurcation point (31).

2. Restenosis

Popma et al. studied restenosis after rotational atherectomy in 210 patients, and showed that symptoms recurred in 46% of patients (36). Angiographic restenosis ($>50\%$ stenosis) was present in 52% of lesions with angiographic follow up. Interestingly, this study showed that restenosis is related to the magnitude of lesion stretch and recoil during the procedure; thus raising the possibility that obtaining the largest, safest diameter by decreasing the plaque burden through albation alone and with minimal stretch induced by PTCA may decrease restenosis. This hypothesis will be tested in a trial designed to study the safety and efficacy of achieving the largest residual lumen possible through rotablation alone on restenosis.

C. Specific Lesion Selection

1. Calcified Lesions

Lesion calcification does not appear to adversely affect the procedural success rates of rotational atherectomy: 82% versus 86% for Rotablator® alone and 95% versus 95% for Rotablator® with adjunctive PTCA (i.e., calcified versus noncalcified, respectively) (37). Major complications (i.e., death, emergency CABG, and Q-wave MI) are also similar for calcified compared with noncalcified lesions. Moreover, the degree of calcification itself does not seem to affect the success or complication rates (38). The Rotablator® is the device of choice in heavily calcified lesions at the Cleveland Clinic.

2. Ostial Lesions

These lesions are associated with a low success rate and a high complication rate when treated with PTCA. Rotational atherectomy appears to improve the results of revascularization of these lesions. Goudreau et al. reported a 97% success rate, with no major ischemic complications in 31 aortoostial and branch ostial lesions (39). Ostial lesions, especially calcified ostial lesions, are solid niches for rotational atherectomy, and the Rotablator® is currently used as a treatment of choice for ostial disease.

3. Diffuse Disease

Diffuse coronary artery disease appears to carry an adverse effect on the results of the Rotablator® (33,40). Whitelow et al. reported on 874 lesions treated with the Rotablator® and found that while the procedural success rate was similar for stenoses < 10 mm in length compared with lesions between 10 to 25 mm in length (95% versus 94%, respectively), the acute major complications (3.6% versus 6.0%, respectively) and the restenosis rates (36% versus 45%, respectively) were higher in patients with diffuse disease (38). In a much smaller population (42 patients) that underwent stand-alone rotablation, Tierstein et al. also found higher complication and restenosis rates with diffuse disease (40). Reisman et al. evaluated the use of rotational atherectomy in the treatment of long lesions (15–25 mm) and found that despite the high initial procedural success rate (92%), these lesions carry a higher rate of Q-wave MI (2.8%) when compared to shorter lesions (41). There was also a statistically nonsignificant trend toward higher procedural complications and restenosis in patients with long lesions. Rotational atherectomy may not improve results in noncalcified stenoses ≥ 25 mm in length, but may still offer a reasonable approach in calcified arteries with long lesions where PTCA results are expected to be suboptimal.

4. Undilatable Lesions

The Rotablator® has been used successfully to treat lesions that failed PTCA. These "undilatable" lesions include lesions that failed to dilate with conventional balloon angioplasty, lesions that could not be crossed with the balloon, and lesions with immediate elastic recoil despite adequate balloon expansion. In a series of 41 such patients, the overall angiographic success rate was impressive: 98% with a final residual stenosis of 25 ± 17%. Acute complications occurred in three patients with a procedural success rate of 90%

Table 5 Rotational Atherectomy

Indications
Ostial stenosis
Calcified lesions
Elastic lesions
Undilatable lesions
Restenotic lesions
Contraindications
Thrombus-containing lesions
Degenerated SVGs
Diffuse disease with large plaque load and limited
distal runoff
Angulation ≥45°[a]
Branch point disease[a]

[a]Relative contraindication.

(42). The Rotablator® or the Excimer laser are our primary choices for such lesions.

Table 5 shows our indications and contraindications for rotational atherectomy.

IV. TRANSLUMINAL EXTRACTION CATHETER (TEC) ATHERECTOMY

A. Methods

1. Description and Technique

The Transluminal Extraction Atherectomy device (Interventional Technologies, Inc., San Diego, CA) consists of two stainless steel blades at the distal end of a rotating hollow flexible tube (Fig. 5). A pressurized flush solution is infused into the guide catheter and around the activated TEC device. When activated, the device functions as a cutting and aspiration system, removing the occluding atherothrombotic plaque inside the blood vessel to an attached vacuum bottle.

During the procedure, a special exchange length guidewire (0.014-in.) with an enlarged olive tip is positioned beyond the stenosis, and the TEC cutter is advanced just proximal to the lesion. With the cutter and vacuum system activated, the rotating cutter (750 rpm) is slowly advanced over the guidewire through the lesion. Several passes are performed until there is little or no re-

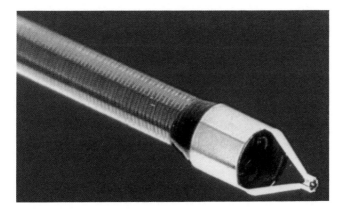

Figure 5 The TEC catheter: Front cutting blades with wide aspiration channel to effectively remove atherosclerotic debris. (Courtesy of InterVentional Technologies, Inc., San Diego, CA.)

sistance. If further intervention is required, the TEC device can be exchanged for a larger cutter or another definitive device (PTCA or DCA catheter).

2. Technical Considerations

Cutter Size. The TEC device is available in 5.5- to 7.5-French sizes. In severely stenotic segments, the smaller cutter (5.5- to 6-French) is begun and gradually upsized until reaching a cutter that is approximately 1 mm smaller than the distal vessel. The same gradual approach is used also when dealing with diffuse disease to attempt to achieve a <20% final residual stenosis, with adjunctive PTCA or DCA in vessels ≥3.0 mm.

Guiding Catheter. We usually perform TEC using the specially designed 10-French tungsten wire-braided, TEC guiding catheter. This relatively large guide provides good support, good opacification, and adequate flushing during cutting.

Guidewire. The TEC guidewire has a stiff shaft and, similar to the Rotablator® guidewire, lacks excellent steerability, and may pose some difficulties when attempting to cross a tight stenosis in tortuous vessels. If this occurs, we preload a traditional 0.014-in. wire into a flexible sheath (Probing Sheath, USCI or Tracker catheter, Target Therapeutics) and steer it into position. The sheath is then tracked over the wire beyond the lesion, and the 0.014-in. wire exchanged for the specialized TEC wire.

B. Clinical Outcome

Unlike standard balloon angioplasty, which improves coronary dimensions by splitting and tearing the obstructive atheroma, TEC exerts its beneficial effect on coronary stenoses by excising the atherosclerotic plaque and extracting the debris by continuous vacuum suction, thus avoiding the potential risks of vascular barotrauma and distal particulate embolization. This technique has potential applications in lesions within saphenous vein grafts, lesions with thrombus, or lesions with marked luminal irregularities. To date, over 2000 TEC atherectomies have been performed in native coronaries and in saphenous vein grafts with procedural success rates exceeding 90% (43).

1. Specific Lesion Selection

Saphenous Vein Grafts. The TEC device has been used in 1114 graft lesions reported in the most recent Coronary TEC Data Registry (43). Success (defined as lesions treated with TEC alone or TEC with adjunctive PTCA, without major complications, with a final stenosis ≤50% and ≥20% improvement from pretreatment) was 89.9% (1001 of 1114 patients). Major complications occurred in 4.8% and minor complications in 28.6% of the cases. However, when the groups were subdivided according to the associated

Table 6 Extraction Atherectomy of Saphenous Vein Graft Stenoses: Results of the 1993 Coronary TEC Registry (43)

Graft lesions	N	Success	Complications	
			Major	Minor
All	1114	89.9%	4.8%	28.6%
Focal, no thrombus	325	94.8%	1.8%	20.9%
Thrombus present	462	87.9%	7.1%	37.7%
Diffuse disease, with thrombus	198	87.9%	6.0%	36.9%

morphological characteristics, it was obvious that the best results are obtained in SVG with discrete lesions and no thrombus (Table 6).

However, on many occasions diseased grafts are degenerated and contain thrombus or other grumous material. It was hoped that the TEC would find a niche in treating this high-risk subgroup of patients. Indeed, TEC has been proposed as a treatment of choice for diseased, degenerated, saphenous vein grafts since its cutting-aspirating technique is thought to be particularly well suited for the treatment of saphenous graft stenosis. However, recent studies indicate that the TEC procedure performed on old, degenerated SVGs that contain thrombus is associated with lower success and higher complication rates than TEC in discrete lesions. Abdelmeguid et al. analyzed 104 lesions in SVGs treated with TEC and compared the results of the procedure in old (>36 months) versus young (≤ 36 months) grafts (44). They found that old SVGs were associated with a lower success rate (86% vs 93%) and a higher residual stenosis (24% vs 12%; $p < 0.05$). There were no major acute ischemic complications in the young SVG group, while the group with old SVGs showed an 8% incidence of death, 1% E-CABG, and 1% Q-wave MI. Follow-up at 6 months revealed a 14% combined incidence of death, MI, and CABG for the old SVG group versus 0% for the group with young SVGs. Hong et al. studied 76 lesions in SVGs treated with TEC, and found that distal embolization occurred in 14% of the patients (45). The group with distal embolization had a 90% incidence of angiographic thrombus versus 33% incidence of thrombus for the group without distal embolization ($p < 0.001$). Embolization was associated with a 50% procedural success (vs 95% in the absence of embolization; $p < 0.001$), a 33% incidence of MI, and a 33% incidence of death (vs 0% and 2%, respectively, for the group without embolization). It was interesting to note that the majority of cases of distal embolization occurred after adjunctive balloon angioplasty, although embolization did occur occasionally after stand-alone TEC. These studies raise some concern about the effectiveness and safety of TEC (or any other device) in old SVGs, especially in the presence of angiographic thrombus and diffuse disease.

These significant complication rates have led to utilization of the TEC in older, degenerated SVGs with unfavorable morphology only in patients who fail medical therapy and who are poor reoperative candidates. Instead, a period of prolonged heparinization or graft thrombolysis may be preferred, with the possible use of new antithrombotic agents (Hirudin) or new antiplatelet agents (7E3), followed by TEC, DCA, or stenting after resolution of the thrombus angiographically. It is possible, though yet untested, that the use of potent antithrombotic or antiplatelet agents before TEC might decrease the complication rate. It is also possible that DCA or stenting after TEC might have a better result compared to adjunctive balloon angioplasty. Obviously, this is an area of great controversy, and advances in interventional cardiology have yet to provide a safe, definitive answer for this high-risk group with degenerated vein graft disease.

Acute Ischemic Syndromes. Kramer et al. reported on 53 patients (62 lesions) with acute coronary syndromes (acute MI, post-MI angina, unstable angina) that underwent TEC atherectomy (46). Over half of these patients had angiographic evidence of thrombus. The overall success was >90%, with two patients undergoing E-CABG and two patients suffering from myocardial infarction. The presence of angiographic thrombus did not seem to have any adverse effect in this study. Clearly, more studies are needed to establish the role of the TEC device in acute ischemic syndromes.

Unfavorable Balloon Lesions. Popma et al. reported on 51 patients with complex lesion morphology undergoing TEC atherectomy and demonstrated a procedural success (angiographic success in the absence of major complications) in 82% of the patients (47). Only lesion-associated thrombus correlated with an unsuccessful outcome. Leon et al. reported on 281 patients who underwent TEC for unfavorable coronary lesions (i.e., diffuse disease,

Table 7 Extraction Atherectomy

Indications
    Thrombus-containing lesions
    Focal saphenous vein graft lesions
    Medically refractory degenerated saphenous grafts
        in poor operative candidates

Contraindications
    Heavily calcified lesions
    Severely angled stenoses
    Small vessels
    Bifurcation lesions
    Dissections

ostial disease, eccentric stenoses, recent MI) with a success rate of >90% achieved for all subsets (48). Complication rates were independent of lesion length, recent MI, but were slightly higher in eccentric lesions (7%). Restenosis rates were similar to standard PTCA, but were unaffected by complex lesion morphology. However, in another study addressing specifically the incidence of restenosis after TEC, Sutton et al. showed that restenosis after TEC is predicted by lesion complexity or ulceration and calcification. Obviously, more studies are needed to better describe the restenosis profile after TEC (49).

Table 7 outlines the current indications and contraindications for extraction atherectomy.

V. CONCLUSIONS

In the past decade, PTCA has been applied to increasingly complex clinical and anatomical situations with simultaneous improvement in success rates and complication rates. However, the incidence of restenosis and abrupt closure, the most common adverse events, has remained relatively high, especially with more complex patient/lesion subsets. It is theoretically possible that these adverse events could be minimized using atherectomy devices that work by fundamentally different techniques. In addition to compressing and reshaping the atheroma, they debulk the plaque. Recent data reviewed in this chapter suggest that atherectomy devices will likely provide more effective treatment in some patient/lesion subsets and extend the indications of percutaneous revascularization in others (Table 8).

The evolution of coronary devices and the strategies optimizing their use will continue over the next few years. Their role will ultimately be determined by the results of randomized trials to establish their merits compared to PTCA, which remains the gold standard at the present time.

Table 8 Morphological Lesion Subsets That Are Likely To Benefit from Atherectomy

Morphology	Atherectomy device	
Proximal LAD	DCA	
Proximal, eccentric stenosis in large vessel	DCA	
Nondegenerated vein grafts	DCA	
Failed PTCA lesion (selected cases)	DCA	my
Moderate to heavy calcification	Rotational atherectomy	
Ostial	Rotational atherectomy, DCA	
Complex lesions (B_2/C)	Rotational atherectomy	
Undilatable lesions	Rotational atherectomy	
Discrete vein graft lesions	DCA, TEC	
Degenerated vein grafts	TEC	

REFERENCES

1. Whitlow PL. Guiding catheters for directional coronary atherectomy. Cathet Cardiovasc Diagn 1993(suppl 1):72–75.
2. Baim DS, Kuntz RE. Directional coronary atherectomy: how much lumen enlargement is optimal? Am J Cardiol 1993;72:65E–70E.
3. Gordon PC, Kugelmass AD, Cohen DJ, Breall JA, Friedrich SP, Carrozza JP, Diver DJ, Kuntz RE, Baim DS. Balloon postdilation can safely improve the results of successful (but suboptimal) directional coronary atherectomy. Am J Cardiol 1993;72:71E–79E.
4. Penny WF, Schmidt DA, Safian RD, et al. Insights into the mechanism of luminal improvement after directional coronary atherectomy. Am J Cardiol 1991; 67:435–437.
5. Umans VA, Strauss BH, Rensing BJ, et al. Comparative angiographic quantitative analysis of the immediate efficacy of coronary atherectomy with balloon angioplasty, stenting, and rotational ablation. Am Heart J 1991;3:836–843.
6. Popma JJ, Topol EJ, Hinohara T, Pinkerton CA, Baim DS, King SB, Holmes DR, Whitlow PL, Kereiakes DJ, Hartzler GO, Kent KM, Ellis SG, Simpson JB. Abrupt vessel closure after directional coronary atherectomy. J Am Coll Cardiol 1992;19:1372–1379.
7. Ellis SG, De Cesare NB, Pinkerton CA, Whitlow P, King SB, Ghazzal ZMB, Kereiakes DJ, Popma JJ, Menke KK, Topol EJ, Holmes DR. Relation of stenosis morphology and clinical presentation to the procedural results of directional coronary atherectomy. Circulation 1991;84:644–653.
8. Hinohara T, Rowe MH, Robertson GC, et al. Effect of lesion characteristics on outcome of directional coronary atherectomy. J Am Coll Cardiol 1991;17:1112–1120.
9. Fishman RF, Kuntz RE, Carrozza JP, Miller MJ, Senerchia CC, Schnitt SJ, Diver DJ, Safian RD, Baim DS. Long-term results of directional coronary atherectomy: Predictors of restenosis. J Am Coll Cardiol 1992;20:1101–1110.
10. Topol EJ, Leya F, Pinkerton CA, Whitlow PL, et al. A comparison of directional atherectomy with coronary angioplasty in patients with coronary artery disease. N Engl J Med 1993;329:221–227.
11. McCluskey ER, Cowley M, Whitlow PL. Multicenter clinical experience with rescue atherectomy for failed angioplasty. Am J Cardiol 1993;72:42E–46E.
12. Leya FS, Lewis BE, Sumida CW, et al. Modified kissing atherectomy procedure with dependable protection of side branches by two-wire technique. Cathet Cardiovasc Diag 1992;27:155–161.
13. Hinohara T, Robertson GC, Selmon MR, Vetter JW, Rowe MH, Braden LJ, McAuley BJ, Sheehan DJ, Simpson JB. Restenosis after directional atherectomy. J Am Coll Cardiol 1992;20:623–632.
14. Pomerantz RM, Kuntz RE, Carrozza JP, et al. Acute and long-term outcome of narrowed saphenous venous grafts treated by endoluminal stenting and directional atherectomy. Am J Cardiol 1992;70:161–167.
15. The CAVEAT II Investigators, North America and Europe. The Coronary Angioplasty versus Excisional Atherectomy Trial (CAVEAT II): Preliminary Results (abstr). Circulation 1993;88:I-594.

16. Abdelmeguid AE, Ellis SG, Whitlow PL, et al. Lack of graft age dependency for success of directional coronary atherectomy and Palmaz-Schatz stenting (abstr). J Am Coll Cardiol 1993;21:31A.

17. Platko WP, Hollman J, Whitlow PL, Franco I. Percutaneous transluminal angioplasty of saphenous vein graft stenosis: long-term follow-up. J Am Coll Cardiol 1989;14(7):1645-1650.

18. Adelman AG, Cohen EA, Kimball BP, Bonan R, Ricci DR, Webb JG, Laramee L, Barbeau G, Traboulsi M, Corbett BN, et al. A comparison of directional atherectomy with balloon angioplasty for lesions of the left anterior descending coronary artery. N Engl J Med 1993;329(4):228-233.

19. Myler RK, Shaw RE, Stertzer SH, et al. Unstable angina and coronary angioplasty. Circulation 1990;82(suppl II):II-88-II-95.

20. DeFeyter PJ, Suryapanata H, Serruys PW, et al. Coronary angioplasty for unstable angina: immediate and late results in 200 consecutive patients with identification of risk factors for unfavorable early and late outcome. J Am Coll Cardiol 1988;12:324-333.

21. Abdelmeguid AE, Sapp SK, Lynch DA, et al. Immediate and follow up results of directional coronary atherectomy for the treatment of unstable angina (abstr). Circulation 1993;88:1-496.

22. Safian RD, Schreiber TL, Baim DS. Specific indications for directional coronary atherectomy: origin left anterior descending coronary artery and bifurcation lesions. Am J Cardiol 1993;72:35E-41E.

23. Lewis BE, Leya FS, Johnson SA, et al. Outcomes of angioplasty (PTCA) and atherectomy (DCA) for bifurcation and non-bifurcation lesions in CAVEAT (abstract). Circulation 1993;88:1-601.

24. Vaska KJ, Franco I, Whitlow PL. Risk of side-branch occlusion following directional coronary atherectomy (abstr). Circulation 1991;84:II-81.

25. Topol EJ, Ellis SG, Fishman J, et al. Multicenter study of percutaneous transluminal angioplasty for right coronary artery ostial stenosis. J Am Coll Cardiol 1987;9(6):1214-1218.

26. Mintz GS, Potkin BN, Keren G, et al. Intravascular ultrasound evaluation of the effect of rotational atherectomy in obstructive atherosclerotic coronary artery disease. Circulation 1992;86:1383-1393.

27. Zotz R, Stahr P, Erbel R, Auth D, Meyer J. Analysis of high frequency rotational angioplasty-induced echo contrast. Cathet Cardiovasc Diagn 1991;22:137-144.

28. Zacca NM, Kleiman NS, Rodriguez AR, et al. Rotational ablation of coronary artery lesions using single, large burrs. Cathet Cardiovasc Diagn 1992;26:92-97.

29. Stertzer SH, Rosenblum J, Shaw RE, et al. Coronary rotational ablation: Initial experience in 302 procedures. J Am Coll Cardiol 1993;21:287-295.

30. Buchbinder M, Warth D, Zacca N, et al. Multicenter registry of percutaneous coronary rotational ablation using the rotablator (abstr). Circulation 1991;84:II-82.

31. Cowley MJ, Warth D, Whitlow PL, et al. Factors influencing outcome with coronary rotational ablation: Multicenter Results (abstr). J Am Coll Cardiol 1993;21:31A.

32. Bertrand ME, Lablanche JM, Leroy F, et al. Percutaneous transluminal coronary rotary ablation with Rotablator (European Experience). Am J Cardiol 1992;69:470–474.
33. Whitlow PL, Buchbinder M, Kent K, et al. Coronary rotational atherectomy: angiographic risk factors and their relation to success/complication (abstract). J Am Coll Cardiol 1992;19:334A.
34. Popma JJ, Satler LF, Pichard AD, et al. Clinical and angiographic predictors of procedural outcome after rotational coronary atherectomy in complex lesions (abstract). J Am Coll Cardiol 1993;21:228A.
35. Whitlow PL, Cowley M, Bass T, et al. Risk of high speed rotational atherectomy in bifurcation lesions (abstr). J Am Coll Cardiol 1993;21:445A.
36. Popma JJ, Satler LF, Pichard AD, et al. A quantitative analysis of factors affecting late angiographic outcome after rotational coronary atherectomy (abstr). J Am Coll Cardiol 1993;21:31A.
37. Leon MB, Kent KM, Pichard AD, et al. Percutaneous transluminal coronary rotational angioplasty of calcified lesions (abstr). Circulation 1991;84:II-521.
38. Altmann DB, Popma JJ, Kent KM, et al. Rotational atherectomy effectively treats calcified lesions (abstract). J Am Coll Cardiol 1993;21:443A.
39. Goudreau E, Cowley MJ, DiSciascio G, et al. Rotational atherectomy for aorto-ostial and branch-ostial lesions (abstract). J Am Coll Cardiol 1993;21:31A.
40. Tierstein PS, Warth DC, Haq N, et al. High speed rotational coronary atherectomy for patients with diffuse coronary disease. J Am Coll Cardiol 1991;18:1694–1701.
41. Reisman M, Cohen B, Warth D, et al. Outcome of long lesions treated with high speed rotational ablation (abstract). J Am Coll Cardiol 1993;21:443A.
42. Brogan WC, Popma JJ, Pichard AD, et al. Rotational coronary atherectomy after unsuccessful coronary balloon angioplasty. Am J Cardiol 1993;71:794–798.
43. The TEC Coronary Registry, November 1993.
44. Abdelmeguid AE, Ellis SG, Whitlow PL, et al. Discordant results of extraction atherectomy in old and young saphenous vein grafts: the NACI experience (abstr). J Am Coll Cardiol 1993;21:442A.
45. Hong MK, Popma JJ, Leon MB, et al. Distal embolization after transluminal extraction catheter treatment of saphenous vein graft lesions (abstr). J Am Coll Cardiol 1993;21:228A.
46. Kramer B, Larkin T, Niemyski P, Parker M. Coronary atherectomy in acute ischemic syndromes: implications of thrombus on treatment outcome (abstr). J Am Coll Cardiol 1991;17:385A.
47. Popma JJ, Leon MB, Mintz GS, et al. Results of coronary angioplasty using the transluminal extraction catheter. Am J Cardiol 1992;70:1526–1532.
48. Leon MB, Pichard AD, Kramer BL, et al. Efficacious and safe transluminal extraction atherectomy in patients with unfavorable coronary lesions (abstr). J Am Coll Cardiol 1991;17:219A.
49. Sutton JM, Gitlin JB, Casale PN, et al. Complex lesions with ulceration or calcification are predictors of restenosis after transluminal extraction atherectomy (abstr). J Am Coll Cardiol 1993;21:442A.

9

Thrombolysis of Occluded Vein Grafts

Joseph R. Hartmann
Good Samaritan Hospital, Downer's Grove, Illinois

I. INTRODUCTION

Coronary artery bypass surgery (CABG) is the most common cardiac surgical procedure, with more than 200,000 cases performed each year in the last 15 years. Despite the excellent initial result of CABG in terms of low morbidity and mortality, the long-term patency of vein grafts has been less than ideal. As our patients age, the scope of this problem is growing, and new approaches must be found to treat a new disease (i.e., new-onset angina in the post-CABG patient).

A. Long-Term Fate of Vein Grafts

There have been several excellent long-term sequential angiographic studies on vein graft patency. In a recent study of 222 patients with 741 venous grafts by Fitzgibbon et al. (1), early (1 month) occlusion occurred in 8% of patients, 13% at 1 year, 20% at 5 years, 41% at 7.5 years, 41% at 10 years, and 45% after 11.5 years (Fig. 1). In addition, 38% of patients had evidence of atherosclerosis, with 14% (5% of all patient grafts) having at least a 50% diameter stenosis of the lumen by the 5-year follow-up angiogram. By 10 years, 35% of patients had >50% stenosis, and 75% of grafts showed some evidence of atherosclerosis. This most recent study agrees with older angio-

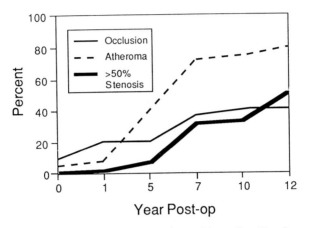

Figure 1   Summary of three long-term angiographic studies. Development of occlusion, atherosclerosis, and >50% stenosis in post-CABG patients. (From Refs. 1–3.)

graphic reports from the Montreal Heart Institute and the Cleveland Clinic. In 1983, Campeau et al. (2) reported that 3.4% of grafts were occluded at 3 weeks, 10% at 6–18 months, 19% at 5–7 years, and 37% at 12 years after CABG. The incidence of graft atherosclerosis increased from 16% (5% with >50% stenosis) at 7 years to 46% (32% with >50% stenosis) by 12 years. Lytle et al. (3) from the Cleveland Clinic reported similar results in 1985. Thirty-six percent of grafts were occluded 7.3 years after CABG, with 18% of patent grafts being stenotic and 45% of these with >50% stenosis.

After the first year, graft patency remains relatively stable with closure rates of only 0.5%–3% per year. In all studies, there appears to be a major increase in closure of approximately 20% at year 7, with only 40–50% of grafts remaining patent between year 7 and year 12. Note the corresponding rise in atherosclerosis in vein grafts and the increase in lesions with >50% stenosis. These lesions frequently lead to complete occlusion.

B. Pathological Changes in Vein Grafts

1. Thrombosis

Trauma to the vein graft at the time of harvesting can produce immediate platelet deposition with subsequent formation of mural thrombus. This along with a small target vessel that results in an already poor blood flow and a poor surgical technique are likely the causes for early graft closure (4).

2. Intimal Hyperplasia

Smooth muscle cell proliferation begins by 1 month and can be either slow or rapid, the latter depending on the amount of mural thrombus produced by platelet deposition (4). This mechanism is probably responsible for graft closure within the first year. Intimal hyperplasia appears to occur to some degree in all patients and reduces luminal dimension by 25% at 1 year (5). Smooth muscle cell proliferation appears to diminish or stop after the first year (6).

3. Atherosclerosis

The development of atherosclerosis is relatively constant between 1 and 5 years after CABG and averages 20%. As noted in Figure 1, there is a dramatic rise in the extent and severity of atherosclerotic changes noted after 7 years post-CABG. This is what Fitzgibbon has called the "7.5 year phenomenon" (1). In a longitudinal study by Bourassa et al. (7), between 5 to 7 years and 10–12 years after CABG the percentage of grafts with atherosclerosis increased from 17 to 46% and the percent of stenoses > 50% rose from 33 to 70%. It is also at this 7.5-year point when the greatest increase in graft occlusions occurs.

4. Summary

Late graft occlusions comprise a combination of the processes summarized above. The degree to which each of these contributes to the occlusion will predict the success or failure of the therapy. For instance, if the main cause of closure is diffuse intimal hyperplasia, it is unlikely that any therapy will be successful.

However, late graft occlusion is likely a combination of thrombosis and atherosclerosis. Walts et al. (8) noted that thrombosis occurring on a ruptured atherosclerotic plaque commonly caused late graft occlusion. In addition, Solymoss et al. reported that late thrombosis was present in 80% of atherosclerotic grafts, 100% of grafts with aneurysmal dilatation, and only 40% of grafts without atherosclerosis (9).

Considering these findings, any therapy directed at recanalizing totally occluded vein grafts must take into account the pathology present in the diseased bypass graft.

C. Anatomical Factors

Anatomical, technical, and histological parameters have an impact on the long-term patency of bypass graft angioplasty (10,11). Bourassa et al. (10) reported that distal artery diameter, intraoperative graft flow, and the surgeon's experience all had a significant effect on early and 1-year patency

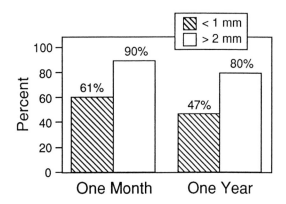

Figure 2 Patency rates 1 month and 1 year after CABG related to size of distal native vessel. (From Ref. 10.)

(Fig. 2). One-year patency was 47% when the grafted artery was <1 mm in diameter, as compared with an 80% patency when the artery was >2 mm ($p < 0.05$). Similarly, there was a 49% 1-year patency when graft flow was <50 ml/min versus 89% patency when flow was >50 ml/min ($p < 0.001$) (Fig. 3). Although these factors appear to have the greatest influence in the first year, it is likely that distal artery diameter and graft flow have an inverse relationship to not only initial success at recanalization, but also long-term patency.

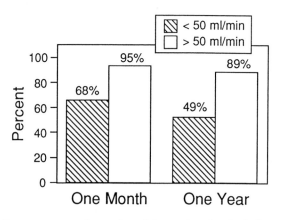

Figure 3 Patency rates at 1 month and 1 year showing the influence of graft flow. (From Ref. 10.)

Bourassa also showed the relationship between quality of distal runoff and surgical experience (10). Comparing their first 300 bypass cases with their last 300 cases, they found that poor distal runoff and little surgical experience resulted in a 30% 1-year patency (Fig. 4). This contrasts with the 90% 1-year patency seen when distal runoff was good and the surgical team was considered experienced.

The histology of the vein graft lesion has an effect on the ability to re-establish flow in these occluded grafts. Chronic total native coronary artery occlusions have either a tapered tip or an abrupt cut-off (Fig. 5) (11). Two types of fibrous tissue were identified with each of the two occlusion morphologies: type 1, a loose network of fibrous tissue continuing throughout the entire length of the occlusion; and type 2, in which the fibrous tissue network did not penetrate the occlusion. In four of five cases with the tapering type, such as that seen in the left of Figure 5, the loose fibrous tissue penetrated the occlusion, which may explain the improved recanalization rate of total occlusions with a tapering type of occlusion. This pattern is more likely to respond to recanalization. However, it is very likely that this pattern changes over time and that the earlier an occlusion is treated, the less dense the fibrous tissue will be and the greater the chance that recanalization will be successful.

D. The Difference Between Native Coronary and Vein Graft Occlusions

Both native coronary and late vein graft occlusions are caused by a rupture of atherosclerotic plaque with luminal narrowing followed by the de-

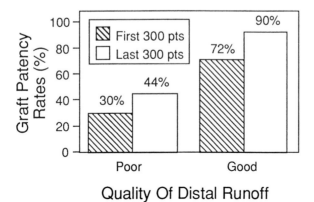

Figure 4 Graft patency rates at 1 year related to distal runoff and surgical experience. (From Ref. 10.)

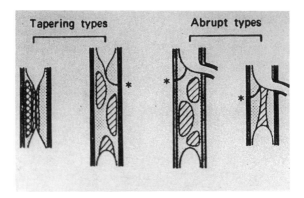

Figure 5 Histology examples of total native coronary occlusions. Chronic total native coronary artery occlusions have two types of occlusions, either a tapered tip or an abrupt flush occlusion. (A) and (D) have loose fibrous tissue penetrating the length of the occlusion. (B) and (C) have a denser fibrous mass without penetration of loose fibrous tissue. The tapering type on the left shows small recanalized areas surrounded by loose fibrous tissue penetrating the occlusion. In four out of five cases of the tapering type, the loss fibrous tissue penetrated the occlusion, which may explain the improved recanalization rate of total occlusions with a tapering type of occlusion. This pattern is more likely amenable to recanalization than examples (B), (C), and (D). These examples were taken from native coronary arteries with occlusion durations of >1 year. (From Ref. 11.)

velopment of a superimposed obstructing thrombus. However, it is after this point that the processes differ. The native coronary occlusion leads to an acute infarction in most cases. There may be some proximal propagation of thrombus, but only back to the next collateral. By and large, an occluded vein graft does not initiate a myocardial infarction. The majority of vein graft occlusions are either asymptomatic or cause a change in the patient's anginal pattern. For example, in a group of post-CABG patients reported by Lambert et al. (12), myocardial infarction accounted for only 22% of late clinical events. This occlusion does not usually result in infarction because the distal vessel has ample collateral vessels. The burden of thrombus in occluded vein grafts is considerably larger than in native coronary arteries because thrombus fills the proximal portion of the vein graft from the inciting lesion back to the origin of the vein graft. It is this burden of thrombus that has not been recognized when attempting to recanalize chronic total vein graft occlusions.

1. Angioplasty in Nonoccluded Vein Grafts

In an excellent review by de Feyter (13) of 16 articles reporting the results of angioplasty in nonoccluded vein grafts on 1571 patients, clinical success was reported in 88% of cases (Table 1). Myocardial infarction occurred in approximately 4% of cases and need for urgent bypass surgery in <2%. Procedure-related death occurred in <1% of patients and distal embolization was seen in <3%. It is not clear whether an enzyme rise was seen in these cases of embolization. Clinical success was less in the proximal portion of the graft (87%) than in the body (94%) or the distal anastomosis (90%).

Angiographic follow-up in 12 articles ranged from 56 to 100% and revealed an overall restenosis rate of 42% with 58% in the proximal graft, 52% in the body, and 28% in the distal site (13).

These studies really represent an excellent result that must be kept as a standard when attempting to recanalize totally occluded grafts.

Long-term follow-up reveals that these patients are at the end-stage of their coronary disease as their 5-year event-free survival is only 26% with a 5-year mortality rate of 26% (14).

2. Angioplasty of Totally Occluded Vein Grafts

Direct angioplasty of totally occluded vein grafts has been fraught with difficulty. de Feyter reported on the results of direct balloon angioplasty in 15 patients with total occlusions of 3- to 6-month duration. Initial clinical success was achieved in 7 (47%) with 5 (30%) procedural myocardial infarctions (15). Only one patient maintained a patent vessel at follow-up. This led de Feyter to state what has become consensus on direct angioplasty in totally occluded vein grafts: it is "a challenge that should be resisted." This result could have been predicted considering the pathology of occluded vein grafts described above.

3. Reoperations

Why not reoperate on everyone who presents with uncontrolled angina after a vein graft occlusion? Table 2 summarizes the results of second bypass op-

Table 1 Initial Results of Angioplasty of Nonoccluded Saphenous Vein Grafts

Patients (no.)	Success (%)	Death (%)	MI (%)	Emboli (%)	Urgent CABG (%)
1571	88	<1	<4	<3	<2

MI = myocardial infarction; CABG = coronary artery bypass grafting.
Source: From Ref. 13.

Table 2 Morbidity and Mortality in CABG Reoperations

Author (Ref.)	Patients (no.)	Mortality (%)	MI (%)	Stroke (%)
Williams (16)	453	3	10	NR
Lytle (17)	1500	3.4	8	2
Carrier (18)	331	12	18	NR
Total (Avg)	2284	4.7%	9.5%	2%

MI = myocardial infarction.

erations in 2284 patients from three institutions with excellent reputations (16–18). Overall operative mortality ranges from 3 to 12% and averages 4.6%. Perioperative myocardial infarctions ranged from 8 to 18% and averaged 9.8%. These results compare with a mortality rate of 1% and a perioperative myocardial infarction rate of 0.6% in patients undergoing a primary procedure (17).

It is apparent that any procedure that hopes to prolong the useful life of a vein graft must exceed the results of direct angioplasty and must approach the success rate and complication rate obtained by repeat operations.

II. RECANALIZATION OF CHRONICALLY OCCLUDED AORTO-CORONARY VEIN GRAFTS: THROMBOLYSIS AND ANGIOPLASTY

It appears that the chronically occluded vein graft is similar to the occluded superficial femoral artery or a femoral-popliteal bypass graft in that there is an offending lesion that occludes the vessel and precipitates thrombosis of the artery or bypass graft back to the next proximal collateral or, in the case of the bypass graft, back to the origin of the graft.

Considering the degree of thrombus identified at the time of graft removal at reoperation, it was expected that it might be possible to turn an old, occluded graft into a younger, nonoccluded graft.

Several assumptions were made:

1. Success rates should approach 70%, considering the fact that 69% of grafts and 72% of patients with occluded vein grafts had thrombotic occlusions.
2. Complications would be less than those for direct balloon angioplasty and bypass surgery since lysis of thrombus should reduce embolization and subsequent myocardial infarction.

3. Long-term patency would be less than that for angioplasty of non-occluded vessels considering the fact that occluded grafts are more likely to have poorer distal runoff and lower graft flow than patent, nonoccluded grafts.

A. Study Patients

Between January 1987 and July 1990, 46 consecutive patients underwent attempted recanalization of a chronically occluded aorto-coronary saphenous vein bypass graft. Patients with an acute Q-wave myocardial infarction were excluded. Age of occlusion varied by history or angiography from 0.2–28 weeks.

B. The Protocol

Detailed descriptions of both the protocol and procedure are included in Appendix I, and a list of equipment is included in Appendix II. In summary, a 7-French angiographic catheter is placed in the origin of the occluded graft. There must be a "nipple" to seat the catheter or the maximum support needed for a prolonged infusion will not be obtained. An 0.038 SOS (145 cm) wire, after removal of the stylet, is passed over an 0.014-in. floppy guidewire into the thrombus. In the event that the floppy guidewire could not be advanced, an intermediate or standard guidewire was substituted. Minimal force was applied when passing the guidewire to reduce the risk of perforation. Once the guidewire was positioned, the SOS wire was passed over the guidewire to a position several centimeters into the graft and the guidewire was then removed (Fig. 6). The farther the thrombus could be penetrated, the greater the chance for success.

A coaxial infusion of urokinase, 50,000 U/h proximally at the origin of the graft through the angiographic catheter and 50,000 U/h distally through the SOS wire (100,000 U/h), was begun. The sheath and angiographic catheter were sutured to the skin and covered with a sterile dressing (Fig. 7). The patient was brought to the critical care unit for continued coaxial urokinase infusion. Average time to lysis was 20–24 h. Longer infusion times are sometimes required.

Urokinase infusion was continued until there was antigrade flow or no further evidence of lysis. Angiography may be performed several times a day to assess progress of lysis. In the ideal case, a precipitating lesion is identified in the graft after establishment of flow into the distal vessel. Balloon angioplasty can then be performed on a "younger looking," nonoccluded vein graft.

Figure 8 shows the progression of lysis in an occluded right coronary vein graft which had been perfused for 24 h. Angioplasty at the anastomosis

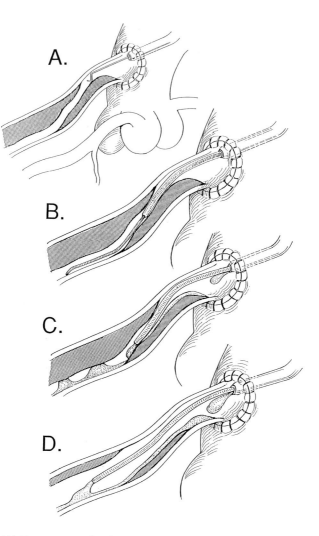

Figure 6   (A) Engagement of ostium of vein graft with passage of guidewire. (B) Advancement of SOS wire. (C) Initiation of coaxial infusion. (D) Successful completion of lysis.

produced an excellent result turning an occluded 8-year-old graft into a younger looking graft amenable to angioplasty.

C. Results

In our first report of 47 grafts in 46 patients, 79% were successfully recanalized (20). Adjunctive balloon angioplasty of a residual lesion was per-

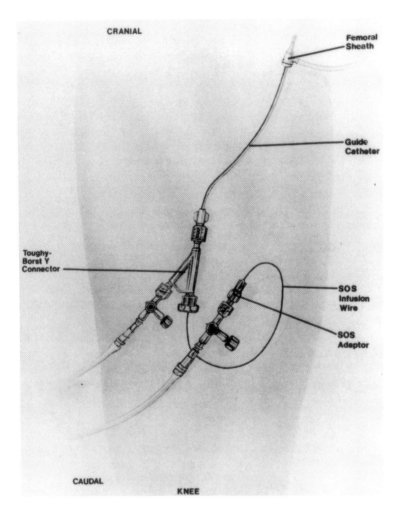

Figure 7 Illustration of limb demonstrating procedural setup.

formed in 35 (95%) of these 37 cases. Two patients had no obvious lesions requiring angioplasty. In 10 cases (21%), graft patency was not achieved. Difficulty in positioning the angiographic catheter or SOS wire, or both, was experienced in five of these unsuccessful cases. In two patients, the procedure was terminated prematurely despite evidence of lysis in the proximal portion of the target graft because of the patient's inability to remain still.

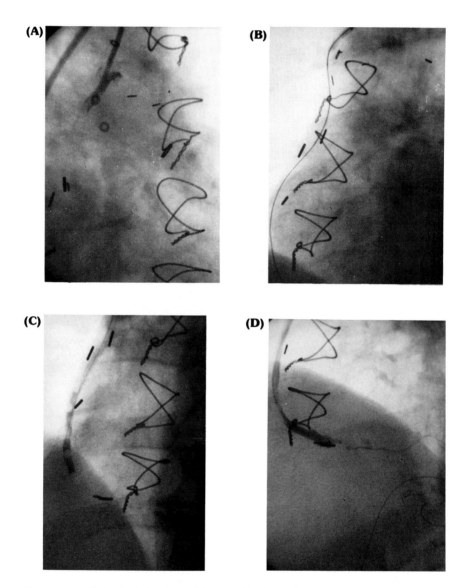

Figure 8   (A) Occluded ostium of 8-year-old vein graft. (B) Placement of SOS wire. (C) 12-h angiogram showing partial lysis with residual thrombus. (D) 24-h angiogram showing lysis of thrombus with antegrade flow into distal native coronary. (E) Balloon angioplasty at anastomotic lesion. (F) Final result. Note the residual thrombus at the 12-h angiogram and the ghost of the distal right coronary at the 24-h angiogram when antegrade flow had been established.

(E) **(F)**

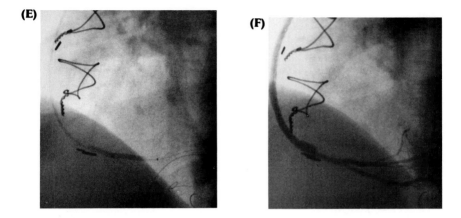

Figure 8 Continued

Complications are listed in Table 3. Q-wave myocardial infarction occurred in two patients (4%) and a non-Q-wave myocardial infarction (defined as a doubling of CPK) occurred in four (8.5%) patients.

When distal embolization occurred, the urokinase infusion was doubled to 200–250,000 U/h which frequently sped up lysis. Because embolization is certainly a sign that antegrade flow has been established, angioplasty should not be performed at this time unless the patient is very unstable as the graft usually has a significant residual clot burden.

While only one patient required a single unit blood transfusion, four additional patients demonstrated a decrease in hemoglobin of approximately 2g/dl for which transfusion was not given.

There were no procedure-related deaths.

D. Clinical Follow-Up

All patients were followed clinically for symptoms of angina pectoris, myocardial infarction, and the need for further intervention. The mean

Table 3 Results of Recanalization in 46 Patients with 47 Aorto-coronary Vein Grafts Using Urokinase Lysis Prior to Angioplasty

Patients	Success	MI	non-Q-wave MI	Stroke	Death
46	79%	4%	8.5%	0	0

follow-up was 27.2 months. Fourteen patients developed angina, two developed congestive heart failure, and four underwent repeat aorto-coronary bypass surgery. There were four deaths during the follow-up period (two sudden, one due to congestive heart failure, and one in which circumstances are unknown). Twenty-two patients (61%) remained free from symptoms during the follow-up.

Twenty (54%) successfully treated patients underwent repeat angiography during the 27-month follow-up period because of recurrent angina. The grafts in 13 patients (65%) were patent, but 2 of the 13 patients required angioplasty for recurrent graft stenosis and the remainder had progression of disease in other vessels.

E. Discussion

The initial study confirmed our assumptions:

1. Considering the pathology of totally occluded vein grafts, our success rate was in the range predicted by our assumptions (i.e., around 70%, actually 79%).
2. With a Q-wave infarction rate of 4%, this approach was less than the 30% reported for direct balloon angioplasty and the 9.8% average reported after reoperation. There were no procedure-related deaths in our group, compared with the average of 4.6% in reoperated patients.
3. Reocclusion occurred in 35% of the patients. Two additional patients had patent grafts but still required angioplasty. This gives a reocclusion/restenosis rate of 45%. Although only 54% of our patients were restudied, this restudy rate is similar to that reported in angioplasty of nonoccluded vein grafts.

It was obvious that this initial approach offered something new to patients returning with angina after bypass surgery. It has permitted some patients to avoid reoperation and to lead a more active lifestyle. The next step was to see if this approach could be duplicated by other clinicians and to get a better angiographic follow-up.

III. ROBUST

Robust (*R*ecanalization of *O*ccluded aorto-coronary *B*ypass grafts *us*ing *U*rokinase—a *S*erial *T*rial) is a larger trial using the same protocol described above with a 6-month follow-up angiogram. Seven centers were chosen because of the expertise of the clinical investigators. Inclusion and exclusion criteria were the same. Patients who had vein graft occlusions for <6 months were enrolled. All patients were encouraged to be kept on aspirin (325 mg) and a therapeutic dose of warfarin until the 6-month angiogram.

Table 4 ROBUST: Baseline Characteristics ($n = 107$)

Mean age	61 years
Male	79%
Caucasian	97%
Smoker	60%
Family Hx CAD	56%
CHF	8%
Diabetes	20%
Exercise angina	65%
Rest angina	68%
Prior AMI	72%
Prior PTCA target CABG	13%
Redo CABG	8%

CAD = coronary artery disease; AMI = acute myocardial infarction; PTCA = percutaneous transluminal coronary angioplasty; CABG = coronary artery bypass grafting.

A. Patient Enrollment and Follow-up

One hundred and seven patients were enrolled. Seventy-three patients complied consistently with the protocol, and 34 patients had protocol violations. Baseline characteristics are included in Table 4.

Angiograms were reviewed by surgeons at the treating institution and at the coordinating center. Reviewing surgeons were blinded as to the clinical status of the patients and any concomitant diseases. Opinions were based soley on the review of angiograms. Cases were ranked as to the surgical difficulty as follows: Class A—technically operable, moderate amount of myocardium at risk, good result expected; Class B—small amount of myocardium at risk, only one vessel disease, PTCA preferable; Class C—difficult, but technically operable, marginal benefit due to small amount of myocardium at risk; Class D—difficult, small, distal vessel, good result not expected; and Class E—inoperable.

Patients were encouraged to return for a 6-month angiogram. Clinical follow-up was performed at the treating institution and, by phone, at the coordinating center.

Table 5 ROBUST: Initial Recanalization Efficacy

	Protocol compliant (73)	Protocol violation (34)	Total sample (107)
Successful	56 (77%)	20 (59%)	76 (71%)
Unsuccessful	17 (23%)	14 (41%)	31 (29%)

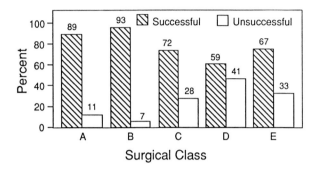

Figure 9   Success rate by surgical classification.

B. Results

Recanalization was successfully achieved in 77% of the protocol-compliant patients and in 59% of patients in whom the protocol was violated (71% success for the group as a whole) (Table 5). Recanalization rates were highest in surgical class A and B and fell as the surgical difficulty increased (Fig. 9).

The mean urokinase dosage in the successfully recanalized patients was 3.7 million units and 4.5 million units in the unsuccessfully recanalized patients. The mean decrease in fibrinogen levels was 93 mg/dl in the successfully recanalized patients and 188 mg/dl in the unsuccessfully recanalized group.

Acute success of recanalization did not appear to be affected by the age of the graft (Fig. 10). Acute success as influenced by TIMI flow after thrombolysis and before PTCA was 100% in TIMI 2 and 3 (Fig. 11). Acute success

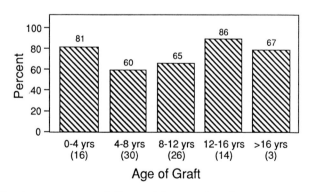

Figure 10   Acute success as influenced by age of graft.

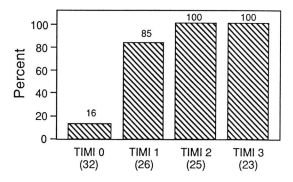

Figure 11 Acute success as influenced by TIMI grade blood flow after thrombolysis prior to PTCA.

did not appear to be related to the duration of occlusion, although there were few patients enrolled who had occlusions beyond 2 months (Fig. 12).

Complications were less in the successfully recanalized patients and in the protocol-compliant patients (Table 6). In the group as a whole, Q-wave myocardial infarction occurred in 5%. Enzyme elevation was seen in 17%. Emergency CABG was required in 4%. Stroke occurred in 3% and in-hospital death in 7%. Cause of in-hospital death is listed in Table 7.

Six-month angiograms were performed for 51% of the successfully recanalized patients. Forty-one percent had a patent graft at follow-up (Fig. 13). If TIMI 3 flow was achieved by thrombolysis at initial recanalization, the 6-month patency was 67% (Fig. 14). Patency did not seem to be affected

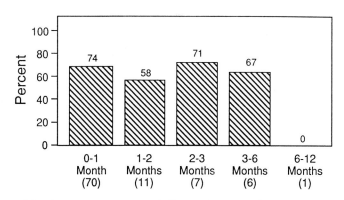

Figure 12 Acute success rate as influenced by duration of occlusion of graft.

Table 6   ROBUST: Acute Adverse Events

	Successful	Unsuccessful	Protocol compliant	Protocol violation	Total
Q-wave MI	1%	13%	4%	6%	5%
Enzyme elevation	16%	19%	15%	21%	17%
Emergent CABG	3%	6%	3%	6%	4%
Stroke	0%	10%	4%	0%	3%
Death	3%	16%	3%	15%	7%

MI = myocardial infarction; CABG = coronary artery bypass grafting.

Table 7   ROBUST: Acute Mortality

Patient ID	Cause of death	Days postenrollment
1003	Intracranial hemorrhage	2
1103	Ruptured ventricle	2
3002	End-stage coronary disease	28
4008	Electrical mechanical dissociation	1
6012	Unknown	21
6014	Ventricular fibrillation	9
7009	Ventricular fibrillation	8

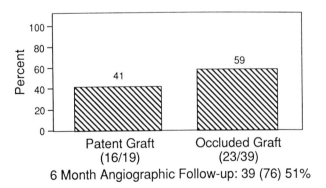

Figure 13   Six-month follow-up on successfully recanalized patients.

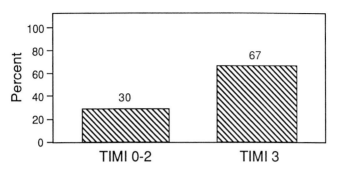

Figure 14   Six-month patency as influenced by TIMI grade blood flow after thrombolysis prior to PTCA.

Table 8   ROBUST: The Effects of Aspirin and Warfarin Therapy on 6-Month Graft Patency

	Patent	Occluded
Aspirin	0%	4%
Warfarin	19%	4%
Both	82%	91%

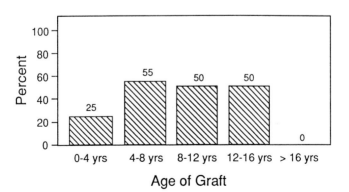

Figure 15   Six-month patency as influenced by age of graft.

by the use of warfarin or aspirin (Table 8). Six-month patency, as influenced by the age of the graft, is shown in Figure 15. Six-month patency was approximately 50% in 4- to 16-year-old grafts and only 25% in grafts younger than 4 years, suggesting that there may be technical or anatomical factors responsible for the early initial closure and the subsequent reduction in 6-month patency.

C. Discussion

This protocol, when followed by experienced interventionalists, results in a reasonable initial success rate. Lower complications can be expected if the protocol is strictly adhered to. In addition, appropriate selection of patients, specifically those patients who are poor candidates for repeat operations because of their underlying anatomy and concomitant diseases, is critical.

Initial success rates may be improved by reviewing both the initial preoperative angiogram to determine the size of the distal vessel and the operative report, with special attention to the graft flow, to ascertain whether recanalization might produce long-term patency.

IV. SUMMARY

The problem of aorto-coronary vein graft occlusion remains a major clinical challenge. Thrombolysis of occluded bypass grafts offers one method of preserving the life of some occluded vein grafts. At the present time, we cannot determine with accuracy who will benefit from this approach. But after much experience, the following can be recommended:

1. This procedure is safe and effective when applied to the subgroup of patients outlined and when the protocol is strictly adhered to.
2. This procedure should only be performed by those cardiologists with extensive interventional experience. It takes a considerable amount of time, patience, and endurance (for both the doctor and the patient).
3. It is a procedure that requires the constant attention of *one* physician who must be available at all times during the treatment period.
4. Reviewing the preoperative angiogram to assess the quality of the distal vessel might give important information as to the likelihood of this procedure being both effective and beneficial.
5. Reviewing the operative report for graft flows will be a helpful clue in determining who might benefit from this procedure.
6. This procedure is intended for patients with only one occluded graft going to viable, ischemic-producing muscle.

7. The earlier a patient is treated after occlusion, the easier it will be to recanalize the vessel. New onset angina or a change in a stable anginal pattern in a postbypass patient should be aggressively investigated.
8. Future technologies may prolong the life of these vein grafts and hopefully reduce the present "Achilles heel" of this procedure, which is restenosis.

APPENDIX I: PROCEDURAL STEPS

1. Using a multipurpose 18-gauge, 2¾-in. thin wall procedure needle without stilet, carefully enter the front wall of the femoral artery. A posterior exit should be avoided.
2. Advance a 0.035-in. (150 cm) guidewire through the needle into the abdominal aorta and remove the needle.
3. Advance a 7- or 8-French arterial sheath and dilator assembly over the guidewire.
4. Slip a plastic luer lock adapter device over a 7- or 8-French angiographic catheter to prepare it for insertion into the introducer sheath. This device will be used to secure the catheter in place at the conclusion of the procedure.
5. Infuse 5000 U of intravenous heparin. This bolus dose should be repeated after 1 h in the event the patient is still in the catheterization laboratory. If heparin therapy has already been initiated, do not infuse the 5000 U but continue the infusion at ordered dose, provided the PTT is therapeutic (>50 s).
6. Advance the angiographic catheter over the guidewire into the ascending thoracic aorta.
7. Connect a Toey-Borst (T-B) adapter to the end of the angiographic/angioplasty guide catheter.
8. Connect the system to a manifold. Purge the system of air and flush it with fluid.
9. Position the angiographic catheter securely into the orifice of the occluded graft. Catheter selection must be appropriate to assure that the catheter seats securely into the stub of the occluded graft.
10. Obtain angiography of the vein graft in at least two projections and record the projection numbers. These projections will be repeated for all subsequent angiography sessions.
11. Monitor vital signs q 15 min $\times$ 4, then q 30 min $\times$ 4, then q 1 h until therapy is completed.

12. Assess all puncture sites as well as the sheath site q 30 min for hematoma or bleeding. Pulse, temperature, sensation, and general appearance of the involved extremity should be monitored hourly.
13. Keep the patient well sedated.
14. Perform interim histories and cardiovascular physical examinations daily for the duration of the infusion.
15. Continue the infusion through both the SOS wire and guiding catheter for approximately 4–8 h.
16. Following this time period, return to the catheterization laboratory and inject dye distally through the SOS wire to determine the degree of thrombus dissolution. Document dissolution of thrombus on cine angiography using the same projections as the baseline angiography.
17. If thrombus dissolution is not satisfactory, increase the urokinase infusion to a total of 250,000 U/h (proximal 125,000 U/h; distal 125,000 U/h). In addition, attempt to advance the SOS infusion wire over a Hi-Torque Floppy wire. Even in the event that TIMI flow is 0, the ability to probe the vessel and advance the SOS wire may indicate softening of the occlusion.
    Note: if the monitored fibrinogen level falls to less than 120, the urokinase dose should be adjusted to an intermediate dose, 180,000 U/h (proximal 90,000 U/h; distal 90,000 U/h).
18. Continue the infusion and restudy the patient approximately 22–26 h from the onset of the urokinase administration using the same initial projections. Once again, if thrombus dissolution is not satisfactory, the urokinase dose may be increased to 360,000 U/h (proximal 180,000 U/h; distal 180,000 U/h), provided that the patient's fibrinogen level is at least 120.
    Note: the urokinase infusion should be continued at the discretion of the cardiologist as long as the thrombus dissolution appears to be progressing. Once lysis begins, it is critical to continue the infusion until the vessel is thrombus free, as interruption of the infusion prematurely will result in almost immediate rethrombosis.
    The infusion, however, should be discontinued when the graft appears open or when no progress is evident. If no thrombolysis is noted, the urokinase infusion should be given for at least 24 h. The total dose of urokinase should not exceed 360,000 U/h or fall below 100,000 U/h.
19. When flow is noted in the distal native coronary artery, perform dilatation of the suspected offending lesion with balloon angioplasty.
    Note: every attempt should be made to dissolve thrombi prior to dila-

tation. Dilatation should be avoided if significant thrombus remains in the vein graft.

APPENDIX II: EQUIPMENT SPECIFICATIONS (PARTIAL LISTING)

B-D multi-purpose procedure needle.
18 gauge, 2¾ in.
Fits 0.032–0.038 guidewires.
Catalogue #8295.
Namic custom angiographic kit.
Three-part manifold, two IV spikes, pressure monitoring tubing.
Catalogue #60070281.
ACS rotating hemostasis valve.
Catalogue #23242.
Cordis emerald guidewire.
Fixed core, Teflon coated, 3 mm J. 150 cm, 0.035 in.
Cook plastic luer lock adapter.
For use with 6.0–8.0 French catheters.
Catalogue #PMILLA-UCC-L.
USCI SOS open-ended, 0.038, 145 cm, straight wire.
Standard taper.
Catalogue #6200.
Namic three-way stopcock with rotating adapter.
Catalogue #70025008.
ACS guidewire.
Hi-Torque Floppy II 0.014, 175 cm.
Catalogue #22339M.
Hi-Torque Intermediate 0.014, 175 cm.
Catalogue #22231 7M.
Hi-Torque Standard 0.014, 175 cm.
Catalogue #22318M
Spectramed dead ender.
Catalogue #MDE-001.
Cordis high-flow 7-French catheters.
3M Tegaderm dressing, 8 in. × 12 in.
Catalogue #1629.

APPENDIX III: SAMPLE STANDING ORDERS

1. Admit to ICU/CCU. Notify Attending and Consultants.
2. Urokinase 1,500,000 U in 250 cc D_5 W to infuse at _____ U/h distally and _____ U/h proximally.

3. Heparin 25,000 U in 500 cc D_5 W to infuse at _____ U/h.
4. Hemoglobin, PTT, Fibrinogen, CPK/isoenzyme and FDP levels q 4 h following the onset of urokinase infusion and notify cardiologist of results.
5. Hemoglobin, PTT, Fibrinogen, CPK/isoenzyme and FDP levels q 8 h during urokinase infusion. Notify N.D. if Hgb drops more than 2 g, if PTT is < 120 mg.
6. Serum creatinine level 24 h following onset of urokinase infusion.
7. Continue q 8 h CPK/isoenzyme levels for 24 h following the discontinuance of the infusion.
8. Type and crossmatch for packed red blood cells, fresh frozen plasma, and cyroprecipitate.
9. If PTT is < 70 s:
   a. Bolus with 2000 units of heparin and increase drip by 100 U/h.
   b. Notify M.D. if heparin drip is increased on > two consecutive q 8 h PTTs or if heparin rate exceeds 2200 U/h.
10. If the PTT is greater than 150 s, hold the heparin for 2 h, then resume drip at 100 U/h less than prior rate.
11. If PTT is > 120 but < 150, decrease the drip by 100 U/h than prior rate.
12. No IM injections while on heparin.
13. No arterial sticks during urokinase infusion. Draw all laboratory specimens from the arterial sheath or an IV site with a stopcock.
14. Guaiac all stools, urine, and emesis. Notify cardiologist of positive results.
15. Complete bed rest with an egg crate mattress. Keep patient flat and avoid all unnecessary activity or turning.
16. Restrain patient as necessary with either soft restraints or a knee immobilizer to keep involved extremity straight.
17. Secure tubing connections and check them q 1 h to maintain proper position.
18. Monitor vital signs q 15 min × 4, then q 30 min × 4, then q 1 h until therapy is completed. Do not use Dinamap.
19. Check all puncture sites as well as the sheath site q 30 min for hematoma or bleeding during therapy.
20. Check the pulse, temperature, sensation, and a general appearance of the involved extremity q 1 h during therapy. Monitor for ecchymosis, petechiae, and swelling.
21. Apply direct pressure to bleeding site and notify M.D.
22. Insert an in-dwelling foley catheter.
23. Keep patient well sedated:
   a. Versed 1–3 mg q/h IV prn.
   b. Nubain 1–3 mg q/h IV prn.

24. Tylenol #3 1 or 2 tablets po q 3 h prn for pain.
25. Diet as tolerated. Advance to low sodium/low cholesterol.
26. Push P.O. fluids.
27. Assess the 12-lead ECG daily for the duration of the infusion and stat with any incidence of chest pain. Have house M.D. read and call cardiologist.

REFERENCES

1. FitzGibbon GM, Leach AJ, Kafka HP, Keon WJ. Coronary bypass graft fate: long-term angiographic study. J Am Coll Cardiol 1991;17:1075-80.
2. Campeau L, Enjalbert M, Lesperance J, Vaislic C, Grondid CM, Bourassa MG. Atherosclerosis and late closure of aortocoronary saphenous vein grafts: sequential angiographic studies at 2 weeks, 1 year, 5 to 7 years, and 10 to 12 years after surgery. Circulation 1983;68(suppl II):II-1-7.
3. Lytle BW, Loop FD, Cosgrove DM, Ratliff NB, Easlay K, Taylor PC. Long-term (5 to 12 years) serial studies of internal mammary artery and saphenous vein coronary bypass grafts. J Thorac Cardiovasc Surg 1985;89:248-58.
4. Fuster V, Chesebro JH. Coronary artery bypass grafting. A model for the understanding of the progression of atherosclerotic disease and the role of pharmacological intervention. In: Neri Scerneri GG, McGiff JC, Paoletti R, Born GVR (eds). Advances in Prostaglandin, Thromboxane, and Leukotriene Research. Vol. 13. New York: Raven Press 1985:285-99.
5. Bourassa MG, Campeau L, Lesperance J, et al. Changes in grafts and coronary arteries after saphenous vein aortocoronary bypass surgery: Results at repeat angiography. Circulation 1982;65(suppl II):II-90.
6. Campeau L, Lesperance J, Corbara F, et al. Aortocoronary saphenous vein bypass graft changes 5 to 7 years after surgery. Circulation 1978;58(suppl):170.
7. Bourassa MG, Fisher LD, Campeau L, et al. Long-term fate of bypass grafts: The Coronary Artery Surgery Study (CASS) and Montreal Heart Institute experiences. Circulation 1985;72(suppl V):V-71.
8. Walts AE, Fishbein MC, Sustaita H, et al. Ruptured atheromatous plaques in saphenous vein coronary artery bypass grafts: A mechanism of acute, thrombotic, late graft occlusion. Circulation 1982;65:197.
9. Solymoss BC, Nadeau P, Millette D, et al. Late thrombosis of saphenous vein coronary bypass grafts related to risk factors. Circulation 1988;78(suppl 1)78:140.
10. Bourassa MG, Campeau L, Lesperance J. Changes in grafts and in coronary arteries after coronary bypass surgery. In: Waters DD, Bourassa MG, eds. Care of the Patient with Previous Coronary Bypass Surgery. Philadelphia: FA Davis, 1991:83-100.
11. Katsuragawa D, Fujiqara H, Miyamae M, Sasayama S. Histology of Chronic Total Coronary Occlusion. J Am Coll Cardiol 1993;21:604-611.
12. Lambert M, Kouz S, Campeau L. Preoperative and operative predictive variables of late clinical events following saphenous vein coronary artery bypass graft surgery. Can J Cardiol 1989;5:87.

13. de Feyter PJ, van Suylen RJ, de Jaegere PP, Topol EJ, Serruys PW. Balloon angioplasty for the treatment of lesions in saphenous vein bypass grafts. J Am Coll Cardiol 1993;21:1539–49.
14. Platkio WP, Hollman J, Whitlow PL, Franco J. Percutaneous transluminal coronary angioplasty of saphenous vein graft stenosis: long-term follow-up. J Am Coll Cardiol 1989;14:1645–50.
15. de Feyter PJ, Serruys PW, van den Brand M, Meester H, Deatt K, Suryapranata H. Percutaneous transluminal angioplasty of a totally occluded venous bypass graft: a challenge that should be resisted. Am J Cardiol 1989;64:88–90.
16. Williams CD, Hoffmann TH, Casali RE, Wright RN, Selby JH. Re-operative coronary artery bypass: adverse effects of emergency procedures (abstr). Circulation(suppl II) 1989;80:II-626.
17. Lytle BW, Loop FD, Cosgrove DM, et al. Fifteen hundred coronary reoperations: Results and determinant of early and late survival. J Thorac Cardiovasc Surg 1987;93:847–59.
18. Carrier M, Perreault L, Pettetier LC. Reoperation for coronary artery bypass grafting. In: Waters DD, Bourassa MG, eds. Care of the Patient with Previous Coronary Bypass Surgery. Philadelphia: FA Davis, 1991:257–263.
19. McNamara TO, Fisher JR. Thrombolysis of peripheral arterial and graft occlusions: improved results using high dose urokinase. AJR 1985;144:769–775.
20. Hartmann JR, McKeever LS, Stamato NJ, et al. Recanalization of chronically occluded aortocoronary saphenous vein bypass grafts by extended infusion of urokinase: initial results and short-term follow-up. J Am Coll Cardiol 1991;18:1517–23.

10

Adjunctive Thrombolysis in Angioplasty

Tyrone J. Collins

Ochsner Medical Institutions, New Orleans, Louisiana

I. INTRODUCTION

There are conflicting reports in the literature regarding the significance of intracoronary thrombus as a harbinger of potential complications associated with coronary angioplasty (1–11). The presence of intracoronary thrombi might reasonably be expected to predispose a traumatized endovascular surface to thrombotic occlusion. It is hypothesized that intraluminal thrombus associated with complex coronary stenosis and additional injury during angioplasty provides a substrate for the development of more thrombus and resultant thrombotic complications (Fig. 1).

Prior studies have demonstrated an increased incidence of angioplasty complications associated with unstable angina and complex coronary lesion morphology (1,3,4,7,10–13). Patients with unstable angina have been shown to have an increased incidence of intracoronary thrombi compared with stable angina patients (14–16).

The awareness that patients with intracoronary thrombus present with increased complications during percutaneous transluminal coronary angioplasty (PTCA) has led to the emergence of strategies to reduce this risk. The most commonly used technique has been the administration of intracoronary thrombolytic agents as an adjunct to balloon angioplasty (17). In this chapter, we will discuss the indications for, common methods of, and clinical

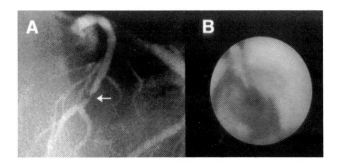

Figure 1 (A) Coronary angiogram demonstrating mid-LAD stenosis. (B) Angioscopic view of the stenotic area revealing thrombus. LAD = left artery descending.

use of adjunctive thrombolysis. We will not address two specific circumstances of adjunctive thrombolysis, namely, the treatment of occluded saphenous vein grafts and salvage therapy after abrupt occlusion, both of which are discussed in detail elsewhere in this book.

II. INDICATIONS

The adjunctive use of thrombolytic agents can either be prophylactic or therapeutic. The prophylactic intracoronary administration of lytics assumes that a high-risk group for intracoronary thrombus has been identified (without angiographic evidence of thrombus) and that treatment of the high-risk group will have a positive clinical outcome. Therapeutic use of intracoronary thrombolytic agents is indicated either before, during, or after angioplasty in patients determined to be at high risk for thrombotic complications. Its indications and clinical outcome can be determined by invasive assessment procedures.

A. Prophylactic Administration

It is important to understand that the mechanism by which lysis can affect clinical benefit is via clot dissolution. Although prophylactic therapy is intended for all patients in the high-risk subgroup, a percentage of these patients will not have thrombus and, therefore, cannot benefit from the thrombolytic therapy. If the percentage of patients without thrombus is high, the beneficial effect achieved in the minority of patients with thrombus will be diluted when the results of the entire group are analyzed. The stratification of patients in a high-risk subgroup to receive thrombolytic therapy (i.e., those with unstable angina) is one area where angioscopy may well have clinical utility to identify a group of patients with intracoronary thrombus much more accurately than angiography.

Another critical element in assessing the utility of prophylactic intracoronary lysis is the delivery of the agent. Successful lysis depends on the drug coming into direct contact with the thrombus over a period of time. Nonselective coronary administration and bolus dosing probably do not effectively deliver the drug to the thrombus and, therefore, are likely to be ineffective.

B. Therapeutic Administration

Therapeutic use of intracoronary thrombolytic agents in routine clinical applications is predicated on the angiographic identification of intracoronary thrombus either before, during, or after angioplasty. The outcome of therapeutic administration can be judged by angiographic improvement and the clinical outcome of the patients. However, angiography is an insensitive tool for identifying intracoronary thrombus, which limits its utility in identifying patients for lytic therapy and in quantifying any benefit achieved. While angioscopy is more sensitive than angiography and therefore a better tool, it is not commonly used.

The presence of intracoronary thrombus in acute ischemic syndromes, acute myocardial infarction, postmyocardial infarction angina, or unstable angina makes these patients at high risk for thrombotic complications of PTCA. The identification of intracoronary thrombus, angiographically or angioscopically, is justification for adjunctive thrombolysis.

C. Contraindications

The absolute contraindications for intracoronary lytic therapy include (1) prior treatment with streptokinase (if streptokinase is to be used again); (2) a known hypersensitivity to the agent; (3) coronary artery perforation; and (4) cardiac rupture or perforation.

Because the doses used for intracoronary thrombolysis are small, systemic thrombolysis usually does not occur. This makes the well-known contraindications to systemic thrombolysis—the increased risk of systemic bleeding complications in patients with a history of stroke, recent surgical procedures, major trauma, recent or active gastrointestinal bleeding, and other medical conditions predisposing the patient to bleeding complications—relative contraindications.

III. METHODS

A. Procedure and Instrumentation

A percutaneous femoral entry is the usual approach to obtain vascular access for PTCA and adjunctive intracoronary thrombolysis. Conventional

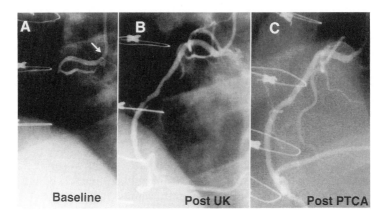

Figure 2   (A) Baseline angiogram. (B) After urokinase infusion via coronary catheter. (C) Final angiogram after PTCA.   UK = urokinase; PTCA = percutaneous transluminal coronary angioplasty.

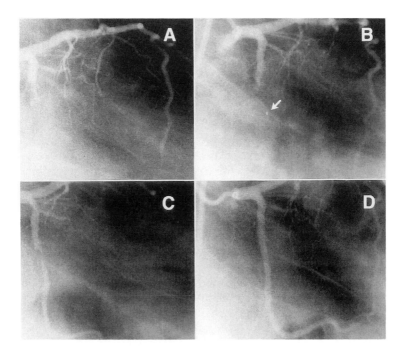

Figure 3   (A) Baseline angiogram. (B) Infusion catheter. (C) Postthrombosis. (D) Final angiogram after PTCA.   PTCA = percutaneous transluminal coronary angioplasty.

angioplasty techniques, premedication, and equipment are used. For native coronary arteries, a diagnostic or guiding catheter may be used to infuse thrombolytic agents (Fig. 2). The drug is administered by hand injection, by an infusion pump, or angiographic injector.

A more selective means of delivering the thrombolytic agent is via the central lumen of the PTCA catheter or an infusion catheter or wire (Fig. 3) placed in the target vessel. Under these circumstances, the proximal holes of the catheter or wire are positioned proximal to the culprit lesion. Position is obtained by advancing the catheter or wire over a 0.014-in. angioplasty wire. At our institution, we have commonly used a multihole 3-French catheter for this approach, but have also employed a hollow 0.035-in. infusion wire and other catheters and wires designed specifically for infusion purposes.

If thrombus has embolized distal to the angioplasty site, the angioplasty balloon catheter may be positioned across the dilated area and the wire removed for selective distal infusion of thrombolytic drug through the central lumen of the balloon. Alternatively, the drug may be given through the guiding catheter, leaving the balloon and/or wire across the lesion in the culprit artery. A third option would be to insert the infusion catheter. This catheter may be used to selectively treat embolization in the culprit artery or neighboring coronary artery.

The coronary angioplasty perfusion balloon catheter (Stack Perfusion, ACS, Mountain View, CA) allows lytic drug infusion through a balloon catheter, including the option of administering the lytic agent during balloon inflation (Fig. 4).

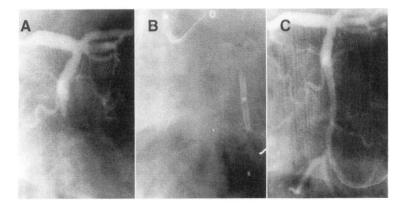

Figure 4   (A) Baseline. (B) Perfusion catheter inflated while r-tPA is administered. (C) Final angiogram.

The duration of the infusion is variable. One approach is to infuse a lytic drug for 20–40 min and then make an angiographic assessment. If the thrombus has been dissolved, the infusion may be terminated. However, in some cases a prolonged infusion (4–24 h) continuing outside of the catheterization laboratory is desirable (Fig. 5). In this case, the catheters must be clearly labeled and secured in place before moving the patient from the catheterization laboratory.

In our laboratory, we first attach 12-in. tubing to all infusion ports to ensure that the catheter bodies remain sterile after they are covered with sterile towels and a clear plastic adherent dressing. We then suture the catheters and sheath in place, taking special care not to kink the catheters. We usually split the infusion between guiding catheter and an intracoronary infusion catheter. The total infusion rate can be delivered in equal amounts via the

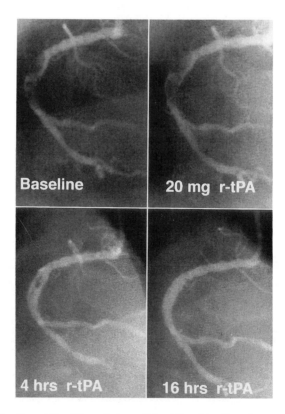

Figure 5   Baseline. After 20-mg bolus r-tPA. After 4 h of continuous r-tPA. After 16 h of continuous r-tPA;angioplasty was not necessary.

catheter and infusion ports or in unequal amounts, with the bulk of the drug being given through the distal (intracoronary) port closest to the thrombus.

Because it is important that patients remain in a supine position to minimize the risk of catheter dislodgement, we liberally prescribe analgesics and sedative/hypnotics for their comfort and sedation. We also administer a heparin infusion to maintain systemic anticoagulation. Patients should be closely monitored in an intensive care setting during the infusion because of the risk for bleeding, including groin hematoma.

B. Administration of the Thrombolytic Agent

The thrombolytic agents available for intracoronary administration are streptokinase, recombinant tissue-type plasminogen activator (rt-PA), and urokinase. The dosage, route, and duration of administration will vary according to the agent used. While early attempts to perform adjunctive thrombolytic therapy were based upon intravenous administration, most investigators now advocate intracoronary administration. The recommendation for intracoronary thrombolysis is based upon increased success rates while using less drug, thereby achieving the desired result faster with less cost and fewer complications.

1. Streptokinase

Streptokinase, the first thrombolytic agent used, is a single-chain polypeptide produced by hemolytic streptococci that must bind with plasminogen to form an activator to convert plasminogen to plasmin. As a foreign protein, it is potentially antigenic, and if a patient has significant levels of streptococcal antibodies present, allergic reactions may result and the streptokinase may be inactivated (18–21).

In 1981, Rentrop and coworkers were among the first to report their experience documenting the efficacy of administering streptokinase directly into the coronary artery during acute myocardial infarction (22). At a mean dose of $67,300 \pm 63,200$ IU of intracoronary streptokinase, Myer and associates reported successful PTCA results in patients with acute myocardial infarction (23). It has been recommended that the total dose of intracoronary streptokinase administered should not exceed 200,000 IU to avoid a systemic lytic effect (22,24). Adjunctive intracoronary streptokinase has been successfully administered in bolus doses of 10,000 to 20,000 IU and a continuous infusion rate of 2000 IU/min (17,22–27).

In comparing intracoronary streptokinase (2000 IU/min) and urokinase (6000 U/min) (28), there was no significant difference in the time to opening thrombosed coronary arteries. There also was no difference in the baseline serum fibrinogen values among the two groups. However, after treatment, 66% of the streptokinase-treated patients had serum fibrinogen levels below

100 mg/dl, compared to only 6% of the urokinase-treated patients ($p<$ 0.001). This appeared to correlate well with bleeding complications, which occurred in 29% of the streptokinase patients compared to only 11% of the urokinase group ($p<0.05$) (28).

2. Recombinant Tissue-Type Plasminogen Activator (rt-PA)

Tissue plasminogen activator, a human protein produced by normal vascular endothelium, is clinically available as a recombinant product (rt-PA). It differs from both urokinase and streptokinase in that it is bound by fibrin and, therefore, potentially acts selectively on clot-bound plasminogen. The recommended dose of intravenous rt-PA (Activase®, Genentech, South San Francisco, CA) for acute myocardial infarction is 100 mg. Selective intracoronary treatment with this drug employs a smaller dose. Adjunctive, intracoronary administration of 10–110 mg of rt-PA has been reported in patients with acute myocardial infarction or unstable angina undergoing PTCA. Bolus doses of 0.5–20 mg have been followed by infusions of 0.04–2.0 mg/min (29–35). It has been calculated that the intracoronary concentration of rt-PA necessary for effective thrombolysis is 2.0 μg/ml plasma concentration (30,35).

3. Urokinase

Urokinase (Abokinase®, Abbott Laboratories, Abbott, IL) is probably the most widely used agent for adjunctive intracoronary thrombolysis. It is a human protein and has no antigenic properties. It differs from streptokinase by acting directly on plasminogen to form plasmin. Infusion rates ranging from 2000 to 20,000 U/min (up to 1,000,000 U total dosage) have been reported (36–41). The drug is administered over 15 min or longer. Our practice has been to administer urokinase at rates of 1000–4000 U/min for 30 min, after an initial intracoronary bolus of 5000–25,000 U. If a longer infusion is necessary, we infuse urokinase through two ports (1000 U/min via the guide or diagnostic catheter, and 1000–3000 U/min via an infusion catheter) (Table 1).

Table 1 Urokinase: Ochsner Method (1,000,000 U/250 cc NS = 4000 U UK/cc)

Mixture (UK U/h)	Rate (cc/h)	Equivalent dosage (U/min)
1000	15	60,000
2000	30	120,000
3000	45	180,000
4000	60	240,000

UK = urokinase.

IV. CLINICAL RESULTS

A. Acute Myocardial Infarction

Intravenous thrombolysis has largely replaced intracoronary lysis as a treatment for acute myocardial infarction, primarily due to the ease and rapidity of administration without the requirement for a catheterization laboratory. However, there is a role for intracoronary thrombolysis as an adjunct to balloon angioplasty in patients with acute myocardial infarction who have angiographic evidence of occlusive or subocclusive thrombus after intravenous thrombolysis or during direct angioplasty.

Early reports of adjunctive thrombolytic therapy demonstrated the efficacy of combined mechanical (PTCA) and lytic (streptokinase or urokinase) therapy in patients with acute myocardial infarction and intracoronary thrombus (42–47). Hartzler and coworkers (44) reported the results of intracoronary streptokinase as an adjunct to PTCA in 41 patients. Total occlusions were present in 29 patients and subtotal occlusions were present in 12 patients undergoing emergency cardiac catheterization. They administered a 10,000-U bolus followed by 2000 U/min for 15–60 min. Successful recanalization was obtained in 85% (35/41) of the patients.

In another early study, 66 consecutive patients with acute myocardial infarction were treated in four treatment arms: (a) PTCA alone ($n = 11$); (2) PTCA followed by intracoronary streptokinase infusion ($n = 15$); (3) intracoronary streptokinase alone ($n = 11$); and (4) intracoronary streptokinase followed by PTCA ($n = 29$) (45). They found that the need for subsequent revascularization was significantly higher in the group receiving streptokinase alone (82%) than those in whom either PTCA or PTCA and streptokinase (<30%) was administered. They found that in patients with large residual clot burdens or those in whom the initial PTCA was unsuccessful, streptokinase resulted in further angiographic improvement in all except one patient.

B. Unstable Angina

Clinical studies have documented the increased risk of occlusive complications when intracoronary thrombus is identified periprocedurally with PTCA (1–3). Using intracoronary angioscopy in 122 patients undergoing PTCA, we found that angiography significantly underestimated the incidence of intracoronary thrombi (48). Intracoronary thrombus was also more commonly associated with the more complex AHA/ACC type B and C lesions compared to the less complex type A lesions. We found that *angioscopic* thrombus was associated with either a major complication or a recurrent ischemic event after PTCA (relative risk 3.11, 95% CI 1.28–7.60, $p = 0.01$) and that *angiographic* thrombi were not associated with these complications (relative risk 0.85, 95% CI 0.36–2.00, $p = 0.91$). When compared with clinical variables (i.e., age, sex, unstable angina, and stable angina) or angiographic morphology (i.e., thrombus or AHA/ACC lesion criteria), angioscopic intracoronary thrombus was most strongly associated with in-hospital adverse events following PTCA (Fig. 6).

The use of intracoronary urokinase as an adjunct to PTCA in patients with unstable angina has proven to be beneficial in several reports (49,50). Pavlides and associates (49) treated 80 patients (before abrupt closure) with intracoronary urokinase and PTCA and compared the results to a matched control group ($n = 167$) that did not receive urokinase. The endpoints that were compared were procedural success rates and the occurrence of a cardiac event. Patients with intracoronary thrombus treated with urokinase infusions benefited most, with cardiac events occurring in 3% of the urokinase-treated group versus 19% in the control group ($p = 0.07$). They noted that patients with intimal dissections had more adverse cardiac events (21%) when treated with urokinase than did the control group (9%) ($p = 0.1$). Surprisingly, more patients in the control group required blood transfusions but the difference did not achieve statistical significance.

In a nonrandomized trial of intracoronary urokinase before and after PTCA in 74 patients with medically refractory acute ischemic syndromes

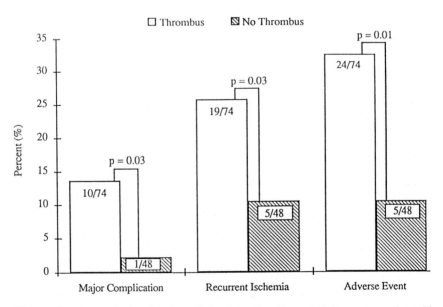

Figure 6 Bar graph showing the relationship of angioscopic intracoronary thrombi to in-hospital adverse angioplasty outcomes.

[crescendo unstable angina ($n = 33$) and early postmyocardial infarction angina ($n = 41$)], Anwar and coworkers (50) reported a 100% procedural success and a 7-month event-free survival of 78%. Their technique was to selectively infuse 250,000 U of urokinase, half before and half after balloon angioplasty. In six patients, an additional infusion of 250,000 U of urokinase was given after balloon angioplasty for the angiographic appearance of intracoronary thrombus. After the procedure, patients were maintained on a heparin infusion for 3 days. There were no serious bleeding complications and the mean nadir fibrinogen level in their patients was 273 ± 47 mg/dL.

C. Intracoronary Thrombus

The therapeutic use of intracoronary thrombolysis as an adjunct to PTCA in the setting of angiographic intracoronary thrombi has been very encouraging. Vaitkus and his associates (51) described 27 patients with angiographic intracoronary thrombi treated with urokinase. They delivered a mean dose of 245,100 U of urokinase over 6–75 min. One of the most important variables in predicting which patients would have successful procedures was the rate at which the urokinase was infused. Patients given at least 140,000 U of urokinase within 50 min had fewer angioplasty-related complications than patients receiving a slower rate of infusion over a longer time.

Excellent results for adjunctive intracoronary thrombolysis were reported in 27 patients with angiographic intracoronary thrombus and nine patients with distal embolization (52). Twenty-seven patients had intracoronary thrombus, 26 of whom had thrombus visualized prior to PTCA. Intracoronary urokinase was administered at a dose of 250,000–1,000,000 U (mean 429,100 U) and complete angiographic lysis was obtained in 23 (88%) of 26 patients. Nine patients with distal embolization after PTCA were treated with an average dose of 472,000 U of urokinase. Successful lysis of the embolus occurred in 8 (89%) of 9 patients.

In another report of adjunctive intracoronary thrombolysis. Chapekis and colleagues (53) reported the results of prolonged infusions of urokinase in 17 patients with native coronary artery thrombus. Urokinase was administered as a bolus dose of 120,000 U followed by a multilevel infusion for 18–24 h. Successful lysis of the intracoronary thrombus occurred in 16 of 17 (94%) patients. There were no major complications associated with this technique of prolonged infusion of intracoronary urokinase.

Finally, there is a report describing the treatment of large (> 2 cm) intracoronary thrombi with adjunctive lysis. Grill and Brinker (54) reported a 50% success rate for intracoronary streptokinase (300,000–500,000 IU) given over 60 min in this unusual group of patients. The average duration of symptoms in these patients suggested that the thrombus had been present for longer than 2 weeks (16 days). The age of the thrombus and the use of streptokinase may be the explanation for the relatively low rate of successful lysis. Another important factor is that these patients had a large volume of intracoronary thrombus, which may not have been completely lysed with only a 60-min infusion and may have achieved a higher rate of success had the infusion been continued longer.

IV. SUMMARY

Elective percutaneous transluminal coronary angioplasty enjoys an excellent primary success rate. However, subgroups of "high-risk" patients, namely, those with acute coronary syndromes such as unstable angina and acute myocardial infarction, have been identified and are associated with the presence of intracoronary thrombus. Selective intracoronary infusions of thrombolytic agents are effective in removing coronary thrombi and appear to increase the success rate of PTCA in these high-risk patients. Intracoronary thrombolysis may be accomplished at lower doses than are required for effective intravenous therapy and, therefore, are associated with fewer bleeding complications.

Further studies are needed to determine the role of prophylactic administration of intracoronary lytic agents in patients at high risk for complications and to determine the optimal therapeutic regime including the thrombolytic agent of choice, dosage level, route of administration, and duration of therapy.

REFERENCES

1. Mabin TA, Homes DR, Smith HC, et al. Intracoronary thrombus: role in coronary occlusion complicating percutaneous transluminal coronary angioplasty. J Am Coll Cardiol 1985;5:198–202.
2. Sugrue DD, Holmes DR Jr, Smith HC, et al. Coronary artery thrombus as a risk factor for acute vessel occlusion during percutaneous transluminal coronary angioplasty: improving results. Br Heart J 1986;56:62–66.
3. Ellis SG, Roubin GS, King SB III, et al. Angiographic and clinical predictors of acute closure after native vessel coronary angioplasty. Circulation 1988;77:372–379.
4. de Feyter PJ, van den Brand M, Jaarman G, et al. Acute coronary occlusion during and after percutaneous transluminal coronary angioplasty. Frequency, prediction, clinical course, management, and follow-up. Circulation 1991;83:927–936.
5. Simpfendorfer C, Belardi J, Bellamy G, et al. Frequency, management and follow-up of patients with acute coronary occlusions after percutaneous transluminal coronary angioplasty. Am J Cardiol 1987;59:267–269.
6. Detre KM, Holmes DR Jr, Holubkov R, et al. Incidence and consequences of periprocedural occlusion. The 1985–1986 National Heart, Lung and Blood Institute Percutaneous Transluminal Coronary Angioplasty Registry. Circulation 1990;82:739–750.

7. de Feyter PJ, Suryapranata H, Serruys PW, et al. Coronary angioplasty for unstable angina: Immediate and late results in 200 consecutive patients with identification of risk factors for unfavorable early and late outcome. J Am Coll Cardiol 1988;12:324–333.

8. Sinclair IN, McCabe CH, Sipperly ME, et al. Predictors, therapeutic options and long-term outcome of abrupt reclosure. Am J Cardiol 1988;61:61G–66G.

9. Bredlau CE, Roubin GS, Leimbruber PP, et al. In-hospital morbidity and mortality in patients undergoing elective coronary angioplasty. Circulation 1985;72: 1044–1052.

10. Ellis SG, Roubin GS, King SB III, et al. In-hospital cardiac mortality after acute closure after coronary angioplasty: analysis of risk factors from 8207 procedures. J Am Coll Cardiol 1988;11:211–216.

11. de Feyter PJ, de Jaegere PPT, Murphy ES, et al. Abrupt coronary artery occlusion during percutaneous coronary angiplasty. Am Heart J 1992;123:1634–1642.

12. Ellis SG, Vandormael MG, Cowley MJ, et al. Coronary morphologic and clinical determinants of procedural outcome with angioplasty for multivessel coronary disease: implications for patient selection. Circulation 1990;82:1193–1202.

13. de Feyter PJ. Coronary angioplasty for unstable angina. Am Heart J 1989;118: 860–868.

14. Ramee SR, White CJ, Collins TJ, et al. Percutaneous angioscopy during coronary angioplasty using a steerable microangioscope. J Am Coll Cardiol 1991; 17:100–105.

15. Sherman CT, Litvack F, Grundfest W, et al. Coronary angioscopy in patients with unstable angina pectoris. N Engl J Med 1986;315:913–919.

16. Mizuno K, Satomura K, Miyamoto A, et al. Angioscopic evaluation of coronary-artery thrombi in acute coronary syndromes. N Engl J Med 1992;326:287–291.

17. Suryapranata H, DeFeyter PJ, Serruys PW. Coronary angioplasty in patients with unstable angina pectoris: Is there a role for thrombolysis? J Am Coll Cardiol 1988;12:69A–77A.

18. Baumgartner TG, Davis RG. Streptokinase induced anaphylactic reaction. Clin Pharmacol 1982;1:470–471.

19. Totty WG, Romano T, Benian GM, et al. Serum sickness following streptokinase therapy. AJR 1982;138:143–144.

20. van Breda A, Katzen BT. Thrombolytic therapy of peripheral vascular disease. Sem Intervent Radiol 1985;2:354–368.

21. Weatherbee TC, Esterbrooks DJ, Katz DA, et al. Serum sickness following selective intracoronary streptokinase. Curr Ther Res 1984;35:433–438.

22. Rentrop P, Blanke H, Karsch KR, et al. Selective intracoronary thrombolysis in acute myocardial infarction and unstable angina pectoris. Circulation 1981; 63:307–317.

23. Meyer J, Merx W, Schmitz H, et al. Percutaneous transluminal coronary angioplasty immediately after intracoronary streptolysis of transmural myocardial infarction. Circulation 1982;66:905–913.

24. Six AJ, Brommer EJP, Muller EJ, et al. Activation of the fibrinolytic system during intracoronary streptokinase administration. J Am Coll Cardiol 1987;9: 189–196.

25. Ambrose JA, Hjemdahl-Monsen C, Borrico S, et al. Quantitative and qualitative effects of intracoronary streptokinase in unstable angina and non-Q wave infarction. J Am Coll Cardiol 1987;8:1156–1165.
26. Grill HP, Brinker JA. Nonacute thrombolytic therapy: an adjunct to coronary angioplasty in patients with large intravascular thrombi. Am Heart J 1989;118: 662–667.
27. Vetrovec GW, Leinbach RC, Gold HK, et al. Intracoronary thrombolysis in syndromes of unstable ischemia: angiographic and clinical results. Am Heart J 1982;104:946–952.
28. Tennant SN, Dixon J, Venable TC, et al. Intracoronary thrombolysis in patients with acute myocardial infarction: comparison of the efficacy of urokinase with streptokinase. Circulation 1984;69:756–760.
29. Berghofer G, Kokott N, Loos D, et al. rt-PA intracoronarily in acute myocardial infarction with and without prior IV application. Fibrinolysis 1990;4(suppl 1):31.
30. Ruocco NA, Currier JW, Jacobs AK, et al. Experience with low-dose intracoronary recombinant tissue-type plasminogen activator for nonacute total occlusions before percutaneous transluminal coronary angioplasty. Am J Cardiol 1991;68:1609–1613.
31. Tiefenbrunn AJ. Tissue-type plasminogen activator: intracoronary applications. Cathet Cardiovasc Diagn 1990;19:108–115.
32. Samaha JK, Quigley P, Kereiakes DJ, et al. Intracoronary thrombolytic therapy in patients with refractory thrombus after intravenous treatment (abstr). J Am Coll Cardiol 1989;13:92A.
33. DiSciascio G, Kohli RS, Goudreau E, et al. Intracoronary recombinant tissue-type plasminogen activator in unstable angina: A pilot angiographic study. Am Heart J 1991;122:1–6.
34. Pitney MR, Cumpston N, Mews GC, et al. Use of twenty-four hour infusions of intracoronary tissue plasminogen activator to increase the application of coronary angioplasty. Cathet Cardiovasc Diagn 1992;26:255–259.
35. Johns JA, Gold HK, Leinbach RC, et al. Prevention of coronary artery reocclusion and reduction in late coronary artery stenosis after thrombolytic therapy in patients with acute myocardial infarction. A randomized study of maintenance infusion of recombinant human tissue-type plasminogen activator. Circulation 1988;78:546–556.
36. Neuhaus KL, Tebbe U, Gottwik M, et al. Intravenous recombinant tissue plasminogen activator (rt-PA) and urokinase in acute myocardial infarction: results of the German activator urokinase study (GAUS). J Am Coll Cardiol 1988;12: 581–587.
37. Verna E, Repetto S, Boscarini M, et al. Management of complicated coronary angioplasty by intracoronary urokinase and immediate re-angioplasty. Cathet Cardiovasc Diagn 1990;19:116–122.
38. Goudreau E, DiSciascio G, Vetrovec GW, et al. Intracoronary urokinase as an adjunct to percutaneous transluminal coronary angioplasty in patients with complex coronary narrowings or angioplasty-induced complications. Am J Cardiol 1992;69:57–62.

39. Jain A, Ramee SR, Mesa J, et al. Intracoronary thrombus: chronic urokinase infusion and evaluation with intravascular ultrasound. Cathet Cardiovasc Diagn 1992;26:212–214.
40. Schieman G, Cohen BM, Kozina J, et al. Intracoronary urokinase for intracoronary thrombus accumulation complicating percutaneous transluminal coronary angioplasty in acute ischemic syndromes. Circulation 1990;82:2052–2060.
41. Cernigliaro C, Sansa M, Bongo AS, et al. Clinical experience with urokinase in intracoronary thrombolysis. Clin Cardiol 1987;10:222.
42. Goldberg S, Urban PL, Greenspon A, et al. Combination therapy for evolving myocardial infarction: intracoronary thrombolysis and percutaneous transluminal angioplasty. Am J Med 1982;72:994–997.
43. Gold HK, Cowley MJ, Palacios IF, et al. Combined intracoronary streptokinase infusion and coronary angioplasty during acute myocardial infarction. Am J Cardiol 1984;53:122C–125C.
44. Hartzler GO, Rutherford BD, McConahay DR, et al. Percutaneous transluminal coronary angioplasty with and without thrombolytic therapy for treatment of acute myocardial infarction. Am Heart J 1983;106:965–973.
45. Holmes DR, Smith HC, Vlietstra RE, et al. Percutaneous transluminal coronary angioplasty, alone or in combination with streptokinase therapy, during acute myocardial infarction. Mayo Clin Proc 1985;60:449–456.
46. Kitazume H, Iwama T, Suzuki A. Combined thrombolytic therapy and coronary angioplasty for acute myocardial infarction. Am Heart J 1985;111:826–832.
47. Yasuno M, Saito Y, Ishida M, et al. Effects of percutaneous transluminal coronary angioplasty: intracoronary thrombolysis with urokinase in acute myocardial infarction. Am J Cardiol 1984;53:1217–1220.
48. White CJ, Ramee SR, Collins TJ, et al. Angioscopically detected coronary thrombus correlates with adverse PTCA outcome (abstr). Circulation 1993;88(suppl IV):IV-3206.
49. Pavlides GS, Schreiber TL, Gangadharan V, et al. Safety and efficacy of urokinase during elective coronary angioplasty. Am Heart J 1991;121:731–737.
50. Anwar A, Myler RK, Nguyen K, et al. Combined coronary angioplasty, urokinase and heparin in the treatment of acute ischemic syndromes. J Invas Cardiol 1991;3:41–48.
51. Vaitkus PT, Hermann HC, Laskey WK. Management and immediate outcome of patients with intracoronary thrombus during percutaneous transluminal coronary angioplasty. Am Heart J 1992;124:1–8.
52. Goudreau E, DiSciasio G, Vetrovec GW, et al. Intracoronary urokinase as an adjunct to percutaneous transluminal angioplasty in patients with complex coronary narrowings or angioplasty-induced complications. Am J Cardiol 1992;69:57–62.
53. Chapekis AT, George BS, Candela RJ. Rapid thrombus dissolution by continuous infusion of urokinase through an intracoronary perfusion wire prior to and following PTCA: results in native coronaries and patent saphenous vein grafts. Cathet Cardiovasc Diagn 1991;23:89–92.
54. Grill HP, Brinker JA. Nonacute thrombolytic therapy: an adjunct to coronary angioplasty in patients with large intravascular thrombi. Am Heart J 1989;118:662–666.

11

Supported Coronary Angioplasty

John S. Wilson and E. Magnus Ohman
Duke University Medical Center, Durham, North Carolina

I. INTRODUCTION

The use of percutaneous revascularization procedures has grown explosively during the last decade. Originally used mostly in patients with relatively stable coronary artery disease, they are now being applied during the acute phase of myocardial infarction and in patients with unstable angina. Because percutaneous interventions are now being used in patients with unstable symptoms and severely reduced left ventricular function, including cardiogenic shock, there is a need to understand the relative strengths and weaknesses of a variety of support devices available to the interventional cardiologist. This chapter will summarize the existing knowledge of percutaneous devices that can be used acutely, prophylactically, or on a standby basis.

II. INDICATIONS FOR PERCUTANEOUS INTERVENTION

The spectrum of clinical instability that the angioplasty operator may encounter stretches from cardiogenic shock and impending death to stable symptoms in "high-risk" patients scheduled for percutaneous interventions. The "high-risk" clinical features include left ventricular dysfunction or dilatation of vessel(s) supplying >50% of viable myocardium. In patients with cardiogenic shock the goal is to stabilize the patient to sufficiently restore patency or blood flow to the infarcted area by either percutaneous transluminal coronary angioplasty (PTCA) or coronary artery bypass grafting (CABG) (2). Although the mortality in cardiogenic shock is approximately 70% (3), the patients in whom revascularization is performed have a substantial improvement in in-hospital survival (2,4). The knowledge of the variety of support devices is critical in this setting.

For patients with scheduled procedures, the relative benefit-to-risk ratio of medical therapy, CABG, or percutaneous interventions can be more easily assessed. Various definitions have been used to describe patients at "high risk" for coronary intervention. In the past, high-risk characteristics included advanced age, multivessel disease, multiple lesions to dilate, prior coronary artery bypass grafting, poor left ventricular function, and left main stenosis as the target lesion (5). Today, the majority of patients considered "high risk" have significantly depressed left ventricular function and/or a lesion(s) in vessels supplying a substantial amount of myocardium. The common thread in all these definitions is that patients would not be expected to tolerate balloon or device occlusion of the vessel or abrupt closure during or following the procedure. A useful analogy can be drawn between ischemia during angioplasty in the high-risk patient and the pathophysiology of cardiogenic shock. Although actual cellular necrosis is not part of the initial insult during PTCA, ischemic left ventricular dysfunction can be quite significant and the dramatic and downward spiral seen in cardiogenic shock may ensue in this high-risk population as well. Once hypotension results, coronary perfusion pressure may be inadequate to restore flow to the ischemic myocardium and further left ventricular dysfunction may occur despite deflation of the balloon.

Unfortunately, it remains difficult to accurately predict which patients will be hemodynamically intolerant of PTCA, develop abrupt closure, or die. In an overview from the literature of approximately 25,000 patients undergoing angioplasty in North America, the overall mortality rate was only 0.7% (6). The patient characteristics that independently correlated with a higher in-hospital mortality were cardiogenic shock or heart failure, older age, and female gender. Anatomical correlates with mortality were depressed left ventricular function and multivessel coronary artery disease. The most important post-PTCA characteristic that has been found to be related to a higher in-hospital mortality is abrupt closure of the dilated coronary artery segment, which had an incidence of approximately 6.7% when data on nearly 9000 patients were combined (6). Unstable angina and multivessel coronary artery disease were independent predictors of abrupt closure, as were certain lesion characteristics, branch point lesion, lesion length >20 mm, thrombus, total occlusion, and multiple lesions dilated. The post-PTCA characteristic associated with a higher rate of abrupt closure was dissection of the coronary artery segment.

Ellis and coworkers (7) have built on the experience of a coronary jeopardy score developed by Califf and colleagues (8). The jeopardy score was derived by ascribing a point score to each segment dilated that supplies an area of equal size myocardium that would become akinetic in the event of abrupt closure. A maximum score is reached when all coronary segments supplying functional myocardium are dilated. Thus, a score >3 would be applied if >50% of viable myocardium were dilated. In Ellis' observations, the in-hospital mortality was >10% with a >2.5 jeopardy score and 4% with an ejection fraction <25%. The latter characteristic did not contribute independently to in-hospital mortality. The National Registry of Elective Supported Angioplasty suggested indications for the use of cardiopulmonary support in high-risk patients (9). These included ejection fractions <25% and/or target vessel supplying >50% of the myocardium. While these appear to be useful and somewhat conservative guidelines, it became clear in subsequent patients that "standby use" of cardiopulmonary support could be prescribed in a large number of patients without serious sequelae (10). Risk stratification before, during, and after the decision to use support devices needs to incorporate many of the described characteristics. The use of the support device would also need to incorporate the relative risks and complications of the device used. In addition, the selection of a support device will depend on the operator experience with each technique.

III. SYSTEMIC SUPPORT TECHNIQUES AND APPLICATIONS

Various methods and devices developed to "support" the heart and patient during interventions are listed in Table 1. The methods of "local" coronary support include those of anterograde support (autoperfusion balloons) (11,12), distal coronary hemoperfusion (13,14), perfluorocarbon perfusion (15,16), and retrograde support via the coronary sinus (17–19). In this chapter we will focus on systemic support techniques and applications. These include intra-aortic balloon pump counterpulsation, percutaneous cardiopulmonary support, the hemopump, and partial left heart bypass.

A. Intra-Aortic Balloon Counterpulsation

Since its development in the early 1960s (20) and introduction into clinical practice in 1968 (21), intra-aortic balloon counterpulsation (IABP) has gained widespread acceptance. Between 75,000 and 80,000 intra-aortic balloon pumps are inserted each year in the United States alone (22). The main advantages over other support devices are its ease of insertion and widespread availability. The IABP is limited, however, by its dependence on a stable rhythm and some basal cardiac output, as well as by the relatively modest

Table 1 Support Strategies

Coronary (local) Support
  Anterograde local support
    Auto perfusion
      Bailout balloon
      Perfusion balloon
      Temporary stent
    Distal coronary hemoperfusion
    Perfluorocarbon coronary perfusion
  Retrograde local support
    Synchronized coronary sinus retroperfusion
Systemic Support
  Intra-aortic balloon counterpulsation (IABP)
  Cardiopulmonary support (CPS)
  Hemopump
  Partial left heart bypass

hemodynamic effects that it produces. In addition, complications occur in 9–43% (22–24), consisting mainly of limb ischemia, vascular damage requiring repair, and embolic phenomena.

The intra-aortic balloon pump, usually placed in the descending aorta percutaneously via the femoral artery, inflates during diastole and deflates during systole, reducing left ventricular afterload and myocardial oxygen consumption. The IABP may also augment diastolic coronary perfusion, though this is somewhat controversial (see below). The overall hemodynamic effects include a decrease in both peak systolic and end-diastolic left ventricular pressure with a rather large increase in overall aortic diastolic pressure and no change or a slight increase in mean aortic pressure. Pulmonary capillary wedge pressure and left ventricular end-diastolic pressure will decrease by 10–20% while cardiac output may rise 10–40% (22). The major advantages and disadvantages of the balloon pump are presented in Table 2.

The ability of the IABP to augment diastolic perfusion of the coronary arteries has been examined extensively. Fuchs and colleagues, in an early clinical study of seven patients with refractory unstable angina and critical proximal LAD stenosis, demonstrated a good correlation between changes in great cardiac vein blood flow and IABP-augmented aortic mean diastolic pressure (25). The investigators were unable, however, to determine how much of this flow was secondary to contribution by collaterals. Williams and coworkers could not ascribe relief of angina in their six patients with IABP to an increase in regional coronary blood flow and felt that the most likely mechanism was reduction in myocardial oxygen consumption by systolic unloading of the ventricle (26). More recently, three studies have examined

Table 2 Intra-Aortic Balloon Counterpulsation

Advantages
  Displacement not catastrophic
  Pulsatile flow
  FDA approved
  Ability to place in >90%
  Full heparinization not required
  Perfusion technician unnecessary
  Long-term use (weeks)
  May augment coronary perfusion
  Percutaneous
  Small size (10.5–9.5 French)
  Rapid insertion
Disadvantages
  Synchronization with rhythm necessary
  Dependent on LV function
  May not augment coronary perfusion with critical stenoses
  Complications in 9–43%
  Relatively modest hemodynamic effects
  May cause hemolysis/thrombocytopenia
  Contraindicated with aortic insufficiency

IABP augmentation of coronary flow after PTCA. Although MacDonald and colleagues failed to show significant coronary perfusion pressure augmentation by IABP distal to a stenosis, the measurements were made through the central lumen of the PTCA balloon catheter, which may itself hamper blood flow (27). Ishihara and colleagues, using a 3-French coronary Doppler catheter, demonstrated no change in mean coronary flow but did show an increase in peak coronary flow (28). They suggested that this increase in peak velocity of flow rather than in mean flow may have a beneficial effect on reducing reocclusion after coronary angioplasty, a clinical finding demonstrated by others. Recently, Kern and coworkers, utilizing a 0.018-in. Doppler-tipped angioplasty guidewire, demonstrated an increase in both mean and peak coronary blood flow velocity after angioplasty, which was further augmented by the IABP (29). Importantly, there was no significant augmentation prior to dilatation of the critical stenoses. While unloading of the ventricle may reduce ischemia somewhat, PTCA is necessary to maximize the effects of the IABP. In combination, these results may in part help to explain the beneficial effects of IABP in patients with acute myocardial infarction in preventing reocclusion after successful reperfusion (26,28,30–32) and in the improved survival in patients with cardiogenic shock treated with both IABP and revascularization as compared with IABP alone (4).

No randomized trials have evaluated the use of intra-aortic balloon pumping to support high-risk angioplasty. There are, however, four small retrospective studies, each with slightly different definitions of high-risk features, that show reasonable success rates with the use of IABP (17,33–35). These are summarized in Table 3. The two earlier studies (17,34) were performed prior to the availability of perfusion balloon catheters which may further enhance the performance of high-risk angioplasty in conjunction with IABP.

An interesting observation about IABP as a support device for angioplasty is its potential benefit following a successful procedure. Although balloon counterpulsation may not alter diastolic coronary blood flow beyond critical stenoses, following reperfusion with thrombolytic therapy or successful angioplasty there may indeed be augmentation of this coronary flow.

Intra-aortic balloon counterpulsation has also been used for hemodynamic support in patients who have had unsuccessful PTCA or abrupt closure following PTCA (36,37). An interesting study by Jones and coworkers reviewed 777 patients undergoing PTCA and 2068 patients who underwent CABG (37). In the group of patients who developed ST-T changes with chest pain after PTCA, all 12 patients who did not have intra-aortic balloon pumping developed Q-waves after coronary artery bypass surgery compared with 2 of 8 in whom IABP support was used prior to surgery. Three other studies showed hemodynamic stabilization and some resolution of EKG changes with the institution of the IABP (34,36). It is important to note that intra-aortic balloon counterpulsation has very little, if any, role in patients with cardiac arrest in the absence of cardiac output or an intrinsic rhythm (38).

Intra-aortic balloon counterpulsation may be useful in patients with hemodynamic instability undergoing interventional procedures. In addition, it may allow for a longer balloon inflation by ventricular unloading and may serve as a useful bridge in patients who have had failed angioplasty or complications of the procedure requiring urgent surgery. It is unclear what the precise role of IABP is in high-risk patients with stable hemodynamics undergoing angioplasty. Patients who have previously demonstrated instability with balloon inflation in the same lesion certainly would be suitable for IABP support. In addition, ventricular unloading may be beneficial in patients with poor left ventricular function. Certainly a reasonable option in many situations is to gain arterial access with a small diameter sheath in the opposite groin prior to any intervention. If the patient has any instability, the balloon pump can be immediately inserted. Present evidence also supports the idea that prophylactic IABP use after successful intervention may decrease the incidence of abrupt closure with an acceptably low complication rate.

Table 3 IABP Before High-Risk PTCA

	n	Mean F/U (months)	Lesion success	IABP Comp (%)		Events (%)			
						Death	MI	CABG	Repeat intervention
Alcan (1983) (34)	9	NA	9/9	33	In-hospital	11	NA	11	NA
					Follow-up			NA	NA
Szatmary (1988) (17)	16	22	27/30	0	In-hospital	6	0	0	0
					Follow-up			6	6
Voudris (1990) (35)	27	13.1	39/39	4	In-hospital	0	0	0	0
					Follow-up			4	22
Kahn (1990) (33)	28	NA	90/94	11	In-hospital	7	0	0	NA
					Follow-up			NA	NA

NA = not available; IABP = intra-aortic balloon counterpulsion; MI = myocardial infarction; CABG = coronary artery bypass grafting.

1. Aortic Counterpulsation Catheter Insertion Technique

Percutaneous insertion of IABP is best performed using the Seldinger technique through the femoral artery. Other access sites can include the left axillary or subclavian arteries, but using these sites usually requires the assistance of a vascular surgeon. In smaller patients or those with some degree of peripheral vascular disease sheathless insertion is preferable. This reduces the access hole and flow limitation in the iliac artery from 10.5–9.5 French. Observational series have suggested that using this technique can reduce the incidence of limb ischemia without increasing the risk for hemorrhagic complications (39). In obese patients, the standard approach using the 10.5-F sheath with the IABP catheter is preferable as kinking of the catheter can otherwise occur through the long subcutaneous path.

2. Advantages and Disadvantages of Aortic Counterpulsation

In experienced hands percutaneous insertions of IABP can be performed in less than 5 min. This is, therefore, the fastest support technique that can be instituted in the cardiac catheterization laboratory or in other acute care facilities. Figure 1 shows the console. Major complications of IABP occur infrequently and reflect the patient's acuity during the insertion. The complication rate from elective insertion varies from 0–11% in more recent series (23,33,40). The complication rate is considerably higher in the setting of cardiogenic shock or other emergencies. This may be due in part to the fact that patients requiring emergency insertions also have a higher prevalence of risk factors that predispose to complications. These risk factors include female gender and the presence of peripheral vascular disease or diabetes mellitus. The rate of major complications in emergency settings including cardiogenic shock has varied from 4–36% (41).

The major complications of IABP include limb ischemia and vascular trauma or laceration with hemorrhage. Other rare complications include aortic dissection, platelet destruction, embolus to renal or peripheral arteries, and balloon rupture with gas embolus. Nonvascular complications tend to occur in < 1% of cases. In patients who have IABP inserted for > 5 days, the incidence of infection increases considerably (42).

3. Clinical Role of Aortic Counterpulsation

In situations where the incidence of abrupt occlusion is high (such as after rescue angioplasty following failed thrombolysis) or would be catastrophic, balloon counterpulsation may have a preventive role. The TAMI group first demonstrated that IABP use was associated with a lower reocclusion rate after successful reperfusion (30,31). Ishihara et al. demonstrated similar

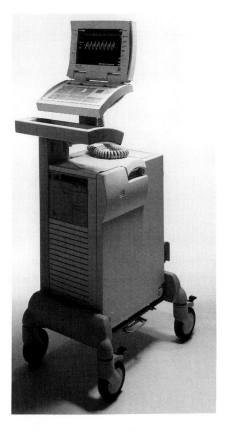

Figure 1 Newer generation intra-aortic balloon pump console. Recent developments of consoles have focused on reducing the size to allow easy transport and occupy less space at the bedside. Technical advances have been made to facilitate rapid gas shuttling for faster inflation and deflation, which allows irregular and rapid heart rates to be better tracked by the intra-aortic balloon pump.

findings in a group of patients undergoing primary angioplasty for acute myocardial infarction (28).

In order to test the hypothesis that IABP reduces the risk of reocclusion without undue vascular or hemorrhagic complications, a randomized trial was performed (32). In this study, 182 patients with acute MI requiring mechanical reperfusion were randomized to 48 h of IABP and IV heparin or heparin alone. The group receiving IABP/heparin ($n = 96$) had a higher patency rate and less recurrent ischemic events than the control group ($n = 86$) with a very low risk of complications. Further analysis of 106 patients undergoing primary PTCA showed no difference in vascular complications or major bleeding between the IABP group and the control group (43). Overall, prophylactic IABP support after successful reperfusion resulted in less recurrent ischemia, less need for repeat intervention, and a lower reocclusion rate.

Another recent series of 56 patients after successful rescue PTCA documented that 36 patients treated with IABP for 24 h had a significantly lower reocclusion rate, better left ventricular (LV) function, and a trend toward a decrease in mortality (44). While this study addressed only patients with acute MI, there may be reason to believe that IABP-augmented diastolic coronary flow after intervention may help to prevent reocclusion in other groups of patients as well. The "high-risk" PTCA group who might not tolerate abrupt closure may be such a group, but further studies are needed to support this claim.

B. Cardiopulmonary Support

One of the recent advances in supporting patients with cardiac decompensation is the use of percutaneous femoral–femoral (i.e., vein to artery) car-

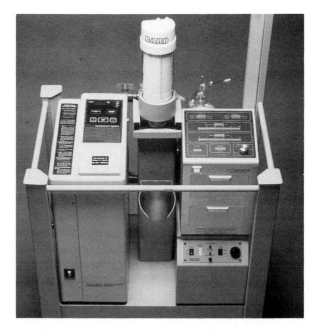

Figure 2 Portable cardiopulmonary support system assembled with centrifugal pump, heat exchanger, and oxygenator. Set-up time is approximately 5–10 min in experienced hands.

diopulmonary bypass, referred to as cardiopulmonary support (CPS). This FDA-approved device (C.R. Bard, Inc.), initially developed for emergent or elective open heart surgery, has gained relatively widespread use over the past few years and the indications for its use have broadened to cardiogenic shock, cardiac arrest, massive pulmonary embolism, hypothermia, drug overdose, and supported elective angioplasty in high-risk patients.

1. Cardiopulmonary Support Technique

The system itself consists of a centrifugal pump, a flow probe, a heat exchanger, and a hollow fiber membrane oxygenator, all connected in closed series with a long femoral vein/right atrial cannula on one end and with a femoral artery cannula on the other. While the system was initially placed via femoral cutdown, it is now routinely placed percutaneously via 18- or 20-French cannulas inserted into the femoral artery and femoral vein. The fact that blood is actively pumped from the right atrium by the centrifugal pump (not relying on gravity as do standard open heart systems) enables the device to generate cardiac output between 4 L/min (18 French) and 6 L/min (20 French). The console, disposable circuit, and cannulae are depicted in Figures 2–4.

After adequate patency of the femoral artery is established by a contrast injection, the cannulas are inserted. The arterial cannula is typically inserted first as it is difficult to gain adequate control of bleeding while dilating the vessel if the venous cannula is already in place. Once the arterial cannula is

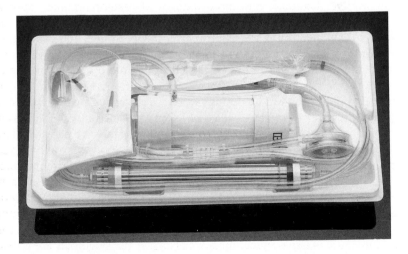

Figure 3 The disposable circuit is preassembled and is ready for mounting and priming with Ringer's lactate or normal saline. Shown are the oxygenator, heat exchanger, and pump head.

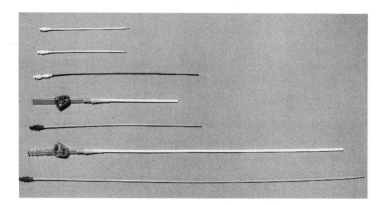

Figure 4   The arterial cannula (shorter) and venous cannula with accompanying stepwise dilators. The 18-French cannulas are shown. For patients weighing >85 kg (200 lbs), the 20-French cannulas should be used. In addition, in cardiac arrests with no spontaneous circulation, the larger cannulas are also recommended.

in place, the venous cannula is placed fluoroscopically over a stiff guidewire into the right atrium. The cannulas are then attached to the tubing connecting it to the centrifugal pump, oxygenation, and heater.

2. Advantages and Disadvantages of Cardiopulmonary Support

The major advantages and disadvantages of cardiopulmonary support are represented in Table 4. There are several technical considerations that deserve special mention. CPS requires extensive personnel and experienced operators for its use. In addition to the cardiologist, a perfusionist and a cardiac anesthesiologist need to be present for initiation and maintenance of CPS. Complications of the procedure are fairly frequent and include vascular complications and bleeding, as well as a risk of air embolism. With regard to the latter, special care must be taken to assure that all unnecessary intravenous lines are clamped during CPS and those that are necessary have all the air removed from the IV solution bag. In addition, central lines such as Swan Ganz catheters should not be opened to air under any circumstances because large amounts of air can be drawn into the system by the negative pressure exerted on the venous side. Also of special note is that the arterial catheter is relatively short and the side holes can be close to the entrance into the femoral artery in obese patients. Even slight withdrawal of the cannula can cause massive subcutaneous bleeding if the side holes are outside the femoral artery. Therefore, meticulous attention must be paid to suturing the cannulas in place and to preventing dislodgement when moving the patient.

Table 4 Cardiopulmonary Support

Advantages
FDA approved
Synchronization with rhythm unnecessary
Provides full circulatory support
Independent of LV function
Decreases myocardial energy consumption
Percutaneous access
Disadvantages
No LV decompression
Large size (18–20 French)
Short-term use (<24–48 h)
Full-dose heparin
Displacement from groin catastrophic
Perfusion technician/cardiac anesthesiologist necessary
Fails to augment myocardial perfusion beyond stenoses
Can cause thrombocytopenia/hemolysis
High complication rate
Nonpulsatile flow

Another technical consideration that also deserves note is in sizing the system to be used in different clinical settings. The larger 20-French cannulas are able to generate flow of up to 6 L/min, which is essential if the CPS is being initiated for cardiac arrest or severe cardiogenic shock. In patients undergoing supported angioplasty who are not already hemodynamically unstable, the smaller 18-French size may be used, as the anticipated flow rates necessary to provide support may be less and complications may be reduced by the smaller size. The weight and height of the patient should always be taken into consideration.

The cannulas can be removed, either surgically or manually with prolonged pressure application, after CPS has been successfully weaned. Some centers continue to use surgical closure for all of their patients feeling that this reduces the vascular complications and allows for uninterrupted heparinization of the patient. Our experience has been that prolonged clamping of the groin can be safely and effectively done, resorting only to·surgical closure in those patients who cannot be taken off anticoagulation, or who fail clamping. Anatomical characteristics such as extreme obesity may preclude percutaneous removal, which is otherwise the preferable method of removal.

The hemodynamic effects of the nonpulsatile pumping of blood consist mainly of systolic unloading of the ventricle and a dramatic reduction of right atrial and pulmonary artery pressures from preload reduction. In addition, there will be a narrowing of the pulse pressure as flow rates are increased and there may be some decrease in mean arterial pressure as well.

This system is capable of maintaining perfusion to vital organs even in the setting of electromechanical dissociation, ventricular fibrillation, or asystole. The main disadvantage in these particular situations is that the device provides no left ventricular decompression (blood still enters passively from the pulmonary circulation), so if cardiac enlargement ensues, decompression may have to be done manually with a pigtail catheter in the ventricle.

3. Clinical Role of Cardiopulmonary Support

The exact effect of CPS on myocardial function remains to be conclusively evaluated. Paulides and colleagues (45) assessed global and regional myocardial function by echocardiography in 20 patients undergoing PTCA with cardiopulmonary support. Wall stress (afterload) was significantly decreased with the initiation of CPS. Global left ventricular function was unchanged when the patients were on CPS but did decrease with balloon inflation. Interestingly, regional wall motion deteriorated in areas supplied by arteries with greater than or equal to 50% stenosis just by going on CPS and a further decrease was seen with balloon inflation. Thus, while many patients will have little or no chest pain or EKG changes on CPS with balloon inflation, CPS may not prevent ischemia in the myocardium supplied by the target vessel or by other vessels with significant stenoses. In addition, CPS does not offer any myocardial protective effect beyond a lesion if abrupt closure occurs.

Cardiopulmonary support was first applied in a portable fashion in 1966 (46), although the bulk of the experience has been in the last few years. Several studies have reported its use in patients suffering from cardiac arrest or cardiogenic shock and are presented in Table 5 (46–55). Although the numbers in the studies are small, in-hospital mortality in this group after cardiopulmonary support, and in some circumstances revascularization, is high, running between 20 and 88%. The bulk of the studies show mortality rates of 70% or higher. Obviously, this group of patients would be expected to do poorly without CPS so it is very difficult to know what role it has in this population. The outcome certainly tends to be better if the arrest happens in the setting where CPS can be initiated almost immediately [i.e., cardiac catheterization laboratory (56)] and if revascularization is an option.

By the late 1980s cardiopulmonary support was being used as a means of supporting high-risk patients in angioplasty. The currently available data are presented in Table 6 (9,57–62). The largest series to date is that of the National Registry of Elective Supported Angioplasty (9,63). The initial series of 105 patients included in the 1988 National Registry was reported in 1990 (9). The suggested criteria for entry were patients with severe or unstable angina and at least one likely dilatable coronary artery stenosis, left ventricular ejection fraction < 25%, and/or a target vessel supplying > half

Table 5 Outcome of Cardiopulmonary Support for Cardiac Arrest or Cardiogenic Shock

	n	Successful weaning (%)	% In-hospital mortality
Kennedy (1966) (46)	8	NR	88
Mattox (1977) (55)	43	67	60
Phillips (1989) (53)	20	NR	70
Shawl (1989) (47)	10	NR	20
Overlie (1990) (48)	35	43	77
Reedy (1990) (50)	38	69	76
Sugimoto (1991) (49)	8	NR	75
Rees (1992) (51)	9	44	56

NR = not reported.

of the viable myocardium. Twenty-nine percent of the patients had dilation of their only patent coronary vessel and 19% of patients were deemed to have inoperable disease. While the angioplasty success rate was 95%, major complications occurred in 39% of patients and overall in-hospital mortality was 8%. It became evident during the 1988 experience that patients may benefit by having cardiopulmonary support available but not necessarily instituted during high-risk angioplasty (the so-called standby support). The 1989 National Registry, which was reported in 1992 (63), included 258 patients who had prophylactic CPS and 98 patients who underwent their high-risk angioplasty with standby support only. Although there was some difference in baseline ejection fraction in the two groups, procedural success was similar, as was the rate of emergency CABG and death between the groups. However, major complications occurred in 41% of the patients who underwent their procedure with CPS and in only 12% of patients who did not. Two other studies have examined prophylactic versus standby cardiopulmonary support and are presented in Table 7 (64,65). Hertz and colleagues reported a series of patients with high-risk features that would have qualified for CPS in the National Registry although none of their patients actually underwent prophylactic CPS (65). They compared their results with the 1988 National Registry and found similar rates of procedural success without the extent of major complications. Unfortunately, there has been no randomized prospective study evaluating the outcome of standby versus prophylactic cardiopulmonary support. The findings of the 1989 National Registry underscore our inability to determine who is at greatest risk and in need of supported angioplasty. Due to the high complication rates and lack of indisputable benefit in patients considered "high risk" for coronary intervention, the ACC/AHA Task Force has suggested that individual use

Table 6 Outcome in High-risk PTCA Utilizing Prophylactic Cardiopulmonary Support

	n	EF mean	Lesion success/attempt (%)	Major[a] complications (%)	Emergency CABG %	Abrupt closure (%)	In-hospital deaths (%)
Vogel (1988) (58)	9	26	11/12	11	0	0	11
Tommaso (1989) (57)	10	25	12/13	40	0	0	10
Taub (1989) (61)	7	32	10/10	86	0	0	14
Freedman (1989) (60)	4	30	9/9	0	0	0	0
Shawl (1989) (59)	51	NR	115/117	?	0	4	6
1988 National Registry (1990) (9)	105	32	173/182	39	4	7	8
Ott (1990) (62)	5	24	12/12	40	0	0	0

[a]Death, myocardial infarction, abrupt closure, CABG, or recent PTCA.
EF = ejection fraction; CABG = coronary artery bypass graft; NR = not reported.

Table 7 Prophylactic Versus Standby Cardiopulmonary Support

		EF (%)	Procedural success (%)	Major[a] complications (%)	Emergency CABG (%)	Death (%)
	n					
Tommaso (1989) (64)						
Prophylactic	14	26	86	14	0	14
Standby	9	25	100	0	0	0
Herz (1990) (65)						
"Standby"[b]	56	NR	95	2	5	0
1989 National Registry (1992) (63)						
Prophylactic	258	28	89	41	2	6
Standby	98	34	88	12	2	6

[a]As in Table 6.
[b]Compared their series with the 1988 National Registry (9).
EF = ejection fraction; CABG = coronary artery bypass graft; NR = not reported.

of CPS as a prophylactic measure remains to be clarified by further clinical investigation.

C. The Hemopump

The Hemopump (Johnson & Johnson, Skilman, NJ) was developed as an alternative to other ventricular assist devices and has the main advantages of being intra-arterial and semipercutaneous, making its insertion relatively easy compared with other ventricular assist devices. This device has been in use since 1988 and remains investigational at the present time.

1. Hemopump Technique

The Hemopump is best described as a catheter-mounted axial flow pump utilizing an Archimedes spiral vein screw that rotates at 15,000–27,000 rpm (66). The device decompresses the left ventricle by pumping blood unidirectionally from the left ventricle to the descending aorta. The assembly itself is made of silicone rubber reinforced by a coil spring and has a beveled tip that is placed in the left ventricle. The pump portion of the assembly is 20 cm long by 7 mm in diameter so that the pump end is 21 French in size and the shaft is 11 French as it traverses the femoral artery. The screw portion

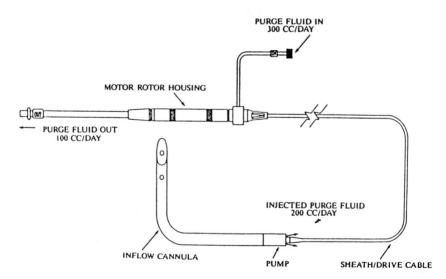

Figure 5 Schematic drawing of the hemopump showing the 21-French device. The motor rotor housing is placed ex vivo, while the sheath and drive cable is placed in the peripheral vasculature with the pump placed in the ascending aorta. A newer 14-French device is currently undergoing clinical evaluations. (Reproduced with permission from Ref. 68.)

in the cannula in the arch of the aorta and is powered via a drive shaft connected to an electromagnetic motor that is outside the body. The Hemopump is capable of delivering 0.5–3.5 L/min of nonpulsatile flow and does not require synchronization with the cardiac cycle or rhythm (67). Figures 5 and 6 depict the Hemopump setup.

The hemodynamic effects of the Hemopump have been described in several studies. Merhige and colleagues demonstrated in dogs that, in the absence of ischemia, the Hemopump reduced left ventricular end-diastolic pressure and resulted in systolic unloading of the ventricle while maintaining mean aortic pressure (68). With ischemia, the same effects were noted with an increase in regional myocardial perfusion with the Hemopump turned on

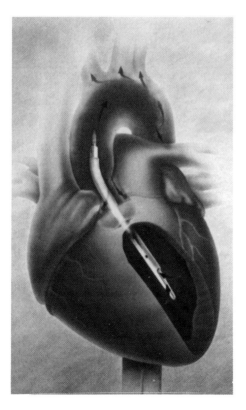

Figure 6 Schematic drawing of the hemopump placed in the left ventricle. Note that the in-flow cannula is placed in the middle of the ventricle and that the pump is in the ascending aorta. The pump can generate approximately 2.5 L/min of continuous output.

as compared with the baseline ischemia. Shiiya and coworkers observed similar findings in six open chest dogs and also showed a reduced O_2 demand and improved blood flow/O_2 demand ratio in the nonoccluded coronaries (69). These hemodynamic effects also appear to be superior to those of intra-aortic balloon pumping in dogs (70). While human correlates are sparse, one small study of four patients with cardiogenic shock after acute myocardial infarction showed the Hemopump increased the cardiac index by 120% and the mean arterial pressure by 48% and reduced the pulmonary capillary wedge pressure by 37% (71).

2. Advantages and Disadvantages of the Hemopump

The major advantages and disadvantages of the Hemopump are presented in Table 8. A few of the major advantages are that the pump does not require synchronization with rhythm, operates independently of left ventricular function, and has both a myocardial protective effect as well as offering decompression for the left ventricle. Unfortunately, in approximately 15–20% of patients the Hemopump cannot be inserted because of size limitations. Smaller devices that are currently under investigation (14 French) may help to allow the Hemopump to be applied to a wider range of patients. The trade-off is that the smaller devices may cause more hemolysis (72) and provide less flow.

Table 8   Hemopump

Advantages
  Decompresses the ventricle
  Decreases myocardial energy consumption
  Augments coronary perfusion
  Perfusion technician unnecessary
  Full heparinization not required
  No significant hemolysis or complement activation
  No synchronization with rhythm necessary
  Works independently of LV function
  May be used up to 14 days
Disadvantages
  Requires arterial cutdown
  Dependent on LV filling
  Limited by size (21 French)
  Inability to place device in 20%
  Smaller devices may cause more hemolysis
  Investigational
  Ventricular arrhythmias
  Displacement from LV could be catastrophic
  Nonpulsatile flow

---

3. Clinical Role of the Hemopump

Initial clinical experience utilizing the device was for postpericardiotomy shock or allograft failure and allowed weaning from cardiopulmonary bypass (73–75). In addition, the device has been used in patients with post-myocardial infarction cardiogenic shock with some limited success (66,74, 76,77). Unfortunately, most of the studies examining the Hemopump have contained small numbers of patients with a wide variety of etiologies of cardiac decompensation. The device appears most beneficial in patients with cardiogenic shock or when used as a bridge in patients awaiting heart transplantation or revascularization. The Hemopump does not appear to have a well-defined role in patients with cardiomyopathy.

The largest clinical trial to date using the Hemopump is a multicenter trial of 123 patients with cardiogenic shock (either postmyocardial infarction or postcardiotomy). Of the 53 patients in whom published data are available (78,79), the Hemopump was successfully inserted in 41 (77%). The 30-day survival of the Hemopump group was 32% and the survival of the "non-insertion group" (those who could not have the device inserted secondary to technical reasons) was 17%. While this trial shows a trend toward improved survival with the Hemopump, it was not randomized and preliminary results of the total 123 patients have found no statistically significant difference in survival between the two groups (22).

The Hemopump seems a likely alternative to other modalities in supporting high-risk PTCA. Loisance and co-workers reported on nine patients with ischemia unresponsive to medical therapy who were felt to be high risk to undergo either surgery or PTCA (80,81). The high-risk surgical characteristics included age >75 years in two patients, ejection fraction <20% in six patients, and no adequate bypass conduit in five patients. The characteristics that were felt to make them high risk for angioplasty included uncontrolled ischemia in seven patients, ejection fraction <20% in six patients, and a target lesion located on the last remaining patent vessel perfusing a major mass of myocardium, with three patients having a lesion located in an unprotected left main coronary artery. The pump was implanted in six of the nine patients. Three patients were not able to receive the Hemopump secondary to small iliac vessels in two and aortoiliac disease in one. In the six patients who had the pump inserted, the cardiac index increased by 25% and pulmonary capillary wedge pressure decreased by 19%. All of them underwent uneventful PTCA without "significant" complications, although three had ventricular tachycardia and one had high degree AV block. Five of the patients remained symptom free at follow-up of 5–15 months, and the remaining patient underwent elective surgical revascularization for persistent angina. The three patients who did not undergo the Hemopump because of size mismatch had significant mortality: one patient died during angioplasty and a second patient died 2 weeks later of uncontrolled myocardial ischemia; the third patient received coronary artery bypass grafting. Unfortunately, there are no other published studies of the Hemopump as a supportive device for high-risk angioplasty. Whether or not it will emerge as a viable option with more widespread applicability remains unclear. The precise role in supported angioplasty will need to be defined in the future.

D. Partial Left Heart Bypass Support

One other area of recent interest as a means of supporting patients during high-risk angioplasty is partial left heart bypass. This particular method is performed percutaneously using a transseptal approach with large bore catheters placed in the left atrium and in the femoral artery (14–20 French). The advantage of this system is that no oxygenator is required since blood is pumped from the oxygenated left atrium to the femoral artery. The disadvantages are that the system is not at the present time widely used and that relatively large catheters are needed for the roller pump to effectively increase the cardiac output (82,83). The exact role of this device in supporting critically ill patients remains to be clarified by further clinical investigation.

IV. CONCLUSIONS

It has become quite clear that proper patient selection for supported angioplasty is the key to maximizing the benefits without increasing the inherent risk with the use of these devices. Intra-aortic balloon pumping appears to have the least risk associated with its use but also has the most modest hemodynamic benefits. By careful clinical investigation, a well-defined role of IABP placement after the procedure to prevent abrupt occlusion and recurrent ischemia, at least in the setting of acute myocardial infarction, has emerged. The other modalities are plagued by higher complication rates and lack of any randomized trials. Future emphasis should be placed on proper patient selection and proper randomized trials.

The decision to use support devices to assist percutaneous interventions is complex. The appropriate selection should be based on patient characteristics, whether complete revascularization or culprit lesion strategy is applied, the area in jeopardy for reduced blood supply, the procedure ischemic duration, and the patient's clinical status. Thus, the selection of support strategy will be different when a discrete (suitable for perfusion balloon angioplasty) culprit lesion in mid-LAD in a patient with an ejection fraction of 20% and stable angina is considered compared with multiple lesions in the mid-LAD, other target lesions in the LCX and the RCA, with an ejection fraction of 20% and unstable angina. In the former scenario the combination of perfusion balloon angioplasty and IABP support may be adequate.

In the latter the prophylactic use of percutaneous CPS may be considered as a better alternative. Ultimately, every case needs to be considered with all the risk factors for procedural mortality, risk of abrupt closure, and technical issues reviewed. For elective procedures, considerations of the laboratory experience with CPS should also be considered. In general, for patients with an ejection fraction of >20%, the IABP is the support device of choice. For patients with an ejection fraction of <20%, IABP with CPS standby or prophylactic CPS should be considered. The decision between these two strategies will depend on the amount of myocardium in jeopardy and the degree of clinical heart failure. Patients with a large area of jeopardy and heart failure should have CPS-supported percutaneous interventions.

Patients requiring hemodynamic support during acute myocardial infarction should have IABP started as soon as possible during the acute cardiac catheterization procedure. Observational data have suggested that the combination of acute angioplasty and IABP use improves in-hospital mortality (4) and can improve sustained coronary artery patency (31). In our experience, the use of CPS should be limited to patients who are undergoing emergency CABG, where IABP cannot fully sustain the patient because of life-threatening arrhythmias. All cardiogenic shock patients who have sustained cardiac arrest or life-threatening arrhythmias in the cardiac catheterization laboratory should have CPS started as soon as possible. Observational data have noted that if CPS can be started within 10 min of cardiac arrest it can be a life-saving procedure (56).

Along with percutaneous interventions, the use of support devices by interventional cardiologists has risen over the last decade. The ultimate challenge has been applying this technology to the right patients and thereby making percutaneous revascularization a safer procedure. In the future, less invasive procedures that combine the physiological benefits of aortic counterpulsation with the considerable peripheral support of CPS will emerge. The challenge for the future will be how such an approach should be developed and, more importantly, in which patients it should be applied.

REFERENCES

1. Saba HI, Saba SR, Morelli GA. Effect of heparin on platelet aggregation. Am J Hematol 1984;17:295–306.
2. Bolooki H. Emergency cardiac procedures in patients in cardiogenic shock due to complications of coronary artery disease. Circulation 1989;79:I-137–I-148.
3. Goldberg RJ, Gore JM, Alpert JS, Osganian V, de Groot J, Bade J, Chen Z, Frid D, Dalen JE. Cardiogenic shock after acute myocardial infarction. N Engl J Med 1991;325:1117–1122.
4. Bengtson JR, Kaplan AJ, Pieper KS, Wildermann NM, Mark DB, Pryor DB, Phillips HR, Califf RM. Prognosis in cardiogenic shock after acute myocardial infarction in the interventional era. J Am Coll Cardiol 1992;20:1482–1489.

5. Hartzler GO, Rutherford BD, McConahay DR, Johnson WJ, Giorgi LV. "High-risk" percutaneous transluminal coronary angioplasty. Am J Cardiol 1988;61: 33–7G.

6. Ohman EM, Phillips HR, Califf RM. An approach to percutaneous revascularization in patients with stable coronary ischemia. In: Roubin GS, Callif RM, O'Neill WW, Phillips HR, Stack RS, eds. Interventional Cardiovascular Medicine: Principles and Practice (Vol 1). New York: Churchill Livingston, 1994: 217–238.

7. Ellis SG, Myler RK, King III SB, Douglas JS, Jr, Topol EJ, Shaw RE, Stertzer SH, Roubin GS, Murphy MC. Causes and correlates of death after unspported coronary angioplasty: Implications for use of angioplasty and advanced support techniques in high-risk settings. Am J Cardiol 1991;68:1447–1451.

8. Califf RM, Phillips HR, Hindman MC, Mark DB, Lee KL, Behar VS, Johnson RA, Pryor DB, Rosati RA, Wagner GS, et al. Prognostic value of a coronary artery jeopardy score. J Am Coll Cardiol 1985;5:1055–1063.

9. Vogel RA, Shawl F, Tommaso C, et al. Initial report of the national registry of elective cardiopulmonary bypass supported coronary angioplasty. J Am Coll Cardiol 1990;15:23–29.

10. Vogel RA, Shawl FA. Report of the National Registry of Elective Supported Angioplasty: comparison of the 1988 and 1989 results (abstr). Circulation 1990; 82(suppl III):III–653.

11. Quigley PJ, Kereiakes DJ, Abbottsmith CW, et al. Prolonged autoperfusion angioplasty: immediate clinical outcome and angiographic follow-up (abstr). J Am Coll Cardiol 1989;13:155A.

12. Hinohara T, Simpson JB, Phillips HR, et al. Transluminal catheter reperfusion: a new technique to reestablish blood flow after coronary occlusion during percutaneous transluminal coronary angioplasty. Am J Cardiol 1986;57:684–686.

13. Snyder R, Wijay B, Angelini P. Percutaneous transluminal coronary angioplasty with hemoperfusion. ASAIO Trans 1991;37:M367–M368.

14. Lehmann KG, Atwood JE, Snyder EL, Ellison RL. Autologous blood perfusion for myocardial protection during coronary angioplasty: a feasibility study. Circulation 1987;76:312–323.

15. Tokioka H, Miyazaki A, Fung P, et al. Effects of intracoronary infusion of arterial blood or Fluosol-DA 20% on regional myocardial metabolism and function during brief coronary artery occlusion. Circulation 1987;75:473–481.

16. Christensen CW, Reeves WC, Lassar TA, Schmidt DH. Inadequate subendocardial oxygen delivery during perfluorocarbon perfusion in a canine model of ischemia. Am Heart J 1988;115:30–37.

17. Szatmary LJ, Marco J, Fajadet J, Caster L. The combined use of diastolic counterpulsation and coronary dilation in unstable angina due to multivessel disease under unstable hemodynamic conditions. Int J Cardiol 1988;19:59–66.

18. Gore JM, Weiner BH, Benotti JR, et al. Preliminary experience with synchronized coronary sinus retroperfusion in humans. Circulation 1986;74:381–388.

19. Nanto S, Nishida K, Hirayama A, Mishima M, Komamura K, Masai M, Sakakibura T, Kodama K. Supported angioplasty with synchronized retroperfusion

in high-risk patients with left main trunk or near left main trunk obstruction. Am Heart J 1993;125:301–309.

20. Moulopoulos SD, Topaz S, Kolff WL. Diastolic balloon pumping (with carbon dioxide) in the aorta—a mechanical assistance to the failing circulation. Am Heart J 1962;63:669–675.

21. Kantrowitz A, Tjonneland S, Freed PS, Phillips SJ, Butner AN, Sherman JL. Initial clinical experience with intraaortic balloon pumping in cardiogenic shock. J Am Med Assoc 1968;203:135.

22. Goldenberg IF. Nonpharmacologic management of cardiac arrest and cardiogenic shock. Chest 1992;102(suppl 2):596S–616S.

23. McCabe JC, Abel RM, Subramanian VA, Gay WA. Complications of intraaortic balloon insertion and counterpulsation. Circulation 1977;57:769–773.

24. Scheidt S, Wilner G, Mueller H, Summers D, Lesch M, Wolff G, Krakaver J, Rubenfire M, Fleming P, Noon G, Oldham N, Killip T, Kantrowitz A. Intraaortic balloon counterpulsation in cardiogenic shock. N Engl J Med 1973;288: 979–984.

25. Fuchs RM, Brin KP, Brinker JA, Guzman PA, Heuser RR, Yin FCP. Augmentation of regional coronary blood flow by intra-aortic balloon counterpulsation in patients with unstable angina. Circulation 1983;68:117–123.

26. Williams DL, Korr KS, Gerwirtz H, Most AS. The effect of intra-aortic balloon counterpulsation on regional myocardial blood flow and oxygen consumption in the presence of coronary artery stenosis in patients with unstable angina. Circulation 1982;66:593–597.

27. MacDonald RG, Hill JA, Feldman RL. Failure of intraaortic balloon counterpulsation to augment distal coronary perfusion pressure during percutaneous transluminal coronary angioplasty. Am J Cardiol 1987;59:359–361.

28. Ishihara M, Sato H, Tateishi H, Kawagoe T, Muraoka Y, Yoshimura M. Effects of intraaortic balloon pumping on coronary hemodynamics after coronary angioplasty in patients with acute myocardial infarction. Am Heart J 1992; 124:1133–1138.

29. Kern MJ, Aguirre F, Bach R, Donohue T, Siegal R, Segal J. Augmentation of coronary blood flow by intra-aortic balloon pumping in patients after coronary angioplasty. Circulation 1993;87:500–511.

30. Ohman EM, Califf RM, Topol EJ, Leimberger JD, George B, Berrios ED, Anderson LC, Keriakes DJ, Stack RS. Aortic counterpulsation with thrombolysis for myocardial infarction: salutary effect on reocclusion of the infarct related artery. J Am Coll Cardiol 1992;19:381A.

31. Ohman EM, Califf RM, George BS, Quigley PJ, Kereiakes DJ, Harrelson-Woodlief L, Candela RJ, Flanagan C, Stack RS, Topol EJ. The use of intraaortic balloon pumping as an adjunct to reperfusion therapy in acute myocardial infarction. Am Heart J 1991;121:895–901.

32. Ohman EM, George BS, White CJ, Kern MJ, Gurbel PA, Freedman RJ, Lundergan C, Hartmann JR, Talley JD, Frey MJ, Taylor G, Leimberger JD, Owens PM, Lee KL, Stack RS, Califf RM, for the Randomized IAPB Study Group. The use of aortic counterpulsation to improve sustained coronary artery patency during acute myocardial infarction: results of a randomized trial. Circulation 1994;90:792–799.

33. Kahn JK, Rutherford BD, McConahay DR, Johnson WL, Giorgi LV, Hartzler GO. Supported "high risk" coronary angioplasty using intraaortic balloon pump counterpulsation. J Am Coll Cardiol 1990;15:1151–1155.
34. Alcan KE, Stertzer SH, Wallsh E, DePasquale NP, Bruno MS. The role of intra-aortic balloon counterpulsation in patients undergoing percutaneous trans-luminal coronary angioplasty. Am Heart J 1983;105:527–530.
35. Voudris V, Marco J, Morice MC, Fajadet J, Royer T. "High-risk" percutan-eous transluminal coronary angioplasty with preventive intraaortic balloon counterpulsation. Cath Cardiovasc Diagn 1990;19:160–164.
36. Margolis JR. The role of the percutaneous intra-aortic balloon in emergency situations following percutaneous transluminal coronary angioplasty. Translum-inal Coronary Angioplasty and Intracoronary Thrombolysis: Coronary Heart Disease IV. Berlin: Springer-Verlag, 1982:145–150.
37. Jones EL, Murphy DA, Craver JM. Comparison of coronary angioplasty in-cluding surgery for failed angioplasty. Am Heart J 1984;107:830–835.
38. Lincoff AM, Popma JJ, Ellis SG, Vogel RA, Topol EJ. Percutaneous support devices for high risk or complicated coronary angioplasty. J Am Coll Cardiol 1991;17:758–769.
39. Nash IS, Lorell BH, Fishman RF, Baim DS, Donahue C, Diver DJ. A new tech-nique for sheathless percutaneous intraaortic balloon catheter insertion. Cath Cardiovasc Diagn 1991;23:57–60.
40. Alcan KE, Stertzer SH, Wallsh E, Bruno MS, DePasquale NP. Current status of intra-aortic balloon counterpulsation in critical care cardiology. Crit Care Med 1984;12:489–495.
41. Scheidt S. Preservation of ischemic myocardium with intraaortic balloon pump-ing: modern therapeutic intervention or *primum non nocere*. Circulation 1978; 58:211–214.
42. Lazar JM, Ziady GM, Dummer SJ, Thompson M, Ruffuer RJ. Outcome and complications of prolonged intraaortic balloon counterpulsation in cardiac pa-tients. Am J Cardiol 1992;69:955–958.
43. Ohman EM, George BS, White CJ, Gurbel PA, Freedman RJ, Lundergan CF, Hartmann JR, Prince CR, Frey M, Taylor G, Leimberger JD, Stack RS, Califf RM for the Randomized IABP Study Group. Reocclusion of the infarct-related artery after primary or rescue angioplasty: effect of aortic counterpulsation. Circulation 1993;88(suppl I):I-107.
44. Ishihara M, Sato H, Tateishi H, Kawagoe T, Yasunobu Y, Shimatani Y, Veda A. Intraaortic balloon pumping following rescue coronary angioplasty after failed thrombolysis. Circulation 1993;88(suppl I):I-107.
45. Paulides GS, Hauser AM, Stack RK, Dudlets PI, Grines C, Timmis GC, O'Neill WW. Effect of peripheral cardiopulmonary bypass on left ventricular size, after-load, and myocardial function during elective supported coronary angioplasty. J Am Coll Cardiol 1991;18:499–505.
46. Kennedy JH. The role of assisted circulation in cardiac resuscitation. JAMA 1966;197:615–618.
47. Shawl FA, Domanski MJ, Hernandez TJ, Punja S. Emergency percutaneous cardiopulmonary bypass support in cardiogenic shock from acute myocardial infarction. Am J Cardiol 1989;64:967–970.

48. Overlie PA. Emergency use of portable cardiopulmonary bypass. Cath Cardiovasc Diagn 1990;20:27-31.

49. Sugimoto JT, Baird E, Bruner C. Percutaneous cardiopulmonary support in cardiac arrest. ASAIO Trans 1991;37:M282-M283.

50. Reedy JE, Swartz MT, Raitnel SC, Szukalski EA, Pennington DG. Mechanical cardiopulmonary support for refractory cardiogenic shock. Heart Lung 1990; 19:514-525.

51. Rees MR, Browne T, Sivanantnay VM, Whittaker S, Hick D, Verma SF, Tan LB, Davies GA. Cardiac resuscitation with percutaneous cardiopulmonary support. Lancet 1992;340:513-514.

52. Phillips SJ, Ballentine B, Slonine D, Hall J, Vandehaar J, Kongtahiwam C, Zeff RM, Skinner JR, Reckmok, Gray D. Percutaneous initiation of cardiopulmonary bypass. Ann Thorac Surg 1983;36:223-225.

53. Phillips SJ, Zeff RH, Kongtahworn C, et al. Percutaneous cardiopulmonary bypass: application and indication for use. Ann Thorac Surg 1989;47:121-123.

54. Shawl FA, Domanski MJ, Wish M, Punja S, Hernandez TJ. Emergency percutaneous cardiopulmonary support in cardiogenic shock: long term follow-up (abstract). Circulation 1989;80(suppl II):II-258.

55. Mattox KL, Beall AC. Application of portable cardiopulmonary bypass to emergency instrumentation. Med Instrum 1977;11:347-349.

56. Overlie PA, Reichman RT, Smith SC, Dembitsky W, Adamson RM, Jaski BE, Marsh DG, Daily PO. Emergency use of portable cardiopulmonary bypass in patients with cardiac arrest. J Am Coll Cardiol 1989;13:160A.

57. Tommaso CL, Gundry SR, Zoda AR, Stafford JL, Johnson RA, Vogel RA. Supported angioplasty: initial experience with high risk patients (abstr). J Am Coll Cardiol 1989;13:159A.

58. Vogel RA. The Maryland experience: angioplasty and valvuloplasty using percutaneous cardiopulmonary support. Am J Cardiol 1988;62:11-4K.

59. Shawl FA, Domanski MJ, Punja S, Hernandez TJ. Percutaneous cardiopulmonary bypass support in high-risk patients undergoing percutaneous transluminal coronary angioplasty. Am J Cardiol 1989;64:1258-1263.

60. Freedman RJ, Wrenn RC, Godley ML, Knoepp JD, Smith C, LaCroix C. Complex multiple percutaneous transluminal coronary angioplasties with vortex oxygenator cardiopulmonary support in the community hospital setting. Cath Cardiovasc Diagn 1989;17:237-242.

61. Taub JO, L'Hommedieu BD, Raithel SC, Vieth DG, Vieth PJ, Barner HB, Vandormael M, Pennington DG. Extracorporeal membrane oxygenation for percutaneous coronary angioplasty in high risk patients. ASAIO Trans 1989; 35:664-666.

62. Ott RA, Mills TC, Tobis JM, Allen BJ, Dwyer ML. ECMO assisted angioplasty for cardiomyopathy patients with unstable angina. ASAIO Trans 1990;36:M483-M485.

63. Tierstein PS. Cardiopulmonary support. Am J Cardiol 1992;69:19F-21F.

64. Tommaso CL, Vogel RA. Supported vs. standby supported angioplasty. Circulation 1980;80(suppl II):II-272.

65. Herz I, Fried G, Feld H, Schulhoff N, Hollander G, Greengart A, Gelbfish J, Lichstein E, Frankel R, Sacchi T, Shani J. High risk PTCA without cardiopulmonary support. Circulation 1990;82(suppl III):III-654.

66. Lincoff AM, Popma JJ, Bates ER, Deck GM, Bolling SF, Meagher JS, Kelly AM, Wampler RK, Nicklas JM. Successful coronary angioplasty in two patients with cardiogenic shock using the Nimbus Hemopump support device. Am Heart J 1990;120:970–972.
67. Wamples RK, Mose JC, Frazier OH, Olsen DB. In vivo evaluation of a peripheral vascular access axial flow blood pump. ASAIO Trans 1988;34:450–454.
68. Merhige ME, Smalling RW, Cassidy D, et al. Effect of the Hemopump left ventricular assist device on regional myocardial perfusion and function: reduction of ischemia during coronary occlusion. Circulation 1989;80(suppl III):III-158–166.
69. Shiiya N, Zelinsky R, Delevze PM, Loisance DY. Effects of hemopump support on left ventricular unloading and coronary blood flow. ASAIO Trans 1991; 37:M361–M362.
70. Smalling RW, Cassidy DB, Merhige M, et al. Improved hemodynamic and left ventricular unloading during acute ischemia using the Hemopump left ventricular assist device compared to intra aortic balloon counterpulsation (abstr). J Am Coll Cardiol 1989;13:160A.
71. Smalling RW, Sweeney MJ, Cassidy DB, et al. Hemodynamics in cardiogenic shock after acute myocardial infarction with the Hemopump assist device (abstr). Circulation 1989;80(suppl II):II-624.
72. Mooney MR, Mooney JF, Van Tassel RA, et al. The Nimbus hemopump: a new left ventricular assist device that combines myocardial protective with circulatory support. J Inv Cardiol 1990;2:169–173.
73. Frazier OH, Wamples RK, Duncan JM, Dear WE, Macris MS, Parnis SM, Fugua JM. First human use of the hemopump, a catheter-mounted ventricular assist device (abstr). J Am Coll Cardiol 1989;13:121A.
74. Frazier OH, Nalcatan T, Duncan JM, Parnis SM, Fuqua JM. Clinical experience with the Hemopump. ASAIO Trans 1989;35:604–606.
75. Burnett CM, Vega JD, Radovancevic B, Conquist JL, Birovljev S, Sweeney MS, Duncan JM, Frazier OH. Improved survival after hemopump insertion in patients experiencing post cardiotomy cardiogenic shock during cardiopulmonary bypass. ASAIO Trans 1990;36:M626–M629.
76. Deeb GM, Bolling SF, Nicklas J, Walsh RS, Steimle CN, Shea MJ, Meagher JS. Clinical experience with the Nimbus pump. ASAIO Trans 1990;36:M632–M636.
77. Phillips SJ, Barker L, Balentine B, Vanderhaar J, Slonine D, Core M, Zeff RN, Kongtahworn C, Skinner JR, Grignon A, Toon RS, Wickemeyer W, Spector M, Wampler R. Hemopump support for the failing heart. ASAIO Trans 1990; 36:M629–M632.
78. Wampler RK, Frazier OH, Lansing AM, Smalling RW, Nicklas JM, Phillips SJ, Guyton RA, Golding L. Treatment of cardiogenic shock with the hemopump left ventricular assist device. Ann Thorac Surg 1991;52:506–513.
79. Wampler RK, Johnson DV, Rutan PM, Riehle RA. Multicenter clinical study of the Hemopump in the treatment of cardiogenic shock (abstr). Circulation 1989;80(suppl II):II-670.
80. Loisance D, Deboise-Rande JL, Deleuze P, Okude J, Rosenval O, Geschwind H. Prophylactic intraventricular pumping in high risk coronary angioplasty. Lancet 1990;335:438–440.

81. Loisance D, Deleuze P, Dubois-Rande JL, Okude J, Shiiya N, Wan F, Geschwind H. Hemopump ventricular support for patients undergoing high risk coronary angioplasty. ASAIO Trans 1990;36:M623–M626.
82. Glassman E, Chinitz L, Levite H, Slater J, Winer H. Partial left heart bypass support during high-risk angioplasty (abstr). Circulation 1989;80(suppl II):II–272.
83. Babic VV, Brojicic S, Kjurisic Z, Vucinic M. Percutaneous left atrial-aorta bypass with a roller pump (abstr). Circulation 1989;80(suppl II):II–272.

12

Reducing Coronary Restenosis After Angioplasty

Robert S. Schwartz and David R. Holmes, Jr.
Mayo Clinic and Mayo Foundation, Rochester, Minnesota

I. INTRODUCTION

Restenosis continues to be the major limitation of all percutaneous interventional coronary revascularization procedures. An estimated 400,000 procedures will be performed during 1993. As the technology for performing these procedures improves, more difficult and higher risk cases are being approached and successfully performed, yielding a primary success rate of >90%.

Improved techniques and methods, combined with the ongoing need to treat recurrent (restenotic) lesions have resulted in the number of catheter-based procedures now exceeding the number of coronary artery bypass operations (1). For some patients the restenosis problem continues to be a major reason for choosing surgery. Solution of this problem would likely increase the overall number of cases being done.

The impact of restenosis on patients can be estimated from the NHLBI PTCA registry from 1985. This study showed that 21% of patients required repeat procedures by the end of 1 year, regardless of whether the primary procedure was single or multivessel in nature. In fact, only 58% of patients were free from death, myocardial infarction, bypass grafting, or repeat angioplasty (2). This "Achilles' heel" has led to an intensive search for answers, but so far with little success.

Many studies have tried to reduce restenosis by employing pharmaco-logical agents already used for angioplasty procedures; unfortunately, all have shown negative or, at best, marginal results (3–14). Newer agents have fared similarly, leading to a series of frustrating, expensive failures.

The advent of new revascularization devices led to hope that new device technology could be employed to reduce the incidence of restenosis. Various potential explanations were advanced, generally founded on the concept that a smoother lumen or "cleaner cut" of the atherosclerotic lesion site might result in less restenosis. Unfortunately, these hypotheses have not been sub-stantiated. This argument was applied to directional and rotational atherec-tomy, excimer laser therapy, and thermal energy applied to the artery. While these technological methods do appear to accomplish the goal of smooth lumen surfaces compared to balloon angioplasty (where plaque fracture is a primary method of therapy), restenosis rates have not diminished. A fea-ture common to these alternative devices is that all create some form of in-jury to the target arterial lesion site in performing the task of reducing lum-inal obstruction. Endothelial denudation is present with each, as is exposure of subintimal atheromatous elements to the flowing bloodstream. The long-term price paid for this arterial injury is increased amounts of neointimal hyperplasia as a direct response. Regardless of type of injury, neointimal thickening appears as a final common pathway in the arterial response to revascularization. Newer concepts regarding some of these devices will be discussed shortly, related to whether the larger initial lumen possible using a specific device might reduce restenosis since there is more lumen in which neointima can grow before causing a recurrent stenosis (15–24).

The failure of both drugs and devices to prevent restenosis suggests that the pathophysiology of neointimal formation is incompletely understood. The incidence, clinical time course, and angiographic correlates of coro-nary restenosis have been well described (2,25–28). Yet these excellent studies represent descriptive features rather than an understanding of neointimal pathophysiology. The formulation of a truly effective therapy thus continues to await better understanding.

II. RESTENOSIS: ANIMAL MODELS

The use of animal models in restenosis has become controversial, since reports of successful animal studies have failed to accurately predict results of human trials using the same agents. There are many potential explana-tions for the differences, but some of the representative models will be dis-cussed first.

A. The Rat Carotid Artery Model

The rat carotid artery was first studied as a model for atherosclerosis (29, 30). It has subsequently been adapted to the study of smooth muscle cell migration and proliferation in restenosis, and has been widely used to test proposed restenosis therapies. This model has become a standard for studying smooth muscle cell response to endothelial injury (31). A major advantage of this model lies in its extensive characterization from a molecular biological perspective (31–37).

The rat carotid artery is injured by air desiccation (38–42) or by balloon inflation and subsequent endothelial denudation (33,43,44). The balloon is inflated and drawn through the artery (while inflated) for multiple passes, generally three or more times (30). The balloon is deflated and removed, and the external carotid artery ligated. Medial smooth muscle cell injury regularly occurs during this process.

Platelet deposition occurs at areas of endothelial denudation, and within 2–3 weeks a smooth neointima covers the injury site. The degree of thickening is typically 50–100 μm. Frequently, the arterial lumen *increases* over baseline. Neointimal thickening results from proliferation and migration of medial smooth muscle cells (45–48). Smooth muscle cell proliferation begins within 1–2 days after denudation, and continues for 14–30 days. Endothelial regrowth is completed by this time. Because neointimal volume is limited, hemodynamically significant stenoses seldom occur in this model.

Many studies have used this model, both from a standpoint of understanding mechanisms (45,49), and for trials to limit neointimal thickening. It is from these studies that the importance of platelet-derived growth factor (PDGF) was established as a stimulant to smooth muscle cell proliferation (45,50–52). One concern about this model is its apparent failure to predict human trial results, most notably using the ACE inhibitor cilazapril. This agent showed marked ability to inhibit neointima in rats, but two well-done human clinical trials showed no effect (53,54).

B. Hypercholesterolemic Rabbit Iliac Model

The rabbit iliac artery has been studied extensively (55,56). Typically, rabbits are begun on a hypercholesterolemic diet of 1–2% cholesterol and 7% peanut oil. This results in blood cholesterol levels of 1000–2000 mg%, and resultant vascular injury. This injury is supplemented by mechanical injury using a 3-French Fogarty balloon catheter inserted into both femoral arteries. This balloon is inflated and successively withdrawn through the artery five or six times. The resulting injury is typically superficial, rarely damaging deep arterial structures, but denuding endothelium.

Six weeks following initial arterial injury, both femoral arteries are examined arteriographically for stenoses. At sites of significant lesions angioplasty is performed with standard balloon dilatation (usually three inflations for 1 min each at 5–10 atm). Four weeks later, angiographic follow-up is performed, the animals are euthanized, and the arterial perfusion fixed at physiological pressures for histopathological examination.

Another method using rabbit iliac arteries uses nitrogen desiccation. The rabbit femoral arteries are exposed bilaterally, and industrial nitrogen gas is infused into the isolated arterial segment through a syringe needle, typically at 80 ml/min for 8–10 min. Following this arterial drying, a hypercholesterolemic diet of 2% cholesterol, 6% peanut oil is fed to the animals and continued for 4 weeks. Angioplasty is then performed using a balloon under fluoroscopic guidance (39,41,42). This model also results in the histopathological appearance of lipid-laden foam cells in the media and outer portions of the neointima. The histopathology of neointima from this technique shows many foam cells (macrophages that have ingested excessive lipid) and voluminous extracellular matrix.

As with rat carotid artery injury, platelet deposition occurs rapidly at sites of balloon-induced plaque fracture. Antiplatelet agents were thus studied early in this model (57) and showed efficacy in reducing neointimal thickness. A wide variety of other agents have been studied in this model and are discussed below.

A variation on the carotid injury process has been reported using electrical stimulation to induce intimal fibromuscular plaques. A recent publication studied the effect of low molecular weight heparin in this model, showing efficacy (58).

C. Rabbit Ear Crush Injury Model

A model also using anesthetized hypercholesterolemic New Zealand rabbits has been described recently (59). The central ear artery is crushed with external pressure in this model. The rabbits are maintained on a diet of 2.4% fat and 1% cholesterol. Neointimal thickening occurs along with smooth muscle cell proliferation (documented by bromodeoxyuridine) for 21 days. Area stenoses appear and measure roughly 40%, with neointimal thickening beginning at day 5. The availability of the central artery makes it accessible for local treatments if desired. The model appears effective in rapidly producing neointima. It is inexpensive and is promising as a model of coronary restenosis.

D. Porcine Carotid Injury Model

Porcine carotid arteries have been studied extensively for arterial thrombus, syndromes of accelerated atherosclerosis (60,61), and restenosis (62,63).

In this model, cutdown is performed on a femoral artery, and a 9-mm balloon advanced into the common carotid arteries. After inflation, the balloon is pulled retrograde to cause endothelial denudation and sometimes deep arterial injury (61,62,64–67).

A vigorous platelet thrombus response to injury is related to vessel injury depth and to other factors such as local shear stress (61,68). With deep vessel injury, exposure of collagen induces platelet aggregation and mural thrombosis, followed by migration and proliferation of smooth muscle cells.

Neointimal formation occurs with deep injury (64,69). Hemodynamically significant stenoses rarely result fron neointima, except in occasional cases of gross thrombus accumulation with subsequent organization (62). Hypercholesterolemia is not required. Platelet deposition occurs early in this model, and has been substantially reduced using the agent hirudin (65,67,70,71). In addition, proliferating cell growth fractions measured by bromodeoxyuridine approach 30%, and have been documented in the first 48 h after injury (69).

E. Porcine Coronary Injury Models

The coronary arteries of domestic crossbred pigs respond similarly to human coronary arteries after sustaining deep injury (72). A hypercholesterolemic diet produces more severe lesions than with standard laboratory diets (73,74). Standard human angioplasty guide catheters and curves fit the por-

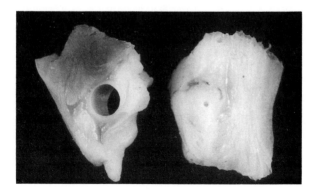

Figure 1 Photograph of severe neointimal thickening in porcine coronary arteries. This section was taken from different sites of the same left anterior descending coronary artery, within 3 mm of each other. The implantation of coil wires is shown in the severely narrowed section while a normal-appearing vessel is seen where there were no coil wires. The neointima induced by the injury has nearly obliterated the lumen of this vessel and resulted in a severe stenosis.

cine aortic root well (20- to 40-kg animals) for engagement of the left main or right coronary arteries. Severe mechanical injury is done to the coronary arteries either by a coronary angioplasty balloon alone (72,75,76), or by delivering an oversized metal coronary stent to the artery for chronic implant. Both methods create injury that results in a thick neointima within 20–28 days. An example of the neointimal thickening at sites of injury is shown in Figure 1. The histopathological features of this neointima are identical to human restenotic neointima (see Fig. 2). Specimens from balloon-only injury typically show a single laceration of media, filled at 28 days by a variable amount of neointima. The oversized stented arteries show multiple injuries in each section, some more severe than others, and resulting in a differential amount of neointima at those sites (Fig. 3). Each injury site may be quantitated in the porcine oversized stent injury model as a mean injury score (Table 1) that is ordinally proportional to injury depth (77,78). The amount of neointimal thickening and corresponding percent stenosis is directly proportional to this score (Fig. 4). This permits creation of an injury-response regression line that can be used to quantitate the response to potential therapies (79).

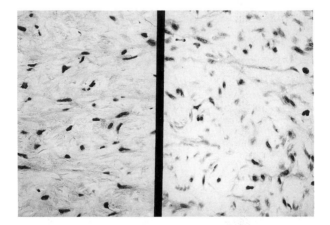

Figure 2 Side-by-side views of human restenotic neointimal hyperplasia (left) compared to tissue resulting from mechanical injury at 28 days from the porcine coronary injury model (right). The cell characteristics, density, and interstitial ground substance are very similar. The neointimal hyperplasia in the pig occurs in a nonatherosclerotic environment and develops rapidly following injury. (Hematoxylin eosin stain, magnification × 300.)

(a)

(b)

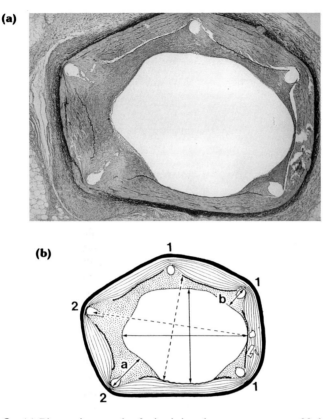

Figure 3 (a) Photomicrograph of wire-injured artery segment at 28 days after injury where different wires created different depths of injury. Neointimal thicknesses for the two wires at the left of the section are greater; the injuries from these wires are correspondingly greater in comparison to those three on the right. Elastic van Gieson stain, magnification × 30. (b) Schematic drawing shows how measurements were made from the above section. The dashed line axes are the native lumen major and minor axes. The solid line axes are the residual lumen major and minor axes. Injury scores for each wire are located on the schematic drawing, outside the vessel (large numerals).

Animal restenosis models have come under increasing criticism for failing to predict clinical trial results. A number of reasons may be invoked to explain the failures. Importantly, the limits of any model must be firmly understood before applying the results to clinical trials. The doses of drug on a per kilogram basis have differed markedly from animal to human trials. For

Table 1 Definition of Injury Score

Description of assigned weight	Injury
0	Internal elastic lamina intact; endothelium typically denuded; media may be compressed but not lacerated.
1	Internal elastic lamina lacerated; media typically compressed but not lacerated.
2	Internal elastic lamina lacerated; media visibly lacerated, external elastic lamina intact but may be compressed.
3	External elastic lamina lacerated. Typically large lacerations of media extending through the external elastic lamina. Coil wires sometimes residing in adventitia.

example, neointimal reduction by ACE inhibition in the rat carotid model has been well documented (80–85). The rats were typically treated with the captopril 100 mg/kg or cilazapril 10 mg/kg body weight per day beginning 6 days before arterial injury and continuing chronologically. Neointima was markedly reduced in both drug treatment groups (42 ± 11% captopril treated versus 111 ± 10% control, and 35 ± 9% cilazapril treated versus 93 ± 5% control), and provided the basis for the two large clinical trials of cilazapril in Europe (MERCATOR) and the United States (MARCATOR).

Both clinical trials showed essentially no effect on restenosis as noted above (53,54). The highest cilazapril dose used in the MARCATOR trial was 20 mg/day for 24 weeks. In a 70-kg patient, this dose is equivalent to 0.29 mg/kg body weight, or 2.5% of the dose reported effective in rats on a body weight basis. Moreover, the 20 mg/day regimen was poorly tolerated in patients due to orthostatic hypotension and other side effects. The dose shown effective in rats was thus 40 times higher than the largest human dose used in MARCATOR. In retrospect, it is not surprising that the clinical trials were negative given this large dose discrepancy.

Another reason that animal models have not shown results comparable to human studies may be in the divergent methods that have been used to assess efficacy. Clinical trials must assess treatment efficacy using angio-

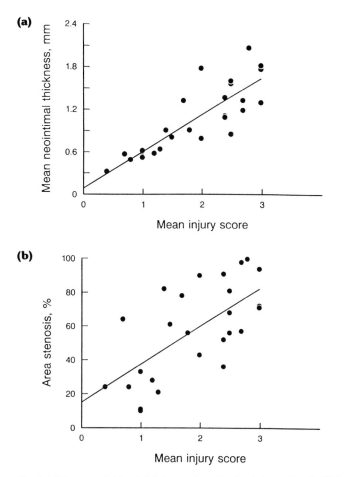

Figure 4 (a) Mean neointimal thickness for all wire injury sites in 26 locations of different porcine vessels is plotted versus mean injury score. A strongly proportional relationship exists ($p < 0.05$), with the plotted regression line. The scatter increases for increasing mean depth of injury. (b) Percent area stenosis (measured from histopathology sections) for the same 26 injury sites plotted versus mean injury score. A similarly strong proportional relationship exists ($p < 0.05$), although the spread is greater. Once again, the scatter increases for increasing mean depth of injury.

graphically derived measures, typically percent stenosis or minimal luminal diameter from the 6-month angiogram. In comparison, animal model studies have the advantage of using histopathological sections for measurement, and response parameters are neointimal volume, percent of medial coverage by neointima, or neointima:media thickness ratios. While these measures may show statistically significant treatment effects, such differences may not translate to quantities that would be observed by angiographic assessments or improvements in clinical outcome.

Substantial differences may exist across species in reaction to arterial injury. These differences may be reflected in both neointimal volume and the response to various therapies. For example, stenosing lesions rarely occur in the dog coronary artery despite significant arterial injury. Clearly, different species develop differing amounts of neointima in response to the same injury.

Model differences confound species differences. For example, the types and severity of injury in the rat carotid artery studies consist of balloon stretch with consequent endothelial denudation only. Major arterial anatomical structures (internal elastic lamina, media, and external elastic lamina) remain intact. This comparatively mild injury contrasts with balloon injury in the rabbit iliac and porcine coronary arteries. In the pig coronary model, it was shown that significant neointimal hyperplasia results only if the internal elastic lamina is fractured (see Fig. 5) (78,86). Neointimal formation rapidly increases as the media and external elastic lamina are damaged (77).

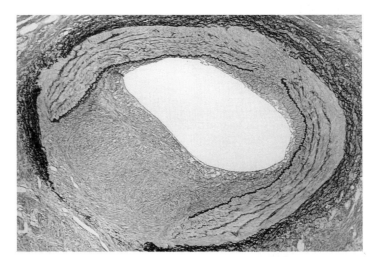

Figure 5   In this section, a porcine coronary artery underwent inflation only, without coil implant. Note the neointimal hyperplasia occurs again only at sites of rupture of the internal elastic lamina. The appearance is proportional in that at the larger laceration of the internal elastic lamina more neointima occurs. Conversely, at the smaller laceration, less neointimal thickening occurs. (Elastic van Gieson stain, magnification × 120.)

Deep arterial injury in both the rabbit and porcine coronary models is quite similar to that occurring in patients during balloon angioplasty, and thus these models may be closer to the types of injury caused by angioplasty balloons.

Recent data suggest that a neointimal proportional response to injury may also exist in balloon angioplasty of human coronary arteries. In this case, the acute gain is a surrogate for vessel injury, as is initial severity of stenosis. Both of these parameters have been shown proportional to angiographic measurement of the late luminal loss in diameter (87). It is uncertain whether neointima that is thick enough to cause angiographically identifiable stenoses would occur in rat carotid arteries if deep arterial injury was accomplished.

The thrombotic response to arterial injury may also differ substantially across species. In the rat carotid model, a thin layer of platelets accumulates at the endothelial denudation site. However, significant fibrin-rich thrombus is virtually never found in this model. Conversely, in the rabbit iliac model, macroscopic thrombus does occur, and has been characterized in a preliminary report (88). In the porcine carotid and coronary models, fibrin-rich mural thrombus also plays a significant role in the response to

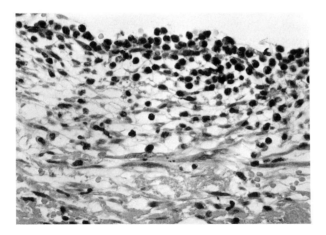

Figure 6 In the porcine coronary injury model, monocytes and lymphocytes appear in dense concentration on both the luminal and mural sides of endothelium, with degenerating thrombus below (amorphous material). These cells begin to accumulate as early as 4 days following arterial injury. The fibrin base, and these cells provide theoretical approaches to solution of the restenosis problem. (Hematoxylin and eosin stain, × 500.)

injury (89,90). In the coronary arteries, fibrin-rich thrombus provides a scaffold for colonization by smooth muscle cells. This scaffold eventually forms the organized neointima, a mechanism suggested in the rabbit also (88). The presence of macrophages, monocytes, and lymphocytes precedes smooth muscle cell infiltration in the pig (Fig. 6). However, this inflammatory response has not been described in rat carotid restenosis studies. The implications of this inflammatory reaction are unclear, but remain to be seen.

III. CLINICAL RESULTS

A. Pharmacological Restenosis Trials

No pharmacological agent has been shown to either consistently or effectively reduce restenosis. A synopsis of the many pharmacological approaches to preventing restenosis is shown in Table 2. Agents from many drug classes and across many different proposed mechanisms are represented in this list of failures. The cost of these failures in both economics and time is quite evident from examining the poor record of results.

The trials themselves provide conflicting results in the case of some agents, while other agents have consistently failed to show efficacy. In the former category, fish oil ingestion in high concentration appears to have some effect, the magnitude of which is unclear. It appears that fish oil must be begun well in advance of the procedure, about 6 days minimum. A meta-analytic review of the fish oil trials shows that of 396 patients from 6 trials with angiographic follow-up, the restenosis rate in treated patients was 26% compared to 32% in the untreated groups.

Trials of aggressive lipid-lowering agents were instituted since this therapy has not proven clearly efficacious in slowing or even causing regression of atherosclerosis. Trials of the lipid-lowering agents lovastatin or probucol have also shown conflicting results. Several large, randomized trials will shortly present data on the efficacy of this therapy against restenosis.

In addition to the ACE inhibitors, conflicting data also exist for calcium channel blockers. Diltiazem has been reported as ineffective (91–93), while some reports of verapamil show reduction (10). These studies are generally not conclusive either due to high overall restenosis rates or because of low angiographic follow-up.

Corticosteroids have generally been considered ineffective against restenosis principally on the basis of a large, well-performed trial from the M-Heart (Multi-Hospital Eastern Atlantic Restenosis Trial) study of 915 patients given steroids in the immediate preangioplasty period (94). Another steroid trial using a dose regimen for 5 days following angioplasty was also negative. The

Table 2 Summary of Pharmacological Restenosis Trials

Class/Agent	Result	Reference
Antiplatelet/PDGF Agents		
Aspirin	Negative	(96)
	Negative	(97)
	Negative	(98)
Aspirin/Dipyridamole	Negative	(99)
Ticlopidine	Negative	(100)
Ciprostene	Negative	(101,102)
Trapidil	Effective	(103)
Thromboxane-A_2	Negative	(104)
Antagonism	Negative	(105)
Anticoagulants		
Coumadin	Negative	(96)
	Negative	(106)
Heparin	Negative	(107)
Low Molecular Weight Heparin		(7)
Anti-inflammatory Agents		
Corticosteroids	Negative	(94)
Colchicine		(9,12,95)
Lipid-Altering Agents		
Fish Oil	Negative	(108)
	Effective	(109)
	Negative	(110,111)
Lovastatin	Negative	(112)
	Effective	(113)
Calcium Channel Blockade		
Diltiazem	Negative	(91)
Nifedipine	Negative	(114)
ACE Inhibitors		
Cilazapril	Negative	(53,54)
Fosinopril		
Miscellaneous		
Prostacyclin	Negative	(115)
Ketanserin		(116)

anti-inflammatory agent colchicine also has been shown to have little effect on restenosis in several clinical trials (9,12,95).

Antiplatelet agents have at best a marginal effect, and have been evaluated for many years. Anticoagulants also have not shown consistent substantial effects against restenosis despite many trials. Such trials include heparin, low molecular weight heparin, and coumadin.

These pharmacological failures do little other than to prove that our understanding of the restenosis process is incomplete. The consistent failures have additionally produced a tough dilemma. Concern about the accuracy of animal restenosis models has recently been voiced. The trial failures imply that more effort must be put into understanding animal model mechanisms, and how they translate to human restenosis pathophysiology. Why have the pharmacological trials failed? It seems that the proper drug or drug combination has not yet been found, that the optimal doses and/or timing have not yet been discovered for an agent already tested, that we have not correctly assessed efficacy in animal models, and that we do not understand the limits of those models.

B. Device Trials and Restenosis

While the majority of clinical trials have shown little or no effect, a pattern appears to be emerging from two important trials of new devices.

1. The CAVEAT Trial

The CAVEAT trial (*C*oronary *A*ngioplasty *V*ersus *E*xcisional *A*therectomy *T*rial) is the first major clinical trial to date showing positive effects on restenosis by directional atherectomy. Thirty-five centers from the United States and Europe participated in this trial, cumulatively enrolling 1012 patients into randomly assigned groups of atherectomy or standard balloon angioplasty of lesions that had been judged suitable for either prior to randomization. Six-month angiographic follow-up was performed, and all coronary angiographic data analyzed using quantitative coronary angiography.

As expected from the randomization process, the two treatment groups at the end of the study were matched for clinical characteristics shown in Table 3. The acute angiographic results of intervention in this trial are shown in Table 4. Despite similar reference diameters and initial lesion minimal luminal diameters, the atherectomy group achieved a larger postprocedural minimal luminen diameter compared to balloon angioplasty (1.05 mm versus 0.87 mm). This occurred at a cost of higher acute complications (DCA:11% vs. PTCA:5%).

Restenosis in this trial was defined as a recurrent lesion of >50% diameter stenosis at a previously successful lesion site. Cumulative minimal lumen diameter analysis was also done to compare each group. Follow-up was available in 862 patients. Using the 50% diameter stenosis binary endpoint definition for restenosis, 50% of patients in the directional atherectomy group versus 57% in the balloon angioplasty group suffered this endpoint ($p = 0.055$). Minimum lumen diameter analysis also showed benefit to the DCA procedure. The most important determinant of final (6-month) minimal lumen diameter was the immediate postprocedure diameter. Two

Table 3 Clinical Characteristics of Patients in CAVEAT I

Angioplasty	Directional atherectomy (512 patients)	Balloon (500 patients)
Mean age (years)	59	59
Male sex	75%	70%
Diabetes	19%	19%
Unstable angina	65%	70%
Ejection fraction	58%	56%
Lesion length (mm)	8.9	8.6
Vessel size (mm)	2.9	2.9
% diameter stenosis	71%	73%

other significant characteristics were preprocedural MLD ($p = 0.0001$) and the presence of diabetes ($p = 0.001$).

The results of this trial have been considered modest by some since a nominal reduction in restenosis rate was achieved at the expense of acute complications. However, the findings should not be minimized: this is the first large trial to show any reduction in restenosis, even if the overall restenosis rates were high by the definition used.

The role of acute postprocedural lumen size appears to be important, possibly suggesting that a larger initial lumen leads to more capacity on the part of the vessel to form neointimal hyperplasia without developing recurrent stenosis. This argument has been termed "bigger is better," and has been argued from both directions. Specifically, the CAVEAT data exemplify the argument well. The larger initial lumen of DCA may have caused the lower restenosis rate. The higher complication rate, though, partially negated the efficacy of the technique.

Deeper resection by DCA may cause more eventual neointimal hyperplasia. At issue is whether there is proportionally more hyperplasia so that the additional acute gain is negated by additional neointima, eventuating in

Table 4 Procedural Characteristics CAVEAT I

Angioplasty	Directional atherectomy (512 patients)	Balloon (500 patients)
Minimal lumen diameter pre (mm)	0.86	0.84
Acute gain (mm)	1.02	0.87
Reference diameter (mm)	2.78	2.78

restenosis. The animal model studies mentioned earlier in this chapter suggest that deeper vessel injury causes more hyperplasia. Whether the differential rate of neointimal formation is higher for deeper resection is currently under investigation.

It is interesting to speculate on the results of tighter initial lesion diameters resulting in higher restenosis rates. This may be because more vessel injury was incurred to open the artery to its final diameter. Animal data clearly show that neointimal hyperplasia is proportional to injury. A 90% diameter stenotic lesion must be expanded fully by a factor of 10 in order to achieve a satisfactory result. This amount of expansion must result in substantial injury to a stenotic vessel segment.

2. The BENESTENT Trial

Preliminary restenosis data now exist comparing balloon angioplasty with coronary stents, termed the BENESTENT trial. This European trial was coordinated by the Thoraxcenter group in Rotterdam and enrolled 260 patients. It was randomized for suitable lesions, with patients receiving either the Palmaz-Schatz slotted tubular stent or balloon angioplasty only. The angiographic endpoints of the trial were 6-month MLD determined using quantitative coronary arteriography. The primary clinical endpoints of this trial were the need for repeat procedures, recurrent angina, or evidence of ischemia, stroke, myocardial infarction, or death. There were 10 subacute occlusions, 6 in the PTCA group and 4 in the stent group.

Using an intention-to-treat analysis, the restenosis rate using this stent was 20% versus 31% for angioplasty. Repeat intervention was required in 13% of stent patients versus 29% of angioplasty patients. The postprocedural MLD for stents was significantly higher, again potentially explaining the difference in restenosis rates (follow-up median MLD: 1.64 mm in the balloon-treated group versus 1.90 mm in the stent group, $p < 0.05$). Further data will be forthcoming for this interesting trial.

The CAVEAT and BENESTENT trials are interesting in that they are the first clinical trials of either drugs or devices to definitively show any impact on restenosis. The mechanistic hypothesis for the demonstrated effect is that the greater acute luminal gains during the procedure yielded larger lumina at 6-month follow-up.

IV. DISCUSSION AND CONCLUSION

The solution to restenosis remains extraordinarily elusive despite much time, effort, and money. Pharmacological interventions have to date proven disappointingly inconsistent.

Mechanical revascularization strategies appear to be offering the first hope toward making an impact. The unifying operational principal of these strategies is that by obtaining as large an initial lumen as possible, more vessel volume can be occupied by neointima without causing luminal reobstruction. While this is indeed a practical solution, it does not address the issue of limiting neointimal growth.

Unfortunately, the mechanical strategies are available at comparatively high cost. For example, not all patients are suitable to undergo directional atherectomy. During the CAVEAT trial, an interventional registry of balloon angioplasty compared to atherectomy procedures was maintained. Results showed that DCA comprised only 11% of all procedures. This number must be artificially low, but nevertheless exemplifies the point that the technique requires larger, proximal, less tortuous vessels that are accessible to the device. The other cost of the DCA technique is the higher acute complication rate.

The use of intracoronary stents also is associated with problems not found in balloon angioplasty. The necessity of anticoagulation is of prime importance, resulting in higher in-patient time and cost, and patient selection issues along with a higher risk of late closure. Not all lesions and coronary anatomy are suitable for stenting as well, with most devices not recommended for vessels < 3.0 mm in diameter. Some stents are also less flexible, making distal access a concern.

All types of revascularization in current use by necessity impose substantial injury on the coronary artery at the site of the stenotic lesion, either by fracturing or removing plaque. The end result is the same: exposure of subintimal tissue structure to flowing blood. Neointimal hyperplasia at the injury site is a good and necessary end in healing the revascularization injury. The problem comes not in eliminating the hyperplastic response, but in modulating it so that only an "appropriate," nonstenosing amount of neointima forms. Neointimal formation appears clearly proportional to the degree of injury.

In summary, hope is finally appearing in limiting restenosis through newer, device-based strategies that provide a larger acute lumen. However, this strategy must be accomplished with the same or fewer complications. It does appear that the larger lumen strategy will not be a complete solution; it will likely ential a combination of pharmacological and mechanical means.

The primary goal for the future is an understanding of vascular response to injury at both cellular and molecular levels. Once the intricacies of this response are better understood, strategic approaches for limiting the response can be better developed.

REFERENCES

1. Bell M, Gersh B. Restenosis: a clinician's perspective. In: Schwartz R, ed. Coronary Restenosis. Boston: Blackwell, 1992:15–54.

2. Holmes DR Jr, Vlietstra RE, Smith HC, Vetrovec GW, Kent KM, Dowley MJ. Restenosis after percutaneous transluminal coronary angioplasty (PTCA): A report from the PTCA registry of the National Heart, Lung, and Blood Institute. Am J Cardiol 1984;53:77C–81C.
3. Austin GE. Lipids and vascular restenosis. Circulation 1992;85:1613–5.
4. Bell L, Madri JA. Original contributions: Effect of platelet factors on migration of cultured bovine aortic endothelial and smooth muscle cells. Circ Res 1989;65:1057–1065.
5. Bowles MH, Klonis D, Plavac TG, et al. EPA in the prevention of restenosis post PTCA. Angiology 1991;42:187–94.
6. Califf R, Ohmann E, Frid D, et al. Restenosis: the clinical issues. In: Topol E, ed. Textbook of Interventional Cardiology. Philadelphia: W.B. Saunders, 1990: 363–94.
7. Faxon D, Spiro T, Minor S, et al. Enoxaparin, a low molecular weight heparin, in the prevention of restenosis after angioplasty: results of a double blind randomized trial (abstr). J Am Coll Cardiol 1992;19:258A.
8. Finci L, Hofling B, Ludwig B, et al. Sulotroban during and after coronary angioplasty. A double-blind, placebo controlled study. Z Kardiol 1989;3:50–4.
9. Grines C, Rizik D, Levine A, et al. Colchicine angioplasty restenosis trial (CART) (abstr). Circulation 1991;84:II-365.
10. Hoberg E, Schwarz F, Schomig A, et al. Prevention of restenosis by verapamil: the verapamil angioplasty study (VAS) (abstr). Circulation 1990;82:III-428.
11. Israel DH, Gorlin R. Fish oils in the prevention of atherosclerosis. J Am Coll Cardiol 1992;19:174–85.
12. O'Keefe J, McCallister B, Bateman T, Kuhnlein D, Ligon R, Hartzler G. Colchicine for the prevention of restenosis after coronary angioplasty. J Am Coll Cardiol 1991;17:181A.
13. Serruys P, Hermans R. The new angiotensin converting enzyme inhibitor cilazapril does not prevent restenosis after coronary angioplasty: the results of the MERCATOR trial (abstr). J Am Coll Cardiol 1992;19:258A.
14. Taylor R, Gibbons F, Cope G, et al. Effects of low dose aspirin on restenosis after coronary angioplasty. Am J Cardiol 1991;68:874–878.
15. Kuntz RE, Safian RD, Carrozza JP, Fishman RF, Mansour M, Baim DS. The importance of acute luminal diameter in determining restenosis after coronary atherectomy or stenting. Circulation 1992;86:1827–35.
16. Kuntz RE, Hinohara T, Safian RD, Selmon MR, Simpson JB, Baim DS. Restenosis after directional coronary atherectomy. Effects of luminal diameter and deep wall excision. Circulation 1992;86:1394–9.
17. Garratt KN, Holmes DR Jr, Bell MR, et al. Restenosis after directional coronary atherectomy: differences between primary atheromatous and restenosis lesions and influence of subintimal tissue resection. J Am Coll Cardiol 1990; 16:1665–71.
18. Hinohara T, Robertson GC, Selmon MR, et al. Restenosis after directional coronary atherectomy. J Am Coll Cardiol 1992;20:623–32.
19. ONeill WW. Mechanical rotational atherectomy. Am J Cardiol 1992;69:12F–18F.

20. Litvack F, Margolis J, Cummins F, et al. Excimer laser coronary (ELCA) registry: report of the first consecutive 2080 patients (abstr). J Am Coll Cardiol 1992;19:276A.
21. Anand RK, Sinclair IN, Jenkins RD, Hiehle JF Jr, James L, Spears JR. Laser balloon angioplasty: effect of constant temperature versus constant power on tissue weld strength. Lasers Surg Med 1988;8:40-4.
22. Buchwald AB, Werner GS, Unterberg C, Voth E, Kreuzer H, Wiegand V. Restenosis after excimer laser angioplasty of coronary stenoses and chronic total occlusions. Am Heart J 1992;123(4 Pt 1):878-85.
23. Ghazzal Z, Burton M, Klein L, et al. Predictors of restenosis following excimer laser: multicenter comprehensive angiographic analysis (abstr). Circulation 1991; 84:II-361.
24. Margolis JR, Litvack F, Kreuthamer D, Trautwein R, Goldenberg T, Grundfest W. Excimer laser coronary angioplasty: American multicenter experience. Herz 1990;15:223-32.
25. Glazier JJ, Varricchione TR, Ryan TJ, Ruocco NA, Jacobs AK, Faxon DP. Factors predicing recurrent restenosis after percutaneous transluminal coronary balloon angioplasty. Am J Cardiol 1989;63:902-5.
26. Black AJR, Anderson V, Roubin GS, Powelson SW, Douglas JR Jr, King SB III. Repeat coronary angioplasty: correlates of a second restenosis. J Am Coll Card 1988;11:714-718.
27. Nobuyoshi M, Kimura T, Nosaka H, et al. Restenosis after successful percutaneous transluminal coronary angioplasty: serial angiographic follow-up of 229 patients. J Am Coll Cardiol 1988;12:616-623.
28. Serruys PW, Luijten HE, Beatt KJ, et al. Incidence of restenosis after successful coronary angioplasty: a time-related phenomenon. A quantitative angiographic study in 342 consecutive patients at 1, 2, 3, and 4 months. Circulation 1988;77:361-71.
29. Clowes A, Reidy M, Clowes M. Kinetics of cellular proliferation after arterial injury: I. Smooth muscle growth in absence of endothelium. Lab Invest 1983; 49:327-332.
30. Clowes AW, Reidy MA, Clowes MM. Mechanisms of stenosis after arterial injury. Lab Invest 1983;49:208.
31. Guyton J, Rosenburg R, Clowes A, Karnovsky M. Inhibition of rat arterial smooth muscle cell proliferation by heparin. In vivo studies with anticoagulant and nonanticoagulant heparin. Circ Res 1980;46:625-634.
32. Clowes AW, Clowes MM, Au YPT, Reidy MA, Belin D. Original contributions: smooth muscle cells express urokinase during mitogenesis and tissue-type plasminogen activator during migration in injured rat carotid artery. Circ Res 1990; 67:61-67.
33. Fingerle J, Au YPT, Clowes AW, Reidy MA. Intimal lesion formation in rat carotid arteries after endothelial denudation in absence of medial injury. Arteriosclerosis 1990;10:1082-1087.
34. Golden MA, Au YP, Kenagy RD, Clowes AW. Growth factor gene expression by intimal cells in healing polytetrafluoroethylene grafts. J Vasc Surg 1990;11: 580-5.

35. Reidy M, Clowes A, Schwartz S. Endothelial regeneration: V. Inhibition of endothelial regrowth in arteries of rat and rabbit. Lab Invest 1983;49:569–575.
36. Simons M, Rosenberg R. Antisense approach to smooth muscle proliferation. Circulation 1991;84:II-342.
37. Simons M, Edelman ER, DeKeyser J, Langer R, Rosenberg RD. Antisense c-myb oligonucleotides inhibit intimal arterial smooth muscle cell accumulation in vivo. Nature 1992;356:62–65.
38. Ragosta M, Gimple L, Haber H, et al. Effectiveness of specific factor Xa inhibition on restenosis following balloon angioplasty in rabbits (abstr). J Am Coll Cardiol 1992;19:164A.
39. Sarembock I, Gertz D, Gimple L, Owen R, Powers E, Roberts W. Effectiveness of recombinant desulphatohirudin in reducing restenosis after balloon angioplasty of atherosclerotic femoral arteries in rabbits. Circulation 1991;84:232–243.
40. Gellman J, Ezekowitz MD, Sarembock IJ, et al. Effect of lovastatin on intimal hyperplasia after balloon angioplasty: a study in an atherosclerotic hypercholesterolemic rabbit. J Am Coll Cardiol 1991;17:251–9.
41. Haber H, Gimple L, Goldstein C, et al. The effect of oral terbinafine on restenosis following balloon angioplasty in rabbits (abstr). Circulation 1991;84:II–332.
42. LaVeau P, Sarembock I, Sigal S, Yang T, Ezekowitz M. Vascular reactivity after balloon angioplasty in an atherosclerotic rabbit. Circulation 1990;82:1790–1801.
43. Au YP, Kenagy RD, Clowes AW. Heparin selectively inhibits the transcription of tissue-type plasminogen activator in primate arterial smooth muscle cells during mitogenesis. J Biol Chem 1992;267:3438–44.
44. Clowes AW, Clowes MM, Vergel SC, et al. The renin-angiotensin system and the vascular wall: from experimental models to man: heparin and cilazapril together inhibit injury-induced intimal hyperplasia. Hypertension 1991;18(Suppl):65–69.
45. Fingerle J, Johnson R, Clowes AW, Majesky MW, Reidy MA. Role of platelets in smooth muscle cell proliferation and migration after vascular injury in rat carotid artery. Proc Natl Acad Sci U S A 1989;86:8412–6.
46. Gerdes J, Li L, Schlueter C, et al. Immunobiochemical and molecular biologic characterization of the cell proliferation-associated nuclear antigen that is defined by monoclonal antibody Ki-67. Am J Pathol 1991;138:867–73.
47. Hanke H, Strohschneider T, Oberhoff M, Betz E, Karsch KR. Time course of smooth muscle cell proliferation in the intima and media of arteries following experimental angioplasty. Circ Res 1990;67:651–659.
48. Hanke H, Strohschneider T, Oberhoff M, Betz E, Karsch KR. Time course of smooth muscle cell proliferation in the intima and media of arteries following experimental angioplasty. Circ Res 1990;67:651–659.
49. Schwartz CJ, Sprague EA, Valente AJ, Kelley JL, Edwards EH. Cellular mechanisms in the response of the arterial wall to injury and repair. Toxicol Pathol 1989;17:66–71.

50. Ferns GA, Raines EW, Sprugel KH, Motani AS, Reidy MA, Ross R. Inhibition of neointimal smooth muscle accumulation after angioplasty by an antibody to PDGF. Science 1991;253:1129–32.
51. Ross R, Harker L. Platelets, endothelium, and smooth muscle cells in atherosclerosis. Adv Exp Med Biol 1978;102:135–41.
52. Ross R. Platelets: cell proliferation and atherosclerosis. Metabolism 1979;28: 410–4.
53. MERCATOR Study Group. Does the new angiotensin converting enzyme inhibitor cilazapril prevent restenosis after percutaneous transluminal coronary angioplasty? Results of the MERCATOR study: a multicenter, randomized, double-blind placebo-controlled trial. Circulation 1992;86:100–10.
54. Faxon DP. Angiotensin converting enzyme inhibition and restenosis: the final results of the MARCATOR Trial (abstr). Circulation 1992;86:I-53.
55. Faxon DP, Weber VJ, Haudenschild C, Gottsman SB, McGovern WA, Ryan T. Acute effects of transluminal angioplasty in three experimental models of atherosclerosis. Arteriosclerosis 1982;2:125–33.
56. Faxon DP, Sanborn TA, Weber VJ, et al. Restenosis following transluminal angioplasty in experimental atherosclerosis. Arteriosclerosis 1984;4:189–195.
57. Faxon DP, Sanborn TA, Haudenschild CC, Ryan TJ. Effect of antiplatelet therapy on restenosis after experimental angioplasty. Am J Cardiol 1984;53: 72C–76C.
58. Hanke H, Oberhoff M, Hanke S, et al. Inhibition of cellular proliferation after experimental balloon angioplasty by low-molecular-weight heparin. Circulation 1992;85:1548–56.
59. Banai S, Shou M, Correa R, et al. Original contributions: rabbit ear model of injury-induced arterial smooth muscle cell proliferation: kinetics, reproducibility, and implications. Circ Res 1991;69:748–756.
60. Ip JH, Fuster V, Badimon L, Badimon J, Taubman MB, Chesebro JH. Syndromes of accelerated atherosclerosis: role of vascular injury and smooth muscle cell proliferation. J Am Coll Cardiol 1990;15:1667–1687.
61. Fuster V, Badimon L, Badimon JJ, Ip JH, Chesebro JH. The porcine model for the understanding of thrombogenesis and atherogenesis. Mayo Clin Proc 1991;66:818–31.
62. Steele P, Chesebro J, Stanson A, et al. Balloon angioplasty, natural history of the pathophysiological response to injury in a pig model. Circ Res 1985;57:105–112.
63. Lam JY, Chesebro JH, Steele PM, et al. Antithrombotic therapy for deep arterial injury by angioplasty. Efficacy of common platelet inhibition compared with thrombin inhibition in pigs. Circulation 1991;84:814–20.
64. Chesebro JA, Lam JYT, Badimon L, Fuster V. Restenosis after arterial angioplasty. a hemorheologic response to injury. Am J Cardiol 1987;60:10B–16B.
65. Ip JH, Fuster V, Israel D, Badimon L, Badimon J, Chesebro JH. The role of platelets, thrombin and hyperplasia in restenosis after coronary angioplasty. J Am Coll Cardiol 1991;17 (suppl B):77B–88B.
66. Lam JYT, Chesebro JH, Steele PM, Dewanjee MK, Badimon L, Fuster V. Deep arterial injury during experimental angioplasty: Relationship to a positive in-

dium-111 labeled platelet scintigram, quantitative platelet deposition and mural thrombus. J Am Coll Cardiol 1986;8:1380–1386.

67. Webster MW, Chesebro JH, Fuster V. Platelet inhibitor therapy. Agents and clinical implications. Hematol Oncol Clin North Am 1990;4:265–89.

68. Adams PC, Badimon JJ, Badimon L, Chesebro JH, Fuster V. Role of platelets in atherogenesis: relevance to coronary arterial restenosis after angioplasty. Cardiovasc Clin 1987;18:49–71.

69. Webster M, Chesebro J, Grill D, Badimon J, Badimon L, Fuster V. The thrombotic and proliferative response to angioplasty in pigs after deep arterial injury: effect of intravenous thrombin inhibition with hirudin (abstr). Circulation 1991; 84:II–580.

70. Heras M, Chesebro JH, Webster MW, et al. Hirudin, heparin, and placebo during deep arterial injury in the pig. The in vivo role of thrombin in platelet-mediated thrombosis. Circulation 1990;82:1476–84.

71. Heras M, Chesebro JH, Penny WJ, Bailey KR, Badimon L, Fuster V. Effects of thrombin inhibition on the development of acute platelet-thrombus deposition during angioplasty in pigs. Heparin versus recombinant hirudin, a specific thrombin inhibitor. Circulation 1989;79:657–65.

72. Schwartz RS, Murphy JG, Edwards WD, Camrud AR, Vlietstra RE, Holmes DR, Jr. Restenosis after balloon angioplasty: A practical proliferative model in porcine coronary arteries. Circulation 1990;82:2190–2200.

73. Rodgers GP, Minor ST, Robinson K, et al. Adjuvant therapy for intracoronary stents. Investigations in atherosclerotic swine. Circulation 1990;82:560–9.

74. Rodgers GP, Minor ST, Robinson K, et al. The coronary artery response to implantation of a balloon-expandable flexible stent in the aspirin- and non-aspirin-treated swine model. Am Heart J 1991;122:640–7.

75. Santoian EC, King SB3. Intravascular stents, intimal proliferation and restenosis. J Am Coll Cardiol 1992;19:877–9.

76. Santoian E, Foegh M, Gravanis M, et al. Treatment with angiopeptin inhibits the development of smooth muscle proliferation in a balloon overstretch swine model of restenosis (abstr). J Am Coll Cardiol 1992;19:164A.

77. Schwartz R, Huber K, Murphy J, et al. Restenosis and the proportional neointimal response to coronary artery injury: results in a porcine model. J Am Coll Cardiol 1992;19:267–274.

78. Schwartz RS, Murphy JG, Edwards WD, Camrud AR, Vlietstra RE, Holmes DR Jr. Restenosis occurs with internal elastic lamina laceration and is proportional to severity of vessel injury in a porcine coronary artery model. Circulation 1990;82:III–656.

79. Schwartz R, Koval T, Edwards W, et al. Effect of external beam irradiation on neointimal hyperplasia after experimental coronary artery injury. J Am Coll Cardiol 1992;19:1106–1113.

80. Powell J, Muller R, Baumgartner H. Suppression of the vascular response to injury: the role of angiotension-converting enzyme inhibitors. J Am Coll Cardiol 1991;17:137B–142B.

81. Powell J, Clozel J, Muller R, et al. Inhibitors of angiotensin-converting enzyme prevent myointimal proliferation after vascular injury. Science 1989;245:186–8.

82. Bilazarian S, Currier J, Haudenschild C, et al. Angiotensin converting enzyme inhibition reduces restenosis in experimental angioplasty. J Am Coll Cardiol 1991;17:268A.

83. Berk B, Vekshtein V, Gordon H. Angiotensin II-stimulated protein synthesis in cultured vascular smooth muscle cells. Hypertension 1989;13:305-14.

84. Brozovich FV, Morganroth J, Gottlieb NG, Gottlieb RS. Effect of angiotensin converting enzyme inhibition on the incidence of restenosis after percutaneous transluminal coronary angioplasty. Cathet Cardiovasc Diagn 1991;23:263-7.

85. Daemen MJ, Lombardi DM, Bosman FT, Schwartz SM. Angiotensin II induces smooth muscle cell proliferation in the normal and injured rat arterial wall. Circ Res 1991;68:450-6.

86. Schwartz RS, Murphy JG, Edwards WD, et al. Coronary artery restenosis and the "virginal membrane":smooth muscle cell proliferation and the intact internal elastic lamina. J Inv Cardiol 1991;3:3-8.

87. Beatt KJ, Serruys PW, Luijten HE, et al. Restenosis after coronary angioplasty: the paradox of increased lumen diameter and restenosis. J Am Coll Cardiol 1992;19:258-66.

88. Wilensky RL, Wong L, March KL, Sandusky GE, Hathaway DR. Immuno-histochemical characterization of arterial injury and restenosis following angioplasty in the atherosclerotic rabbit (abstr). J Am Coll Cardiol 1992;19:169A.

89. Schwartz RS, Edwards WD, Murphy JG, Camrud AR, Holmes DR Jr. Restenosis develops in four stages: serial histologic studies in a coronary injury model. J Am Coll Cardiol 1991;17:52A.

90. Schwartz R, Edwards W, Camrud A, Holmes DJ. Developmental stages of restenotic neointimal hyperplasia following porcine coronary artery injury: a morphologic review. J Vasc Med Biol 1993 (in press).

91. Corcos T, David PR, Bal PG, et al. Failure of diltiazem to prevent restenosis after percutaneous transluminal coronary angioplasty. Am Heart J 1985;109: 926-931.

92. O'Keefe JHJ, Giorgi LV, Hartzler GO, et al. Effects of diltiazem on complications and restenosis after coronary angioplasty. Am J Cardiol 1991;67:373-6.

93. Unverdorben M, Kunkel B, Leucht M, Bachmann K. Reduction of restenosis after PTCA by diltiazem? Circulation 1992;86:I-53.

94. Pepine CJ, Hirshfeld JW, Macdonald RG, et al. A controlled trial of corticosteroids to prevent restenosis after coronary angioplasty. M-HEART Group. Circulation 1990;81:1753-61.

95. OKeefe JHJ, McCallister BD, Bateman TM, Kuhnlein DL, Ligon RW, Hartzler GO. Ineffectiveness of colchicine for the prevention of restenosis after coronary angioplasty. J Am Coll Cardiol 1992;19:1597-600.

96. Thornton MA, Grunetzig AR, Hollman J, King SB 3rd, Douglas JS Jr. Coumadin and aspirin in prevention of recurrence after transluminal coronary angioplasty: a randomized study. Circulation 1984;69:721-727.

97. Ellis S, Roubin G, Wilentz J, Lin S, Douglas J Jr, King S 3rd. Results of a randomized trial of heparin and aspirin vs. aspirin alone for prevention of acute closure (AC) and restenosis (R) after angioplasty (PTCA) (abstr). Circulation 1987;76:IV-213.

98. Mufson L, Black A, Roubin G, et al. A randomized trial of aspirin in PTCA: Effect of high vs. low dose on major complications and restenosis (abstr). J Am Coll Cardiol 1988;11:236A.

99. Schwartz L, Bourassa MG, Lesperance J, et al. Aspirin and dipyridamole in the prevention of restenosis after percutaneous transluminal coronary angioplasty. N Engl J Med 1988;318:1714–9.

100. White C, Knudson M, Schmidt D. Neither ticlopidine nor aspirin-dipyridamole prevents restenosis post PTCA: results from a randomized placebo-controlled multicenter trial (abstr). Circulation 1987;76:IV–213.

101. Darius H, Nixdorff U, Zander J, Rupprecht HJ, Erbel R, Meyer J. Effects of ciprostene on restenosis rate during therapeutic transluminal coronary angioplasty. Agents Actions Suppl 1992;37:305–11.

102. Raizner A, Hollman J, Demke D, et al. Beneficial effects of ciprostene in PTCA: a multicenter, randomized controlled trial (abstr). Circulation 1988; 78:II–276.

103. Okamoto S, Inden M, Setsuda M, Konishi T, Nakano T. Effects of trapidil (triazolopyrimidine), a platelet-derived growth factor antagonist, in preventing restenosis after percutaneous transluminal coronary angioplasty. Am Heart J 1992;123:1439–44.

104. Serruys PW, Rutsch W, Heyndrickx GR, et al. Prevention of restenosis after percutaneous transluminal coronary angioplasty with thromboxane A2-receptor blockade. A randomized, double-blind, placebo-controlled trial. Coronary Artery Restenosis Prevention on Repeated Thromboxane-Antagonism Study (CARPORT). Circulation 1991;84:1568–80.

105. Savage MP, Goldberg S, Macdonald RG, et al. Multi-Hospital Eastern Atlantic Restenosis Trial. II: A placebo-controlled trial of thromboxane blockade in the prevention of restenosis following coronary angioplasty. Am Heart J 1991;122:1239–44.

106. Urban P, Buller N, Fox K, Shapiro L, Bayliss J, Rickards A. Lack of effect of warfarin on the restenosis rate or on clinical outcome after balloon coronary angioplasty. Br Heart J 1988;60:485–8.

107. Ellis SG, Roubin GS, Wilentz J, Douglas JS Jr, King SB III. Effect of 18- to 24-hour heparin administration for prevention of restenosis after uncomplicated coronary angioplasty. Am Heart J 1989;117:777–82.

108. Grigg LE, Kay TW, Valentine PA, et al. Determinants of restenosis and lack of effect of dietary supplementation with eicosapentaenoic acid on the incidence of coronary artery restenosis after angioplasty. J Am Coll Cardiol 1989; 13:665–72.

109. Dehmer G, Popma J, van den Berg E, et al. Reduction in the rate of early restenosis after coronary angioplasty by a diet supplemented with n-3 fatty acids. N Engl J Med 1988;319:733–40.

110. Reis GJ, Pasternak RC. Fish oil and restenosis rates. Lancet 1989;2:1036.

111. Reis GJ, Boucher TM, Sipperly ME, et al. Randomised trial of fish oil for prevention of restenosis after coronary angioplasty. Lancet 1989;2:177–81.

112. Hollman J, Konrad K, Raymond R, Whitlow P, Michalak M, van Lente F. Lipid lowering for the prevention of recurrent stenosis following coronary angioplasty (abstr). Circulation 1989;80:65.

113. Sahni R, Maniet AR, Voci G, Banka VS. Prevention of restenosis by lova-statin after successful coronary angioplasty. Am Heart J 1991;121:1600–8.
114. Whitworth HB, Roubin GS, Hollman J, et al. Effect of nifedipine on recur-rent stenosis after percutaneous transluminal coronary angioplasty. J Am Coll Cardiol 1986;8:1271–6.
115. Knudtson M, Flintoft V, Hansen J, Duff H. Effect of short-term prostacyclin administration on restenosis after percutaneous transluminal coronary angio-plasty. J Am Coll Cardiol 1990;15:691–7.
116. Heik S, Bracht M, Benn H, Erlemeier H, Kupper W. No prevention of re-stenosis after PTCA with ketanserin. A controlled prospective randomized doubleblind study (abstr). Circulation 1992;86:I-53.

13

Saphenous Vein Bypass Graft Angioplasty

Stephen R. Ramee
Ochsner Medical Institutions, New Orleans, Louisiana

Christopher J. White
Health Care International Medical Center, Glasgow, Scotland

I. INTRODUCTION

More than 3 million coronary bypass procedures have been performed since the inception of the procedure in 1968. While coronary bypass surgery is an important advance in the treatment of atherosclerotic coronary artery disease, it does not offer a "cure," but rather a palliative form of therapy for atherosclerotic coronary artery disease (1–3). The durability of these bypass conduits is highly variable. Although the longest patency is associated with internal mammary artery grafts (4), segments of saphenous vein which, unfortunately, have proven to be not as durable, continue to be used in patients requiring multiple grafts.

Percutaneous treatment of stenotic coronary artery saphenous vein grafts poses unique and challenging problems to the interventionalist. Salvage therapy of occluded or thrombosed grafts is discussed in a prior chapter and will not be repeated. Rather, this chapter will discuss strategies aimed at the percutaneous revascularization of diseased or stenotic vein grafts.

A. Pathology of Saphenous Vein Grafts

The age of a bypass graft, the time from surgical placement to the subsequent intervention, appears to correlate with the pathophysiology of graft failure. In general, early closure of a graft (within 1 month) is usually associated with a technical error at either the proximal or distal anastomosis or with poor distal flow in the native artery (5). Saphenous vein grafts, however, placed into the coronary circulation undergo a process, over time, of "arterialization," manifested by diffuse fibrointimal thickening that may result in focal or discrete stenoses (6). Histological studies of saphenous vein bypass graft stenoses demonstrate the progression from fibrointimal proliferation in early graft lesions (<1 year old) to typical atherosclerotic plaque (in grafts >3 years old) that is rich in cholesterol crystals, necrotic debris, blood elements, and foam cells (5,7,8). These plaques are generally soft and bulky, not densely fibrotic or calcified, and may be more likely to fragment and embolize during angioplasty (5).

B. Natural History of Vein Grafts

Angiographic follow-up studies of saphenous vein coronary bypass grafts have demonstrated that 11–25% of grafts will fail within the first year after surgery (9). Graft closure occurs at about 2% per year over the first 6 years and then increases to 4% per year over the next 5 years. Approximately 50% of saphenous vein grafts will be occluded at 11 years after bypass surgery, and the majority of the remaining patent grafts will show some evidence of narrowing (10,11).

As the vein grafts become dysfunctional or fail, patients are again at risk for coronary ischemic events. The risks of performing a second or third coronary bypass must then be weighed against the risks of choosing medical therapy or angioplasty. Repeat coronary bypass has been estimated to carry approximately twice the mortality risk as the initial surgery and, statistically, is not as effective in relieving symptoms as the original procedure (12–14).

II. BALLOON ANGIOPLASTY

A. Indications and Contraindications

The decision to perform balloon angioplasty on a patient with a failing bypass graft is a complex one. Generally, the decision to proceed with a revascularization procedure in a patient with prior bypass surgery is reserved for those with documented coronary ischemia and symptoms refractory to medical therapy. Should a complication occur during angioplasty, emergency bypass surgery poses more risks than an elective operation (15,16). There is a possibility that reoperation through a median sternotomy will compromise or damage existing patent bypass grafts seriously, compromising an already ischemic heart. This is particularly important when one considers how vulnerable the functioning internal mammary graft, which may otherwise be expected to remain patent indefinitely, is to injury during second and third bypass operations.

Other factors to consider when considering angioplasty include the age of the bypass graft, the location of lesion within the graft, and the angiographic appearance of the graft. Some patients, such as those without suitable veins, the elderly, those with severe lung disease, those with severely depressed left ventricular function, or patients with any other medical condition making reoperation a high risk, may be poor candidates for another surgical procedure.

There are few absolute contraindications to performing bypass graft angioplasty other than severe contrast allergy and lack of vascular access. In general, relative contraindications to the procedure are those lesion-specific variables that increase the risk of the procedure, such as diffuse long lesions, the presence of intragraft thrombus or friable plaque, heavy calcification of the lesion, totally occluded grafts, and grafts with poor distal runoff to the native circulation. The level of risk that is acceptable to the patient and operator must be determined individually, weighing the potential for benefit against the consequences of failure.

B. Acute Results and Complications

In general, the acute results of balloon angioplasty in patients with prior bypass surgery (17–26) and, specifically, the results of saphenous vein graft angioplasty have been quite good and comparable to those of native vessel angioplasty (27–29). Waters and Cote (30) pooled results of 10 prior studies of angioplasty in patients with prior bypass. Their combined results from >900 patients (1299 vessels) revealed a success rate per vessel of 90% and a total complication rate of only 6.3%. Major complications included death in 1.0%, myocardial infarction in 4.5%, and the need for emergency coronary bypass surgery in 2.2%.

Although these acute results and complication rates are excellent (Table 1), they probably reflect a selection bias in which higher risk lesion morphologies have been excluded from treatment. These high-risk lesion morphologies have been described as (1) the location of a lesion within the body of the graft; (2) diffuse lesions; and (3) intravascular filling defects consistent with intravascular thrombus (28,31,32).

The angiographic appearance of "friable" or "shaggy" lesions in saphenous vein coronary bypass grafts has been suggested to be a relative contraindication to balloon angioplasty due to the increased risk of distal embolization of atherosclerotic material (28,32). There are reports in the literature that angioplasty of older saphenous vein bypass grafts may be associated with an increased risk of distal embolization (5,31–33). Other investigators, however, have not confirmed the association of acute angioplasty complications with any specific angiographic lesion morphology in bypass grafts or that of older vein grafts with an increased risk of procedural complications (18,25,34–36).

Table 1 Acute Results and Complications of Vein Graft Angioplasty

Author (Ref.)	Year	Patients (n)	Success (%)	QMI (%)	CABG (%)	Death (%)
Plokker (27)	1991	454	90.0	2.8	1.3	0.7
Cote (28)	1987	82	85.0	3.6	1.2	0
Webb (29)	1990	158	85.0	4.0	1.0	0
Reeves (31)	1991	57	95.3	3.5	1.8	1.8
Morrison (26)	1994	75	93.0	3.0	1.0	3.0
Platko (33)	1989	98	91.8	1.0	1.0	2.0

QMI = Q-wave myocardial infarction; CABG = emergency coronary artery bypass graft surgery.

This uncertainty regarding the risk for potential embolization of atherosclerotic material and the questionable ability of angiography to identify a high-risk group for distal embolization during bypass graft angioplasty may be related to the insensitivity of angiography for detecting "friable" lesions within the bypass graft (Fig. 1). We and others (37,38) have demonstrated that coronary angioscopy, the direct visualization of the endoluminal surface, is more sensitive than angiography for identifying complex atherosclerotic plaques and intracoronary thrombi in native coronary arteries. Angioscopy also yields information regarding subtle details of plaque morphology (e.g., presence or absence of pigmentation) as well as specific details of the surface contour of atherosclerotic plaque (i.e., smooth, ulcerated, or friable) (39).

We performed angioscopy of the "culprit" lesion in 21 patients undergoing balloon angioplasty of a saphenous vein coronary bypass graft (40). The age of the saphenous vein bypass grafts averaged 10.1 years and ranged from 5–15 years. All of the ptients had a successful angioplasty procedure reducing the "culprit" stenosis >20% with a residual diameter stenosis of <50% without a major complication. None of the patients had clinical or angiographic evidence of distal embolization following balloon angioplasty.

Angioscopy demonstrated the presence of thrombus in 15 of 21 (71%) grafts compared to only four (19%) detected by angiography ($p < 0.001$) (Fig. 2). Dissection was seen either before or after angioplasty in 14 (66%) grafts by angioscopy versus two (10%) grafts by angiography ($p < 0.01$). Friable or loosely adherent plaque was detected before angioplasty by angioscopy (Fig. 3) in 11 (52%) versus only 4 (19%) grafts by angiography ($p < 0.05$). Interestingly, the age of the bypass graft did not correlate with the presence of friable plaque.

None of our patients exhibited clinical or angiographic evidence of distal embolization associated with angioplasty of these older vein grafts, including

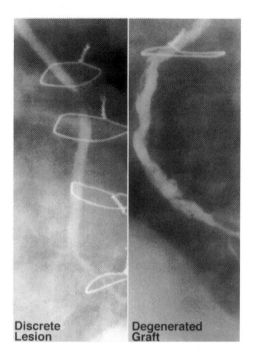

Discrete
Lesion

Degenerated
Graft

Figure 1 Left: Angiography of a discrete lesion in the midbody of a saphenous vein graft. Right: Angiography of a diffusely diseased saphenous vein graft, with irregular borders suggesting "friable" plaque.

the 11 patients with demonstrable friability of the plaque surface by angioscopy. We concluded that the incidence of intravascular thrombi, dissection, and plaque friability was underestimated by angiography in saphenous vein bypass grafts. We also demonstrated that the presence of friable plaque did not preclude an uncomplicated angioplasty procedure, and that in these older grafts ($\geq$5 years old) there was no correlation between their age and the presence of friable plaque. Whether the angioscopic appearance of plaque can predict the grafts in which atheroembolism is more likely to occur will require a larger number of patients to be studied.

C. Long-Term Results

The "Achilles heel" of vein graft angioplasty is the high restenosis rate. Meester and coworkers reported an overall acute success rate of 89% for angioplasty in 133 patients with prior bypass surgery, and an 86% success rate for dilating bypass grafts alone. However, after a mean follow-up of

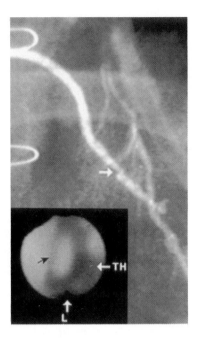

Figure 2 Angiography of an eccentric lesion in the distal portion of a saphenous vein graft. Angioscopy inset shows the lesion in the bypass graft to be associated with thrombus (not seen angiographically) and bulky yellow plaque.

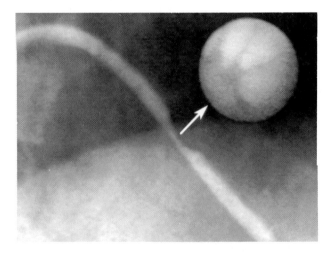

Figure 3 Angiography of a midbody graft lesion with smooth margins. Angioscopy inset shows bulky, friable, yellow plaque present before angioplasty.

2.1 years, only 48% of the patients with successfully dilated grafts were alive, free of myocardial infarction, and had not undergone repeat angioplasty or bypass surgery (41). They observed that normal left ventricular function (EF > 55%) and younger bypass grafts were associated with improved long-term results.

Reeves et al. (31) reported on the long-term clinical (100%) and angiographic (94%) follow-up (mean 32 months, range 18–68 months) of 50 patients who had had successful bypass graft angioplasty. Over that time, 23 (46%) patients remained event-free, with follow-up angiography in 20 patients demonstrating no restenosis. A cardiac event occurred in 27 (54%) patients, including two patients with sudden death and 25 patients with angiographic restenosis. They determined that three factors — lesion location, angiographic lesion morphology, and graft age — predicted restenosis.

The rate of restenosis was 36% for distal anastomosis lesions, 64% for proximal anastomosis lesions, and 63% for midbody lesions ($p < 0.05$). Shorter lesions (< 10 mm) had a restenosis rate of 38% compared to a 100% incidence of restenosis in multiple lesions, diffuse disease, or total occlusions ($p < 0.001$). It was also found that the mean age of the grafts in which restenosis occurred was 62 ± 6 months versus 49 ± 10 months for those grafts free of restenosis ($p < 0.05$).

Graft age had a significant impact on the long-term outcome in 90 patients with successful bypass graft angioplasty performed at the Cleveland Clinic (33). The event-free survival after successful angioplasty of bypass grafts > 3 years old was only 36% compared to 67% in patients with grafts 3 years old or less. However, in contrast to the findings of Reeves et al. (31), they found no association between clinical or angiographic restenosis and lesion site. However, angiographic follow-up was available in only 49 of 90 (54%) patients.

The Dutch experience with 454 patients undergoing saphenous vein graft angioplasty has been that the 5-year survival, after successful bypass graft angioplasty, was 78% compared to 58% in those whom angioplasty was unsuccessful ($p < 0.001$) (27). For all patients, the 5-year event-free survival was only 26%. In patients with successful bypass graft angioplasty, the 5-year event-free survival was 27% compared to only 3% in patients with unsuccessful angioplasty ($p < 0.0001$). When the age of the bypass graft was considered, it was clear that bypass grafts < 1 year were associated with a better 5-year event-free survival (45%) than grafts between 1 and 5 years old (25%) or those > 5 years old (19%) ($p < 0.005$).

In summary, the data on long-term benefits suggest that better results can be achieved with balloon angioplasty in grafts that have discrete lesions that are not total occlusions and in lesions located at the distal anastomosis of the bypass graft. While the majority of reports have agreed that the shorter the duration between bypass surgery and angioplasty (i.e., the younger the age of the bypass graft) the better the long-term result, two series (35,36) have not shown any correlation with bypass graft age and long-term outcome.

III. NEW DEVICES

New technologies such as atherectomy, laser angioplasty, and endovascular stenting are currently in clinical trials to determine what effect, if any, they may have on reducing the incidence of acute complications (e.g., atheroembolism and abrupt occlusion), and improving the long-term patency of saphenous vein graft angioplasty. At this time, no randomized studies have been performed to allow direct comparison with balloon angioplasty results or to compensate for any possible selection bias in patients undergoing treatment with the newer devices.

A. Atherectomy

Two atherectomy procedures, directional coronary atherectomy (DCA) and transluminal extraction catheter (TEC) plaque removal, have been reported in saphenous vein grafts. Directional atherectomy is particularly well suited to eccentric lesions in bypass grafts. The ability to position the cutting chamber window against the lesion allows the operator to "direct" the removal of the plaque against an eccentric plaque while avoiding the less involved portion of the graft. A multicenter trial of DCA in saphenous vein bypass grafts documented a success rate of 88% in 162 bypass grafts (42). Of note, 67% of the lesions selected for directional atherectomy in this trial were classified as eccentric. The overall major complication rate in this series was 1.2%, and no long-term follow-up was reported.

In a series comparing the results of DCA to those of stent placement, Pomerantz et al. (43) reported the results of DCA in 28 patients with 35 vein graft lesions. The average age of the vein grafts treated was 8.3 years. The lesion morphology of the selected lesions included 14 (40%) aorto-ostial lesions and 21 (60%) eccentric lesions. The immediate success rate was 94% (33 of 35 lesions). There were no major complications (i.e., death, Q-wave myocardial infarction, or emergency bypass surgery) associated with the DCA procedure, although one instance of distal embolization and one non-Q-wave myocardial infarction occurred. Angiographic follow-up demonstrated restenosis (>50% diameter narrowing) in 28% of the patients treated with DCA.

The TEC device excises plaque with a rotating cutting blade and then extracts the material by continuous suction. It was theorized that this device could minimize the risk of embolization of debris in saphenous vein grafts.

The results of TEC atherectomy have been reported in a series of 29 vein grafts by Popma and associates (44). They successfully treated 23 of 29 (79%) vein grafts with the TEC device; however, a majority of the patients required balloon angioplasty after the TEC procedure to optimize the final result. Of the treated lesions, 22 (76%) were classified as "degenerated" vein grafts and 18 (62%) had irregular lumen contours by angiography suggesting friable plaque. Disappointingly, five of the 22 (23%) patients classified as having "degenerated" vein graft disease had the procedure complicated by distal embolization despite the use of the extraction catheter.

B. Laser Angioplasty

Laser angioplasty, the use of a highly collimated beam of light transmitted through a fiberoptic catheter to ablate tissue, has been reported as a method of treating both native coronary and saphenous vein graft lesions (45–49). The laser has the potential to ablate and remove plaque which may offer some advantage in saphenous vein graft lesions. A persistent difficulty with all laser systems has been the relative small "neolumen," or channel, created by the relatively small laser cathether. Consequently, the majority of lesions treated require additional dilation with adjunctive balloon angioplasty to successfully complete the procedure.

One potential niche for laser angioplasty in the treatment of saphenous vein grafts is for aorto-ostial lesions. These lesions, at the proximal anastomosis of the vein graft and the aorta have traditionally been difficult to treat with balloon angioplasty and plagued by high rates of restenosis. Eigler and coworkers (50) reported the results of a multicenter registry of 206 excimer laser angioplasty procedures in 200 patients with aorto-ostial lesions. Of these lesions, 59 (28%) involved saphenous vein grafts. Procedural success was 90% in the vein graft lesions (laser and balloon). At 6 months, angiographic follow-up had been obtained in approximately 50% of the patients and the restenosis rate (> 50% diameter stenosis) was found in 35% of the vein graft lesions.

To identify predictors of acute success and long-term patency of treated arteries, Bittl and Sanborn (51) reviewed 200 consecutive excimer laser angioplasty procedures. Interestingly, they found that acceptable results were obtained in saphenous vein grafts older than 3 years old (94%), in ostial lesions (100%), and in lesions longer than 10 mm (94%). Follow-up angiography revealed that, of all lesions, only those in saphenous vein grafts were associated with decreased rates of restenosis (20%).

C. Stents

The use of endovascular stents is an attractive therapy for improving the safety and efficacy of aortocoronary bypass angioplasty. In general, vein grafts have larger lumen diameters than native coronary arteries which makes them favorable candidates for stent implantation. Also, saphenous vein grafts have no side branches, eliminating the problem of "stent jail," the isolation of a side branch when a stent is placed across its origin, that may occur when stenting native coronary arteries.

The initial experience with endovascular stent placement in stent grafts was reported in 1989 by Urban and coworkers (52). They placed a self-expanding stainless steel mesh stent (Wallstent®, Schneider, Minneapolis, MN) into 14 saphenous vein bypass grafts of 13 patients. Successful stent placement was accomplished in all 13 patients with placement of the stent in the body of the graft in 13 grafts and at the aortocoronary anastomosis in one vein graft. At a mean of 7 months, 7 patients remained clinically asymptomatic, 2 patients developed restenosis within the stent, 3 patients developed stenoses outside of the stent, and 1 patient died of progressive heart failure.

In a larger series of saphenous vein grafts stented with the Wallstent, de Scheerder and others (53) reported on the placement of 136 stents in 69 patients. After stent placement, patients were treated with antiplatelet agents and oral anticoagulation. Successful stent implantation was accomplished in all patients. The reference vessel minimal lumen diameter (MLD) was 3.3 mm and the post-stent MLD was only 2.7 mm. Complications included acute thrombotic events in 10% of the patients which resulted in death in three patients, myocardial infarction in five patients, and coronary artery bypass surgery in four patients. Bleeding complications, including 2 fatal intracranial bleeding episodes, 1 retroperitoneal hematoma, 2 cases of gastrointestinal bleeding, 18 access site hematomas that required blood transfusions, and 7 pseudoaneurysms that required surgical repair, occurred in one-third of the patients.

Angiographic follow-up at 4.9 months was obtained in 53 of 59 (90%) patients with successful stenting and no major in-hospital complications. Restenosis (>50% diameter stenosis) was found in 25 of 53 (47%) patients. Three patients were found to have occluded stents. The investigators (53) concluded that although the acute success for stent implantation was excellent, caution should be used when placing stents into a thrombotic environment (e.g., acute myocardial infarction, unstable angina with angiographic thrombi) to minimize the risk of acute thrombosis. Second, meticulous anticoagulation is necessary to avoid bleeding complications.

Experience with a stainless steel, balloon expandable slotted-tubular (Schatz-Palmaz, Johnson & Johnson Interventional Systems, Warren, NJ) coronary stent has been reported in 84 saphenous vein graft lesions of 69 patients (43). The initial success rate for stent placement was 99%. The reference vessel MLD was 3.62 mm and the post-stent MLD was 3.57 mm by quantitative angiography. There were no major in-hospital complications (e.g., death, Q-wave myocardial infarction, or emergency coronary bypass surgery) associated with stent placement, although 1 patient had distal embolization, 9 (13%) patients had non-Q-wave myocardial infarctions, and 5 (7.2%) patients had access site complications. Follow-up angiography demonstrated restenosis (>50% diameter narrowing) in only 25% of patients.

We and others (54,55) have had experience implanting larger, balloon-expandable, tubular slotted peripheral vascular stents (Fig. 4) in saphenous vein grafts. At the Ochsner Clinic, we have placed a total of 111 stents (Palmaz 104 and 154, Johnson & Johnson Interventional Systems, Warren, NJ) in 67 saphenous vein coronary grafts in 62 patients. Indications for stent placement included restenosis lesions in 12 (18%) patients, an unsatisfactory angioplasty result (dissection or residual stenosis >30%) in 29 (43%), abrupt occlusion in 1 (1%) patient, and de novo lesions in 25 (37%) patients with visually estimated graft lumen diameters of ≥3.5 mm. All of the patients were pretreated with antiplatelet agents and maintained on warfarin for 3 months after stent placement (54).

The mean number of stents placed per graft was 1.6, ranging from one to four stents in any given patient. Quantitative angiography revealed a reference MLD of 3.6 ± 0.6 mm. After stent placement, the lesion site MLD was measured to be 3.7 ± 0.5 mm. All patients had immediate angiographic success (≤30% residual stenosis) without stent embolization or abrupt occlu-

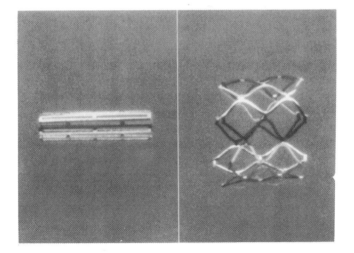

Figure 4 Left: Undeployed Palmaz® 104 stent (Johnson & Johnson Interventional Systems, Warren, NJ). Right: Expanded stent.

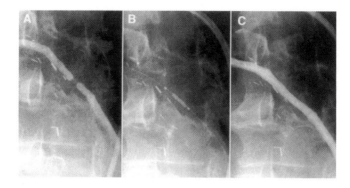

Figure 5 (A) Baseline angiography of a discrete midbody graft stenosis; (B) pre-deployment positioning of the balloon mounted Palmaz® 104 stent; (C) final angiogram following stent deployment.

sion (Figs. 5–7). Complications included death (3%), stent thrombosis (3%), myocardial infarction (6%), bleeding (10%), and access site complications (13%). Follow-up angiography was performed for recurrent ischemia or routinely at 4–6 months in 25 (40%) patients. Angiographic restenosis was present in 8 of 25 (32%). Interestingly, restenosis was associated with a smaller post-stent MLD of 3.41 mm versus 4.01 mm in those without restenosis ($p < 0.006$).

We concluded that placement of stents in these saphenous vein graft lesions had the potential to significantly improve the long-term outcome of bypass graft angioplasty. The current state-of-the-art requires intensive anti-

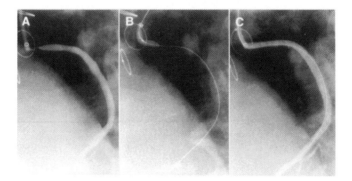

Figure 6 (A) Baseline angiogram showing tight aorto-ostial lesion; (B) balloon inflation and stent deployment; (C) final angiogram poststent deployment.

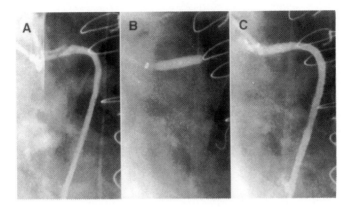

Figure 7 (A) Occlusive dissection following balloon dilation of a proximal stenosis in a vein graft; (B) stent deployment with balloon inflation; (C) final angiogram following stent placement.

coagulation of these metallic stents which requires longer hospital stays and meticulous monitoring of IV/oral anticoagulation to minimize the risk of stent thrombosis or bleeding. While it appears that the acute benefit achievable with stent placement is superior to that of balloon angioplasty alone, it remains to be proven that restenosis in saphenous vein grafts is lower with stent placement than with atherectomy or balloon angioplasty (Table 2).

Stent placement is also associated with an increased incidence of bleeding and thrombotic complications when compared to historical balloon angioplasty data (Table 3). Currently, efforts are underway to assess the results of less aggressive anticoagulation regimens. In view of the large residual lumen diameters obtained in vein grafts after stent placement, a less intensive anticoagulation scheme should suffice and contribute to a lower com-

Table 2 Results of Saphenous Vein Graft Stent Placement

Author	Stent	Patients (*n*)	Success (%)	Ref MLD (mm)	Stent MLD (mm)	Rest (%)
de Scheerder (46)	Wallstent	69	100	3.3	2.7	47
Urban (45)	Wallstent	13	100	NR	NR	38
Pomerantz (43)	JJIS (Coro)	69	99	3.6	3.6	25
White (47)	JJIS (Periph)	67	100	3.6	3.7	32

Ref = reference segment; MLD = minimal lumen diameter; Rest = restenosis; JJIS = Johnson & Johnson Interventional Systems; Coro = coronary; Periph = peripheral.

Table 3   Saphenous Vein Graft Stent Complications

Author	Stent	Patients (n)	Death (%)	Bleed (%)	MI (%)	Thrombosis (%)
de Scheerder (46)	Wallstent	69	4.3	33	6	10
Urban (45)	Wallstent	13	0	8	0	0
Pomerantz (43)	JJIS (Coro)	69	0	7	13	0
White (47)	JJIS (Periph)	67	3.2	10	6.4	3.2

Bleed = bleeding complications; MI = myocardial infarction; JJIS = Johnson & Johnson Interventional Systems; Coro = coronary; Periph = peripheral.

plication rate. Stent placement, therefore, is an attractive therapy for difficult saphenous vein graft lesions, particularly in those saphenous vein grafts of larger diameter.

IV. SUMMARY

The clinical demand for a safe, reliable, nonsurgical approach to the treatment of failed or failing saphenous vein bypass grafts is great. Although the immediate angiographic and clinical success rates in carefully selected patients are very good for balloon angioplasty, the underlying theme seems to point to the fact that some of the newer technologies may allow more patients to be considered candidates for percutaneous revascularization, and also may offer improved long-term patency. Of particular merit is the use of stents, which potentially will dramatically alter our treatment strategy. Currently, stents appear to offer improved immediate results over balloon angioplasty, although comparative trials have yet to be performed. These potential benefits must be balanced against the potential bleeding complications and risk of "subacute" stent thrombosis. As newer delivery techniques are developed it may be possible to avoid anticoagulation in these larger vessels, thereby decreasing the bleeding complications associated with the procedure.

REFERENCES

1. Seides SF, Borer JS, Kent KM, et al. Long-term anatomic fate of coronary-artery bypass grafts and functional status of patients five years after operation. N Engl J Med 1978;298:1213–1217.
2. Campeau L, Lesperance J, Hermann J, et al. Loss of the improvement of angina between 1 and 7 years after aortocoronary bypass surgery. Circulation 1979;60 (suppl I):I-1–I-15.

3. Lawrie GM, Morris GC, Calhoon JH, et al. Clinical results of coronary bypass in 500 patients at least 10 years after operation. Circulation 1982;66(suppl I): I-1-I-5.

4. Cameron A, Green GE, Kemp HG. Role of internal mammary artery in reoperations for coronary artery disease. Adv Cardiol 1988;36:84-89.

5. Saber RS, Edwards WD, Holmes DR, et al. Balloon angioplasty of aortocoronary saphenous vein bypass grafts: A histopathologic study of six grafts from five patients, with emphasis on restenosis and embolic complications. J Am Coll Cardiol 1988;12:1501-1509.

6. Kalan JM, Roberts WC. Morphologic findings in saphenous veins used as coronary arterial bypass conduits for longer than one year. Am Heart J 1990;119: 1164-1184.

7. Waller BF, Rothbaum DA, Gorfinkel JH, Ulbright TM, Linnemeier TJ, Berger SM. Morphologic observations after percutaneous transluminal balloon angioplasty of early and late aortocoronary saphenous vein bypass grafts. J Am Coll Cardiol 1984;4:784-792.

8. Garratt KN, Edwards WD, Kaufmann UP, Vlietstra RE, Holmes DR. Differential histopathology of primary atherosclerotic and restenotic lesions in coronary arteries and saphenous vein bypass grafts: Analysis of tissue obtained from 73 patients by directional atherectomy. J Am Coll Cardiol 1991;17:442-448.

9. Chesebro J, Fuster V, Elveback L, et al. Effect of dipyridamole and aspirin on late vein-graft patency after coronary bypass operation. N Engl J Med 1984; 310:581-588.

10. Campeau L, Enjalbert M, Lesperance J, et al. Atherosclerosis and late closure of aortocoronary saphenous vein grafts: Sequential angiographic studies at 2 weeks, 1 year, 5 to 7 years, and 10 to 12 years after surgery. Circulation 1983; 68:111-117.

11. Fitzgibbon GM, Leach AJ, Kafka HK, et al. Coronary bypass graft fate: Long-term angiographic study. J Am Coll Cardiol 1991;17:1075-1080.

12. Foster ED. Reoperation for coronary artery disease. Adv Cardiol 1988;36:162-164.

13. Cameron A, Kemp HG, Green GE. Reoperation for coronary artery disease, ten years of clinical follow-up. Circulation 1988;78(suppl I):I-158-162.

14. Laird-Meeter K, Vandomburg R, Vanden Brand MJ, et al. Incidence, risk and outcome of reintervention after aortocoronary bypass surgery. Br Heart J 1987; 57:4;27-435.

15. Weintraub WS, Cohen CL, Curling PE, et al. Results of coronary surgery after failed elective coronary angioplasty in patients with prior coronary surgery. J Am Coll Cardiol 1990;16:1341-1347.

16. Celermajer DS, Bailey DP, Beetson R, et al. Emergency coronary artery bypass surgery following coronary angioplasty—favourable medium term outcome after eight years' experience. Austr N Z J Med 1991;21:211-216.

17. Dorros G, Janke LM. Complex coronary angioplasty in patients with prior coronary artery bypass surgery, in situations utilizing multiple coronary angioplasties, and in coronary occlusions. Cardiol Clin 1985;3:49-71.

18. Dorros G, Lewin RF, Mathiak LM, et al. Percutaneous transluminal coronary angioplasty in patients with two or more previous coronary artery bypass grafting operations. Am J Cardiol 1988;61:1243–1247.

19. Dorros G, Lewis RLM. Percutaneous transluminal angioplasty in patients ≥5 years after their last coronary bypass graft surgery. Clin Cardiol 1990;13:403–408.

20. Cooper I, Ineson N, Demirtas E, et al. Role of angioplasty in patients with previous coronary artery bypass surgery. Cathet Cardiovasc Diagn 1989;16:81–86.

21. Corbelli J, Franco I, Hollman J, et al. Percutaneous transluminal coronary angioplasty after previous coronary artery bypass surgery. Am J Cardiol 1985; 56:398–403.

22. Morrison DA. Coronary angioplasty for medically refractory unstable angina in patients with prior coronary bypass surgery. Cathet Cardiovasc Diagn 1990; 20:174–181.

23. Tabbalat RA, Haft JI. Coronary angioplasty in symptomatic patients after bypass surgery. Am Heart J 1990;120:1091–1096.

24. Unterberg C, Buchwald A, Wiegand V, et al. Coronary angioplasty in patients with previous coronary artery bypass grafting. Angiology 1992;43:653–660.

25. Jost S, Gulba D, Daniel WG, et al. Percutaneous transluminal angioplasty of aortocoronary venous bypass grafts and effect of the caliber of the grafted coronary artery on graft stenosis. Am J Cardiol 1991;68:27–30.

26. Morrison DA, Crowley ST, Veerakul G, et al. Percutaneous transluminal angioplasty of saphenous vein grafts for medically refractory unstable angina. J Am Coll Cardiol 1994;23:1066–1070.

27. Plokker HWT, Meester BH, Serruys PW. The Dutch experience in percutaneous transluminal angioplasty of narrowed saphenous veins used for aortocoronary arterial bypass. Am J Cardiol 1991;67:361–366.

28. Cote G, Myler RK, Stertzer SH, et al. Percutaneous transluminal angioplasty of stenotic coronary artery bypass grafts: 5 years' experience. J Am Coll Cardiol 1987;9:8–17.

29. Webb JG, Myler RK, Shaw RE, et al. Coronary angioplasty after coronary bypass surgery: initial results and late outcome in 422 patients. J Am Coll Cardiol 1990;16:812–820.

30. Waters D, Cote G. Angioplasty of bypass grafts and native arteries. Cardiol Clin 1991;21:241–256.

31. Reeves F, Bonan R, Cote G, et al. Long-term angiographic follow-up after angioplasty of venous coronary bypass grafts. Am Heart J 1991;122:620–627.

32. Block PC, Cowley MJ, Kaltenbach M, et al. Percutaneous angioplasty of bypass grafts or of bypass graft anastomotic sites. Am J Cardiol 1984;53:666–668.

33. Platko WP, Hollman J, Whitlow PL, et al. Percutaneous transluminal angioplasty of saphenous vein graft stenosis: Long-term follow-up. J Am Coll Cardiol 1989;14:1645–1650.

34. Marquis JF, Schwartz L, Brwon R, et al. Percutaneous transluminal angioplasty of coronary saphenous vein bypass grafts. Can J Surg 1985;28:335–337.

35. Reeder GS, Bresnahan JF, Holmes DR Jr, et al. Angioplasty for aortocoronary bypass graft stenosis. Mayo Clin Proc 1986;61:14–19.

36. Ernst SM, van der Felts TA, Ascoop CA, et al. Percutaneous transluminal coronary angioplasty in patients with prior coronary artery bypass grafting: Long-term results. J Thorac Cardiovasc Surg 1987;93:268–275.
37. Ramee SR, White CJ, Collins TJ, et al. Percutaneous angioscopy during percutaneous coronary angioplasty using a steerable microangioscope. J Am Coll Cardiol 1991;17:100–105.
38. Sherman CT, Litvack F, Grundfest W, et al. Coronary angioscopy in patients with unstable angina pectoris. N Engl J Med 1986;315:912–919.
39. White CJ, Ramee SR, Mesa J, et al. Percutaneous coronary angioscopy in patients with restenosis after coronary angioplasty. J Am Coll Cardiol 1991;17:46B–49B.
40. White CJ, Ramee SR, Collins TJ, et al. Percutaneous angioscopy of saphenous vein coronary bypass grafts. J Am Coll Cardiol 1993;21:1181–1185.
41. Meester B, Samson M, Suryapranata H, et al. Long-term follow-up after attempted angioplasty of saphenous vein grafts: the Thoraxcenter experience 1981–1988. Euro Heart J 1991;12:648–653.
42. Ghazzal Z, Douglas J, Holmes D, et al. Directional coronary atherectomy of saphenous vein grafts: recent multicenter experience (abstr) J Am Coll Cardiol 1991;17:219A.
43. Pomerantz RM, Kuntz RE, Carrozza JP, et al. Acute and long-term outcome of narrowed saphenous venous grafts treated by endoluminal stenting and directional atherectomy. Am J Cardiol 1992;70:161–167.
44. Popma JJ, Leon MB, Mintz GS, et al. Results of coronary angioplasty using the transluminal extraction catheter. Am J Cardiol 1992;70:1526–1532.
45. Bittl JA, Sanborn TA, Tcheng JE, et al. Clinical success, complications and restenosis rates with excimerlaser coronary angioplasty. The Percutaneous Excimer Laser Coronary Angioplasty Registry. Am J Cardiol 1992;70:1533–1539.
46. Geschwind HJ, Nakamura F, Kvasnicka J, et al. Excimer and holmium yttrium aluminum garnet laser coronary. Am Heart J 1993;125:510–522.
47. Litvack F, Eigler N, Margolis J, et al. Percutaneous excimer laser coronary angioplasty: results in the first consecutive 3,000 patients. The ELCA Investigators. J Am Coll Cardiol 1994;23:323–329.
48. Litvack F, Grundfest WS, Goldenberg T, et al. Percutaneous excimer laser angioplasty of aortocoronary saphenous vein grafts. J Am Coll Cardiol 1989;14:803–808.
49. Heuser RR, Mehta SS. Holmium laser angioplasty after failed coronary balloon dilation: use of a new solid-state, infrared laser system. Cathet Cardiovasc Diagn 1991;23:187–189.
50. Eigler NL, Weinstock B, Douglas JS Jr, et al. Excimer laser coronary angioplasty of aorto-ostial stenoses. Results of the excimer laser coronary angioplasty (ELCA) registry in the first 200 patients. Circulation 1993;88:2049–2057.
51. Bittl JA, Sanborn TA. Excimer laser-facilitated coronary angioplasty. Relative risk analysis of acute and follow-up results in 200 patients. Circulation 1992;86:71–80.
52. Urban P, Sigwart U, Golf S, et al. Intravascular stenting for stenosis of aortocoronary venous bypass grafts. J Am Coll Cardiol 1989;13:1085–1091.

53. de Scheerder IK, Strauss BH, de Feyter PJ, et al. Stenting of venous bypass grafts: a new treatment modality for patients who are poor candidates for re-intervention. Am Heart J 1992;123:1046–1054.

54. White CJ, Ramee SR, Collins TJ, et al. Placement of "biliary" stents in saphenous vein coronary bypass grafts. Cathet Cardiovasc Diagn 1993;30:91–95.

55. Friedrich SP, Davis SF, Kuntz RE, et al. Investigational use of the Palmaz-Schatz biliary stent in large saphenous vein grafts. Am J Cardiol 1993;71:439–441.

14

Salvaging Failed Coronary Angioplasty

John R. Laird and Dale C. Wortham
Walter Reed Army Medical Center, Washington, DC

I. INTRODUCTION

Acute coronary artery closure following percutaneous transluminal coronary angioplasty (PTCA) is the most common reason for failed angioplasty and remains the major cause of death, myocardial infarction (MI), and emergency coronary artery bypass surgery (CABG) complicating this procedure. Despite significant improvements in angioplasty equipment, technique, and operator experience, acute closure continues to occur with a frequency of 3.6–8.3% (1–7). This complication is associated with a mortality of 2–8% and a need for emergency bypass surgery in 20–55% of cases (Table 1). Approximately 50–80% of all acute closures occur while in the cardiac catheterization laboratory (2,6). The remainder are likely to occur within 6 h of the procedure, with acute closure rarely occurring after 24 h.

Acute closure can best be defined as a complete or critical reduction in coronary blood flow at the dilated segment, occurring during or shortly after the angioplasty procedure. Generally this corresponds to thrombolysis in

The opinions expressed are those of the authors and are not to be construed as official or as reflecting the views of the Department of the Army or the Department of Defense.

317

Table 1 Incidence and Complications of Acute Closure After Percutaneous Transluminal Coronary Angioplasty

Author (Ref.)	Patients	Acute closure (%)	MI (%)	Death (%)	CABG (%)
Detre (1)	1801	6.8	40	5.0	35
deFeyter (2)	1423	7.3	36	6.0	30
Lincoff (3)	1319	8.3	20	8.0	20
Ellis (4)	4772	4.4	54	1.9	55
Sinclair (5)	1160	4.7	35	1.9	33
Ellis (6)	8207	3.6	NR	4.4	NR

NR = not reported in the study; MI = myocardial infarction; CABG = emergency coronary bypass grafting.

myocardial infarction (TIMI) grade 2 or less flow following the initial establishment of TIMI grade 3 flow. The clinical and angiographic predictors of
an increased risk for acute closure have been well described (2,4). Acute
closure is often heralded by the sudden onset of chest discomfort with associated clinical and electrocardiographic evidence of ischemia. The severity
of presentation depends on the extent of myocardium supplied by the PTCA
vessel, the degree of collateral circulation, concomitant disease in other vessels, and baseline ventricular function. The exact mechanism of acute closure may vary from case to case, but the primary cause appears to be occlusive dissection at the site of dilation with or without associated thrombus.
Other factors that may play a role include: elastic recoil, coronary vasospasm, and subintimal hemorrhage. In some cases, platelet aggregation and
thrombus formation may be the major mechanism (Fig. 1).

An important aspect of the management of acute closure is prevention.
Calcium channel blockers and intracoronary nitroglycerin may help prevent coronary vasospasm during the procedure. Preprocedural antiplatelet
therapy with aspirin and possibly dipyridamole is essential. Aspirin has been
shown to reduce the incidence of acute coronary occlusion by 50–75% (8).
In the aspirin-allergic patient, the use of ticlodipine or dextran can be considered. Heparin should be administered during the procedure in a dose sufficient to prolong the activated clotting time (ACT) to >300 s. Previous work
has demonstrated that the standard bolus of 10,000 U will not accomplish
this in up to 15% of cases (9). Additional heparin is given during the procedure as needed to maintain the ACT at >300 s. For patients who present
with an acute ischemic syndrome or who have a suboptimal PTCA result
due to dissection or thrombus, an additional 48–72 h of heparin may be
indicated. The avoidance of hypotension in the postprocedural period is

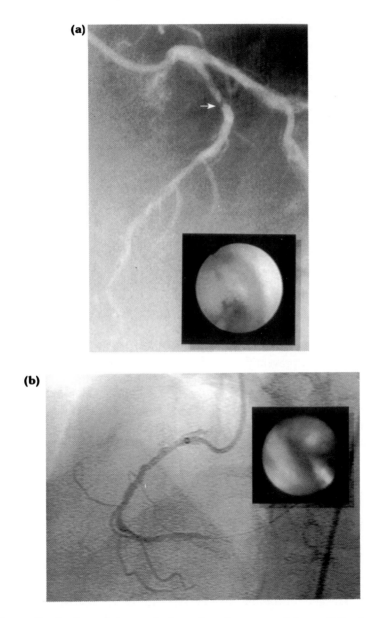

Figure 1 Angioscopic images in the setting of acute vessel closure following PTCA. (a) Intimal dissection is present and appears to be the primary mechanism of acute closure. (b) Acute occlusion of the proximal RCA. Red thrombus is present and is responsible for occlusion of the vessel. (Courtesy of Christopher J. White.) RCA = Right coronary artery.

important. Adequate hydration to counteract the effect of decreased oral intake by the patient and the diuretic effect of the contrast agent is helpful in this regard. It has been suggested that the incidence of out of lab closure may be decreased by observing the patient in the catheterization laboratory for 10–15 min following the final dilation to document any loss of the initial improvement following angioplasty. Repeat PTCA can then be performed as needed (5,10).

The conventional treatment of acute closure has included intracoronary nitrates, additional heparin, thrombolytic therapy, and redilatation of the occluded vessel with prolonged balloon inflation. The success of redilatation is dictated by the ability to recross the area of total occlusion with a guidewire. In general, redilatation with a standard balloon can be expected to be successful in approximately 40% of cases (2,3,5,7). If acute closure is refractory to pharmacological therapy and attempts at redilatation, and the area of myocardium at risk is significant, an autoperfusion catheter is placed and the patient is sent for emergency coronary artery bypass surgery. Intraaortic balloon counterpulsation is commonly employed to help stabilize the patient during transport to the operating room. Even with prompt surgical revascularization, the risk of periprocedural myocardial infarction is as high as 50% (11–15).

Given the nature of the problem, many new devices have been investigated with a goal of preventing or successfully treating acute vessel closure. Important advances include: the perfusion balloon catheter, laser balloon angioplasty, stents, and atherectomy catheters. This chapter will focus on management strategies for acute closure in the new device era, including techniques for use of these new devices and the use of adjunctive pharmacological therapy. A perspective will be provided on the potential for success with these new devices relative to surgery.

II. PROLONGED BALLOON INFLATIONS

Prolonged balloon inflations are the mainstay of the routine management of acute vessel closure. The reason for the angiographic improvement obtained after prolonged balloon inflation has not been extensively studied. Prolonged application of pressure to the injured vessel wall may contribute to the reattachment of intimal tears and may reduce immediate elastic recoil. Any associated thrombus may also be compacted with an overall improvement in vessel flow. With standard balloon catheters the ability to perform prolonged inflations is limited by the patient's tolerance to chest pain and the onset of significant myocardial ischemia with hemodynamic or electrical instability. Techniques to limit distal ischemia during balloon inflation have been proposed, such as the concomitant infusion of oxygenated blood or blood substitutes like the perfluorocarbons (16). These methods have several drawbacks and have not gained widespread acceptance.

The design and development of the autoperfusion or passive perfusion balloon catheter has been a major advance in the treatment of abrupt closure (17). Erbel et al. (18) reported the first human use of a passive perfusion catheter. In 8 of the 11 patients, the average time to the onset of ischemia was delayed. With a different catheter design, Turi et al. (19) documented passive antegrade perfusion of blood and a reduction in myocardial ischemia in dogs. The first commercially available and widely used perfusion balloon catheter is the Stack Perfusion Catheter™ (Advanced Cardiovascular Systems, Temecula, CA). Its use and the results will be described.

A. Perfusion Balloon Catheter Technique

The Stack Perfusion Catheter™ is a 4.5-French double lumen, over-the-wire catheter, with 14 side holes arranged in a linear pattern over the distal 10 cm of the catheter. Four of these side holes are located distal to the 2-cm-long balloon segment which allows for the passive transfer of blood from the proximal holes distal to the balloon. Newer generations of this catheter were designed in an attempt to decrease the shaft size and improve the overall trackability and flexibility of the device. The Stack 40-S™ catheter is a 3.9-French over-the-wire catheter. The RX Perfusion™ and Flowtrack™ catheters are monorail versions of this device with a smaller, more flexible shaft. They allow for more rapid exchange of the perfusion catheter and facilitate single operator use.

It is essential in acute vessel closure that coronary guidewire position be maintained distal to the site of obstruction. The perfusion catheter can then be advanced over a 0.014-in. to 0.018-in. extended or exchange coronary wire and positioned across the site of obstruction (Fig. 2). Following balloon inflation, the wire can then be withdrawn proximal to the side holes to allow for maximum distal coronary perfusion. In addition, careful withdrawal of the guiding catheter out of the coronary ostium may enhance proximal coronary artery inflow. Table 2 shows in vitro flow rate specifications provided by the manufacturer for the different catheter types, wire sizes, and wire positions. Adequacy of distal myocardial perfusion during balloon inflation can be determined by hand injections of contrast through the guiding catheter. Balloon inflation pressures up to 8 atm generally do not result in reduced distal flow by central lumen compression. The number of inflations and the duration of the balloon inflations have varied from study to study. Typical balloon inflation times to treat abrupt closure have been from 3–30 min with the duration determined by protocol, operator discretion, or the adequacy of distal perfusion. As with standard balloon angioplasty,

(a)

(b)

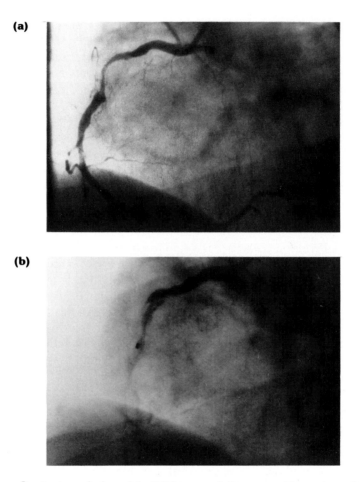

Figure 2 Acute occlusion of the RCA successfully managed by prolonged balloon inflations with a perfusion balloon catheter. (a) Baseline angiogram of the RCA. (b) Acute occlusion with extensive dissection at the site of dilation. (c) Perfusion balloon catheter inflated at the site of occlusion. (d) Successful restoration of patency of the RCA with an acceptable angiographic result. (Courtesy of Andrew J. Carter.) RCA = Right coronary artery.

balloon inflation times may be limited by chest pain, severe hemodynamic or electrocardiographic evidence of ischemia, or significant arrhythmias. During prolonged balloon inflations, some operators have administered additional heparin or thrombolytics through the central lumen of the catheter. Patients with abrupt closure who are successfully treated by perfusion

(c)

(d)

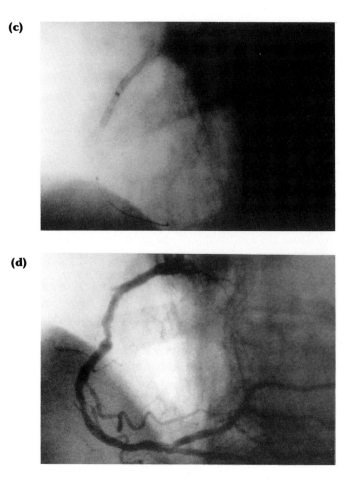

Table 2 Perfusion Catheter Flow Rates

	Flow rates (cc/min)[a]				
	ACS RX flowtrack	ACS RX perfusion	Stack perfusion long	Stack perfusion	Stack 40S
No wire	40	60	55	60	40
0.010″	25	45	40	45	25
0.014″	20	40	35	40	20
0.018″	15	30	25	30	15

[a]Determined with 38% glycerol at room temperature using a pressure of 80 mm Hg.

balloon angioplasty are then carefully monitored for recurrent ischemia and are often maintained on a continuous infusion of heparin for 24–48 h.

B. Perfusion Balloon Catheter Results

Published data support that, in selected cases, use of prolonged inflations with a perfusion balloon catheter will result in improved success rates for the treatment of acute vessel closure refractory to conventional balloon angioplasty (20–22). Saenz et al. (20) reported a successful outcome in 21 of 22 patients with acute closure treated with the perfusion balloon catheter. Twenty of these patients had failed conventional balloon inflations. Leitschuh et al. (21) reported on 36 patients with major dissections that were managed with the perfusion balloon catheter. These patients were compared to 46 consecutive patients with similar dissections treated in a conventional manner immediately before the availability of the perfusion balloon catheter. Use of the perfusion balloon catheter permitted longer inflation times (average 18 min) and a higher angiographic success rate (84% versus 64% for conventional therapy). In a similar study, Van Lierde et al. (22) reported on 37 of 1003 consecutive patients undergoing angioplasty who developed acute vessel closure that could not be redilated by conventional balloon angioplasty. Thirteen (35%) of these patients were sent for immediate emergency bypass surgery. The remaining 24 of the 37 patients were treated by prolonged perfusion balloon inflation (average 28.8 min) with success in 16 patients (67%). The benefit of prolonged balloon inflations greater than 20 min was reported by Jackman et al. (23). Prolonged inflations of 30 ± 9 min (mean ± standard deviation) in 40 patients who had failed extensive PTCA attempts resulted in procedural success in 32 (80%). The authors concluded that in some patients inflations greater than 20 min may be desirable before resorting to emergency CABG or stenting. The use of perfusion balloon catheters for inflations of extremely long duration has been reported. Case reports of inflations from 5–15 h combined with intracoronary thrombolysis have demonstrated the ability of the perfusion balloon to successfully act as a temporary "splint" (24,25).

Although the perfusion balloon catheter is an effective adjunct to the management of abrupt closure, it cannot be universally used. Perfusion catheters, particularly earlier models, are large diameter catheters with a higher deflated balloon crossing profile than standard balloon angioplasty catheters. This can make placement difficult or impractical in small or tortuous vessels, or in arteries with large occlusive dissection flaps. Guidewire access distal to the occlusion must be achieved. This cannot always be accomplished, particularly with guidewire-induced dissection or delayed out of catheterization laboratory acute closure. Since the perfusion system is passive there must be adequate mean central aortic pressure and proximal coronary blood flow. Prolonged balloon inflation across major side branches can result in important myocardial ischemia and chest pain. Conflicting results have been reported on the rate of restenosis following successful perfusion balloon angioplasty for acute closure (26–28). Finally, no randomized concurrent studies have been performed to better define the role of the perfusion balloon catheter and other new devices for the optimal management of acute closure. Despite these limitations, the perfusion balloon catheter is a major, important advance in the management of acute vessel closure complicating PTCA.

III. INTRACORONARY STENTS

The theoretical advantages of stents in the management of acute or threatened closure include the ability to scaffold the arterial wall and improve the caliber of the true lumen after dissection, limit elastic recoil or local vasospasm, and optimize blood flow (Fig. 3). Potential adverse effects include subacute stent thrombosis, bleeding complications, femoral arterial complications, late restenosis, and procedural delays due to difficulties in stent placement. Several different types of stents have been used in the management

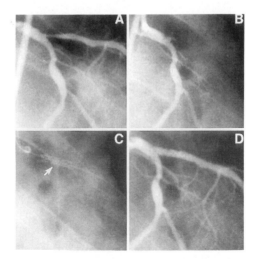

Figure 3 Acute occlusion of the proximal LAD successfully treated with a Wiktor™ coronary stent. (A) Baseline angiogram demonstrating severe proximal LAD stenosis; (B) acute occlusion of the LAD; (C) following stent deployment (white arrow), the tantalum is readily visualized fluoroscopically; (D) follow-up angiogram demonstrating a widely patent vessel. (Courtesy of Christopher J. White.) LAD = Left anterior descending coronary artery.

of acute or threatened closure (29–37). This section will focus on the use of the Gianturco-Roubin Flex-Stent™ (Cook, Inc., Bloomington, IN). The Gianturco-Roubin Flex-Stent was marketed specifically for the management of acute closure (Fig. 4).

A. Gianturco-Roubin Stent Technique

An important aspect of the care of the patient who is receiving a stent is the preprocedural and procedural medical regimen. Preprocedure medications should include soluble aspirin, dipyridamole, and a calcium channel blocker. During the procedure, the patient should receive heparin to maintain the ACT > 300 s, and intracoronary nitroglycerin. Upon determination that a stent is to be placed, the patient should be immediately started on an infusion of dextran 40, 10% solution. A 100- to 200-ml intravenous bolus can be given, followed by a continuous infusion at 50–75 ml/h.

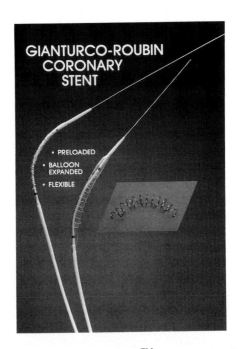

Figure 4 The Gianturco-Roubin Flex-Stent™. The stent consists of a single 0.15-mm filament of surgical stainless steel wrapped in a cylindrical shape with bends adopting an inverted "U" every 360°. The stent is 20 mm in length. (Courtesy of Cook, Inc., Bloomington, IN.)

Important technical considerations include the choice of guidewire and guiding catheter. To increase the chances of successful delivery of the stent, an 0.018-in. guidewire is preferable. This will allow for improved tracking and catheter support during passage through tortuous coronary vessels. An 8-French large lumen guiding catheter is adequate for stent sizes up to 3.5 mm. If a 4.0-mm stent is needed, a 9-French large lumen guiding catheter may be required. This can be problematic if the case was started with an 8-French sheath and guiding catheter, and acute closure occurs. Proper planning and anticipation is required in high-risk cases. If necessary, techniques have been described for exchange of the guiding catheter over a coronary guidewire (38).

In general, the stent size should be chosen to match the diameter of the vessel. When uncertain, slight undersizing is preferable to oversizing. The Gianturco-Roubin stent is mounted on a balloon with an inflation diameter 0.5 mm larger than the final expanded stent diameter; therefore oversizing can lead to dissection of the distal vessel. The importance of proper stent positioning cannot be overemphasized. High-resolution fluoroscopy is necessary to visualize the stent coils and to ensure that the stent was not damaged during positioning. Optimal placement requires that the proximal end of the stent be deployed a few millimeters proximal to the beginning of the arterial segment needing stenting. In the setting of a long dissection, it is essential to identify the distal end of the dissection prior to stent placement. If the end of the dissection and distal run-off cannot be clearly identified, use of a stent should be avoided. If more than one stent is required to cover the area of dissection, the more distal area should be stented first. Passage of another balloon and stent through a previously deployed stent may damage or dislodge either stent.

Following stent deployment, the patient should be observed in the catheterization laboratory for up to 30 min with repeat angiography prior to termination of the procedure. If the initial angiographic result is suboptimal, the stent may be further expanded using a low-profile, noncompliant balloon catheter. If thrombus is visualized within the stent or the region of the stented segment, a prolonged intracoronary infusion of thrombolytic therapy is strongly recommended. The presence of angiographically visible thrombus has been associated with an increased risk of subacute stent thrombosis (34).

After the procedure, the heparin should be discontinued or decreased until the ACT has decreased to $\leqslant 150$ s. The sheath is removed and pressure maintained on the groin for 1 h. Compression devices such as the C-clamp or Femostop (RADI Medical Systems, Uppsala, Sweden) are helpful when prolonged compression is required. The heparin infusion is then restarted with a goal of maintaining the partial thromboplastin time (PTT) at 50–80 s. The Dextran 40 infusion should be continued until the PTT is in the therapeutic range. The patient is started on coumadin and when the prothrombin time (PT) rises to greater than 17 s the heparin infusion can be discontinued. Strict bedrest for 48 h following the procedure is mandatory to reduce the risk of groin complications. The patient is discharged from the hospital on coumadin, soluble aspirin, and dipyridamole. The coumadin and dipyridamole can be discontinued after 2 months if the patient has remained stable.

B. Results of Stenting

There have been several published reports of intracoronary stenting for the management of acute or threatened closure following PTCA (29–37). No randomized comparisons between intracoronary stenting and the conventional therapy of acute closure with prolonged balloon inflations and emergency bypass surgery have been reported. Comparisons between the published results of intracoronary stenting with the results of conventional therapy are difficult given the inclusion of a high percentage of patients with "threatened closure" in the stent population. In addition, the stent literature includes work with three different stents and differing anticoagulant regimens.

The technical success rate for stenting in the setting of acute or threatened closure is 94–100% with a clinical success rate of 87–93% (29–37). The reported incidence of MI varies from 0–32%, with emergency CABG and death occurring in 0–6.7% and 0–6.7% of patients, respectively. Angiographic restenosis in those patients who have undergone restudy has occurred in 28.6–54.0% of cases (29–37). The largest and most comprehensive study to date is the multicenter investigation of the Gianturco-Roubin stent for the treatment of acute or threatened closure after PTCA (37). This study included 518 patients, of whom 494 underwent successful implantation of one or more stents. Thirty-two percent of patients received stents for acute closure and 68% for threatened closure. In-hospital MI occurred in 5.5% of cases and emergency CABG and death occurred in 4.3 and 2.2%, respectively. Subacute stent thrombosis subsequently developed in 8.7% of cases. The incidence of subacute thrombosis decreased over the course of the study, with a thrombosis rate of 5% for the last 202 patients. Of the patients who developed subacute thrombosis, 40% had angiographically evident thrombus in the vessel.before stenting. Follow-up angiography was performed on 336 of 384 eligible patients (87.5%) with a finding of restenosis in 39% of cases.

If one analyzes only those patients who received stents for acute closure ($n = 156$), the incidence of MI was 7.6%, and the incidence of emergency CABG and death was 7.7% and 2.6%, respectively. These numbers compare very favorably with the reported incidence of MI, emergency CABG, and death following acute closure treated with standard balloon angioplasty and prolonged balloon inflations. The only study that has attempted to compare the results of intracoronary stenting with conventional therapy for acute or threatened closure was a matched case-control study reported by Lincoff et al. (35). In this study, 61 patients treated with intracoronary stents for acute or threatened closure were compared with 61 patients treated with conventional therapy prior to the availability of stents. When compared to conventional treatment, stenting was associated with less residual stenosis, better flow in the treated vessel, and a reduced need for emergency CABG. However, there was no difference in the incidence of Q-wave MI or death. The incidence of Q-wave MI in the stent group was much higher in this study than the multicenter study (32% versus 7.6%). This is most likely a reflection of increased time from the onset of acute closure to stent implantation. The incidence of procedure-related Q-wave infarction in patients who underwent stenting within 45 min of closure was very low (3.9%). The authors point out that the results of stenting for acute closure may be improved by the prompt triage of patients to stent placement without prolonged attempts using conventional balloon therapy.

Subacute stent thrombosis remains the main limitation of stenting for the treatment of acute closure. The two major risk factors appear to be the presence of angiographically visible thrombus in the stented segment before or after stenting, and the presence of residual dissection post-stent implantation. The use of small stents may also be associated with an increased risk of subacute thrombosis (37).

In summary, the use of intracoronary stents for the treatment of acute closure is associated with a high initial technical success rate. Strict adherence to the aggressive anticoagulant regimen is crucial for the success of this technique. Subacute stent thrombosis continues to be a limitation of this technique; however, the incidence appears to be declining with greater experience. Every attempt should be made to completely cover and treat dissection when present. Angiographic thrombus should be aggressively treated with prolonged infusions of thrombolytic therapy. When compared to previous results with conventional techniques for acute closure, stenting appears to have a favorable impact on the incidence of MI and the need for emergency bypass surgery. Further studies are needed to define when patients should be triaged to stent placement rather than continuing attempts with conventional techniques including prolonged balloon inflation.

IV. DIRECTIONAL CORONARY ATHERECTOMY

Directional coronary atherectomy (DCA) with the Simpson Atherocath™ has become an accepted therapy for obstructive coronary artery disease. The technique and equipment required for this procedure have been described elsewhere (39–43). DCA can be expected to result in success and complication rates similar to those reported with PTCA. The use of DCA

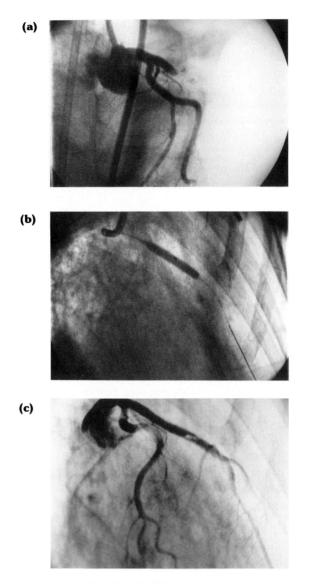

Figure 5 Acute occlusion of the LAD. (a) Baseline angiogram; (b) balloon inflated across occlusion; (c) vessel successfully reopened but with a persistent dissection flap at the site of dilation; (d) directional atherectomy catheter positioned in
vessel; (e) follow-up angiogram demonstrating marked improvement. Several small
fragments of atherosclerotic tissue were removed from the catheter nosecone.

(d)

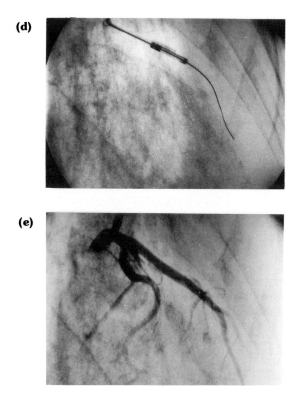

(e)

for the treatment of acute coronary artery occlusion following PTCA has been described (44–51). The theoretical advantage of DCA in this setting is the ability to resect and remove the culprit intimal dissection flap along with the associated atheroma or thrombus (Fig. 5). This can result in improved vessel flow and thereby decrease the likelihood of thrombus formation at the treatment site.

A. Directional Coronary Atherectomy Technique

When acute closure occurs, DCA is most likely to be successful in the setting of a short occlusive dissection. In general, DCA can be considered when the dissection is less than 20 mm in length, not extending beyond the length of a standard balloon. The vessel to be treated needs to be anatomically suitable for the procedure. DCA may not be an appropriate choice in the presence of severe proximal coronary angulation, tortuosity, or heavy calcification. The device should be carefully sized for the artery and low-pressure inflations performed. Device oversizing or high-pressure inflations may increase the risk of vessel perforation in the setting of significant medial dissection. An exchange-length coronary guidewire should be used so that the device can be readily removed to empty the nosecone. If too many cuts are made without emptying the nosecone, the guidewire may become bound and loss of guidewire position could occur during withdrawal of the device. An important shortcoming of DCA for acute occlusion is that it requires upsizing to a larger guiding catheter and sheath. This may also result in loss of guidewire position across the area of coronary occlusion. A technique for exchange of the guiding catheter while maintaining guidewire position in the distal vessel is described in Table 3. Such exchanges can be technically challenging, particularly in the setting of severe ischemia and hemodynamic instability.

Guiding catheters for DCA are available in sizes from 9.5–11 French. Most cases can be successfully performed using the 9.5- or 10-French guides. Newer guiding catheter curves are available from Devices for Vascular Intervention (Redwood City, CA) and Medtronic (Minneapolis, MN) (52). The newer Simpson EX Atherocath™ has a more flexible nosecone, which increases the trackability of the device and lowers the risk of nosecone trauma. These improvements in equipment have increased the chance for success when DCA is employed as a bailout technique after failed PTCA.

B. Directional Coronary Atherectomy Results

There have been several single case reports and small studies of DCA in the setting of failed or suboptimal PTCA (44–51). Several of these published

Table 3 Technique of Exchanging to DCA Guiding Catheter Without Losing Guidewire Position During Acute Vessel Closure

Step 1.	Maintain guidewire in coronary by looping guidewire in aorta.
Step 2.	Pull guide back while maintaining loop in aorta.
Step 3.	Once PTCA guide is removed, place 0.025″ guidewire beside 0.014″ guidewire in PTCA sheath and remove PTCA sheath.
Step 4.	Advance DCA sheath over 0.014″ and 0.025″ guidewires.
Step 5.	Place 125-cm 7-French multipurpose A2 catheter inside DCA guiding catheter.
Step 6.	Advance DCA guide and multipurpose catheter over 0.014″ wire to level of coronary ostium.
Step 7.	Pull out guidewire loop. Advance DCA guide over multipurpose catheter into the coronary ostium.

reports include DCA for patients with acute closure as well as DCA for ineffective dilatation or dissection after PTCA. When analyzing only those cases with acute closure, DCA was successful 75–88% of the time with a need for emergency CABG in 12–25% of cases. There were no deaths reported for bailout DCA in these small studies.

McKeever et al. (51) recently reported their experience with bail-out DCA following failed PTCA in 16 patients. They were successful in 14 of 16 cases (88%), with two patients requiring emergency CABG. Subsequent complications included two cases of acute closure requiring repeat DCA and one non-Q-wave myocardial infarction. At a mean follow-up of 9.9 months, 10 patients were symptom free. Four patients presented with recurrent angina. One patient died of progressive congestive heart failure. Hofling (50) reported on 60 patients who underwent DCA for failed PTCA or for lesions that were felt to be unsuitable for PTCA. This included 23 patients with acute closure. DCA was successful in 20 of 23 cases (87%) with three patients (13%) requiring emergency CABG. One patient was found to have asymptomatic occlusion at 24-h follow-up angiography.

A limitation of this technique is its unsuitability for tortuous or distal vessels due to the rigid, high-profile nature of the catheter. The device is cumbersome and requires considerable operator experience for its safe usage. The need for larger femoral sheaths may increase the risk of bleeding or femoral arterial complications. There is potential for guiding catheter-induced trauma or dissection during these procedures. In addition, there have been reports of coronary perforation or pseudoaneurysm formation when DCA has been used in the setting of acute closure (48,49,53). The greatest risk for coronary perforation appears to occur when treating long or spiral dissections.

In summary, DCA appears to be a very successful technique for bail-out in selected cases of acute closure following PTCA. This procedure appears to be most useful for short occlusive dissections in vessels lacking severe proximal tortuosity. Caution should be exercised when using this technique in the setting of long or extensive coronary dissections.

V. THROMBOLYSIS

The importance of thrombus and thrombus formation in the pathogenesis of evolving myocardial infarction, unstable angina, and acute vessel closure after coronary angioplasty strongly suggests a role for intracoronary thrombolytics in the management of acute closure related to coronary angioplasty (54–57). Thrombus formation may be the primary mechanism for acute closure, or may occur in the setting of extensive coronary dissection. Intracoronary thrombolytics have become part of the conventional treatment of abrupt closure after coronary angioplasty. Unfortunately, in most of the published literature, intracoronary thrombolytics have been administered at the discretion of the operator and without a uniform protocol. This makes the interpretation of published data regarding the efficacy of concomitant intracoronary thrombolysis difficult at best.

A. Thrombolysis Technique

The safety of using intracoronary streptokinase, urokinase, or recombinant tissue-type plasminogen activator (rt-PA) in the treatment of angioplasty-related acute closure has been reported (56,58,59). Streptokinase and urokinase are approved by the FDA for intracoronary administration in the treatment of acute myocardial infarction, while rt-PA is not. None of the agents have a specific labeled indication for intracoronary administration as an adjunct to coronary angioplasty. The intracoronary thrombolytic agent is typically administered slowly by hand injection over 20 min (range 5-90 min) through the angioplasty guiding catheter. Prolonged intracoronary infusions of thrombolytic therapy can be administered for several hours or longer. In particular, this has been used for occluded saphenous vein grafts or in the setting of residual coronary thrombus following stent implantation. The Tracker-18 Soft Stream Catheter™ (Target Therapeutics, Fremont, CA) is useful for this purpose. Balloon inflations with either a standard or autoperfusion balloon catheter may be performed before, during, or after thrombolytic administration, depending on the clinical scenario. In cases of closure of intermediate morphology or mixed dissection and thrombus, balloon inflations are often performed prior to thrombolytic therapy to "tack up" the dissection flap and improve antegrade coronary blood flow. Redilatation may be performed intermittently during the thrombolytic infusion to maintain coronary blood flow at TIMI grade 2 to 3. More selective or distal thrombolytic infusion may be accomplished through the balloon catheter, an infusion catheter, or through an infusion wire. The optimal method of delivery, timing of therapy, best thrombolytic agent and dosage remain unknown. Intracoronary urokinase is administered in a dosage of 100,000–500,000 U in a volume of 30–60 ml (59,60). In some cases, additional urokinase has been administered intravenously in the range of 250,000–3,000,000 U over 30 min (59). Intracoronary streptokinase is administered in a dosage of 250,000–750,000 U, although doses as large as 1,500,000 U have been used (2,61). Intracoronary rt-PA has been used for persistent thrombus following thrombolytic therapy in acute myocardial infarction (62), for reocclusion (63), for chronic coronary artery thrombi prior to coronary angioplasty (64), and for threatened or abrupt closure post-PTCA (58,65). Generally, intracoronary rt-PA is administered in doses of 20–30 mg over

5–15 min or by constant infusions of 0.2 mg/min to 0.4 mg/min for 60–90 min preceded by a 0.5- to 1.0-mg bolus.

B. Thrombolysis Results

The utility of coronary thrombolysis alone or in conjunction with repeat balloon dilation for acute closure has been investigated. Suryapranata et al. (61) reported on 200 consecutive patients with unstable angina who had attempted angioplasty. Acute closure occurred in 21 (11%) of the 196 patients in whom the culprit lesion was crossed and dilated. Redilatation was performed and intracoronary streptokinase (250,000 U) administered to 12 patients who were thought to have thrombotic occlusion. A successful outcome was achieved in 9 of these 12 patients. Similar results were published by Schieman et al. (60) where intracoronary urokinase (100,000–250,000 U) was used to treat 48 patients who developed intracoronary thrombus accumulation related to angioplasty performed in acute ischemic syndromes. The overall angiographic success rate was 90% and on follow-up angiography (obtained in 79% of patients) there was no evidence of reocclusion. This, however, is in sharp contrast to a series of 447 patients reported by Gulba et al. (58), where 27 patients (6%) had acute thrombotic occlusion following angioplasty. While still in the catheterization laboratory, intracoronary (20 mg over 5 min) and intravenous (50 mg over the next 60 min) rt-PA was combined with repeat low-pressure balloon inflations. Reopening of the vessel was achieved in 22 of 27 patients (81.5%) but follow-up angiography 24–36 h later revealed reocclusion in 12 (54.5%). Until follow-up angiography, all patients were maintained on aspirin 250 mg per day and a continuous infusion of heparin at 1250 U/h. Selection bias or the use of rt-PA might in part account for the large discrepancy in reocclusion rates seen between the Schieman and Gulba studies. Verna et al. (66) reported on 33 patients with complicated angioplasty treated with intracoronary urokinase and immediate reangioplasty. The 23 patients who received urokinase had a higher success rate than the 10 patients treated with redilatation only (65% versus 10%).

Specific complications related to the intracoronary use of thrombolytics appear to be infrequent. The systemic effects of intracoronary thrombolytics administered as described above are minimal and do not result in the clinically significant depletion of fibrinogen unless supplemented by additional intracoronary or intravenous doses. Based upon experience with angioplasty following intracoronary (67) and intravenous (68) streptokinase for acute myocardial infarction, concern has been expressed over the potential for exacerbating the thrombotic process or creating subintimal hemorrhage by combining intracoronary thrombolytics and balloon angioplasty. This remains an unresolved issue.

In summary, intracoronary thrombolytics have been used prior to and during coronary angioplasty in patients with acute myocardial infarction, stable and unstable angina, and abrupt closure complicating PTCA. In selected cases of acute coronary artery closure following coronary angioplasty, intra-coronary thrombolysis would appear to be safe and useful adjunctive therapy.

VI. OTHER MODALITIES

Previous work has demonstrated the efficacy of laser balloon angioplasty for the treatment of acute closure (69,70). Laser energy is used to heat vascular tissue, seal dissections by thermal welding, and reduce elastic recoil. A high restenosis rate was reported with this technique, however, leading to withdrawal of this device from investigation. Newer techniques for heating angioplasty balloons with microwave (71) and radiofrequency (72,73) energy are in the early phases of investigation. Radiofrequency thermal balloon angioplasty involves heating the balloon to a lower temperature (60–70°C) than laser balloon angioplasty. This technique has been shown to be effective for sealing dissections and perforations in an animal model of severe arterial wall damage (74). In an attempt to avoid some of the complications of permanent intracoronary stent implantation, temporary stents have been developed for the management of acute closure. Early results with a proto-type temporary stenting device have been reported (75).

Intra-aortic balloon counterpulsation (IABP) has been shown to be effective for reducing the incidence of reocclusion following successful PTCA or thrombolysis for acute myocardial infarction (76,77). In addition, IABP has been reported to be effective for the treatment of recurrent acute closure after coronary angioplasty (78). Recent work with coronary Doppler catheters and the Doppler flow wire has documented an increase in coronary flow during IABP, which may decrease the likelihood of coronary thrombus formation at the dilation site (79).

New pharmacological treatment strategies for acute closure are being in-vestigated actively. Platelet-rich thrombi are commonly observed in patients with occlusion. A monoclonal antibody directed against the platelet glyco-protein IIb/IIIa receptor has been developed and recently approved for use (80). This antibody binds to the glycoprotein IIb/IIIa receptor, thereby block-ing fibrinogen binding. Newer antithrombin agents such as hirudin and its derivative hirulog appear promising. These agents are potent, selective in-hibitors of clot-bound thrombin (81).

VII. SUMMARY

In the new device era, the interventionalist has a variety of options for the treatment of acute coronary closure following PTCA, each with distinct advantages and disadvantages. The challenge is to develop a rational approach for the use of these new technologies. Based on the excellent success rates reported with prolonged balloon inflations, this strategy remains the mainstay of therapy for acute closure and should continue to be the first treatment employed. The highest success rates are achieved with very prolonged inflations, sometimes in excess of 20 min. If prolonged inflations are successful, coronary stenting with its attendant complications can be avoided. Situations in which prolonged balloon inflations may not be the best option, or in which this approach should be abandoned early include: long or spiral dissections, inadequate distal perfusion during balloon inflations, or when a large side branch at the site of dilation results in significant ischemia in that vascular bed during balloon inflations. If prolonged balloon inflations are unsuccessful, and the occlusion is relatively short (<20 mm), DCA is an excellent bail-out option.

When the above measures fail, intracoronary stenting can be employed with a high success rate. Strict adherence to the anticoagulant/antiplatelet regimen and post-stent routine will lower the risk of stent complications. If there is persistent dissection or thrombus following stent implantation, the risk of subacute thrombosis is higher and the use of the stent as a temporrary bridge to CABG should be considered. This is particularly true for the patient in whom sudden occlusion of the stent might result in hemodynamic collapse.

Thrombus plays an important role in acute vessel closure following coronary angioplasty. The concomitant use of intracoronary thrombolytic therapy with repeat balloon dilation is an effective treatment strategy. Newer antithrombotic and antiplatelet agents will improve our ability to treat refractory coronary thrombus. With the use of combined pharmacological and mechanical intervention, acute closure will be successfully managed in the great majority of cases without major complications or the need for emergency CABG.

REFERENCES

1. Detre KM, Holmes DR Jr, Holubkov R, et al. Incidence and consequences of periprocedural occlusion. The 1985–1986 National Heart, Lung, and Blood Institute percutaneous transluminal coronary angioplasty registry. Circulation 1990; 82:739–750.
2. de Feyter PJ, van den Brand M, Jaarman G, et al. Acute coronary artery occlusion during and after percutaneous transluminal coronary angioplasty. Frequency, prediction, clinical course, management, and follow-up. Circulation 1991;83: 927–936.
3. Lincoff AM, Popma JJ, Ellis SG, et al. Abrupt vessel closure complicating coronary angioplasty: clinical, angiographic, and therapeutic profile. J Am Coll Cardiol 1992;19:926–935.

4. Ellis SG, Roubin GS, King SB III, et al. Angiographic and clinical predictors of acute closure after native vessel coronary angioplasty. Circulation 1988;77: 372–379.

5. Sinclair IN, McCabe CH, Sipperly ME, Baim DS. Predictors, therapeutic options and long-term outcome of abrupt reclosure. Am J Cardiol 1988;61:61G–66G.

6. Ellis SG, Roubin GS, King SB III, et al. In-hospital mortality after acute closure after coronary angioplasty: analysis of risk factors from 8,207 procedures. J Am Coll Cardiol 1988;11:211–216.

7. Kuntz RE, Piana R, Pomerantz RM, et al. Changing incidence and management of abrupt closure following coronary intervention in the new device era. Cathet Cardiovasc Diagn 1992;27:183–190.

8. Barnathan ES, Schwartz S, Taylor L, et al. Aspirin and dipyridamole in the prevention of acute coronary thrombosis complication coronary angioplasty. Circulation 1987;76:125–134.

9. Ogilby JD, Kopelman HA, Klein LW, et al. Adequate heparinization during PTCA: Assessment using activated clotting time (abstr). J Am Coll Cardiol 1988;11:237A.

10. Satler LF, Leon MB, Kent KM, Pichard AD. Strategies for acute occlusion after coronary angioplasty. J Am Coll Cardiol 1992;19:936–938.

11. Reul GJ, Cooley DA, Hallman GL, et al. Coronary artery bypass surgery for unsuccessful percutaneous transluminal coronary angioplasty. J Thorac Cardiovasc Surg 1984;88:685–694.

12. Cowley MJ, Dorros G, Kelsey SH, et al. Emergency coronary bypass surgery after coronary angioplasty: The NHBLBI institute's percutaneous transluminal coronary angioplasty registry experience. Am J Cardiol 1984;53:22C–26C.

13. Killen DA, Hamaker WR, Reed WA. Coronary artery bypass following percutaneous transluminal coronary angioplasty. Ann Thorac Surg 1985;40:133–138.

14. Golding LAR, Loop FD, Hollman JL, et al. Early results of emergency surgery after coronary angioplasty. Circulation 1986;74(suppl III):26–29.

15. Talley JD, Jones EL, Weintraub WS, King S. Coronary artery bypass surgery after failed percutaneous transluminal coronary angioplasty. Circulation 1989; 79(suppl I):126–131.

16. Jaffe CC, Wohlgelernter D, Cabin H, Bowman L, Deckelbaum L, Remetz M, Cleman M. Preservation of left ventricular ejection fraction during percutaneous transluminal coronary angioplasty by distal transcatheter coronary perfusion of oxygenated Fluosol DA 20%. Am Heart J 1988;115:1156–1163.

17. Ciamppricotti R, Dekkers P, El Gamal M, van der Krieken A, Relik RH. Catheter reperfusion for failed emergency coronary angioplasty without subsequent bypass surgery. Cathet Cardiovasc Diagn 1989;18:159–164.

18. Erbel R, Clas W, Busch U, von Seelen W, Brennecke R, Blomer H, Meyer J. New balloon catheters for prolonged percutaneous transluminal coronary angioplasty and bypass flow in occluded vessels. Cathet Cardiovasc Diagn 1986; 12:116–123.

19. Turi ZG, Campbell CA, Gottimukkala MV, Kloner RA. Preservation of distal coronary perfusion during prolonged balloon inflation with an autoperfusion catheter. Circulation 1987;6:1273–1280.
20. Saenz CB, Schwartz KM, Slysh SJ, Palenca K, Curry CR. Experience with the use of the coronary autoperfusion catheter during complicated angioplasty. Cathet Cardiovasc Diagn 1990;20:276–278.
21. Leitschuh ML, Mills RM, Jacobs AK, Ruocco NA, LaRosa D, Faxon DP. Outcome after major dissection during coronary angioplasty using the perfusion balloon catheter. Am J Cardiol 1991;67:1056–1060.
22. Van Lierde JM, Glazier JJ, Stammen FJ, Vrolix MC, Sionis D, De Geest H, Piessens JH. Use of an autoperfusion catheter in the treatment of acute refractory vessel closure after coronary balloon angioplasty: immediate and six month follow up results. Br Heart J 1992;68:51–54.
23. Jackman JD Jr, Zidar JP, Tcheng JE, et al. Outcome after prolonged balloon inflations of >20 minutes for initially unsuccessful percutaneous transluminal coronary angioplasty. Am J Cardiol 1992;69:1417–1421.
24. Brenner AS, Browne KF. Five-hour balloon inflation to resolve recurrent reocclusion during coronary angioplasty. Cathet Cardiovasc Diagn 1991;22:107–111.
25. Little T. Prolonged coronary splinting in the management of acute coronary closure. Cathet Cardiovasc Diagn 1992;25:213–217.
26. Ba'albaki HA, Weintraub WS, Tao X, et al. Restenosis after acute closure and successful reopening: implications for new devices (abstr). Circulation 1990;82 (suppl III):III–134.
27. Landau C, Jacobs AK, Currier JW, Bilazarian SD, Leitschuh ML, Ryan TJ, Faxon DP. One year followup of PTCA induced dissection treated with a perfusion balloon catheter. Circulation 1991;84(suppl II):II–131.
28. Tenaglia AN, Fortin DF, Frid DJ, Gardner LH, Nelson CT, Tcheng JE, Califf RM. Restenosis and long-term outcome following successful treatment of abrupt closure during and after angioplasty. Circulation 1991;84(suppl II):II–131.
29. Sigwart U, Urban P, Golf S, et al. Emergency stenting for acute occlusion after coronary balloon angioplasty. Circulation 1988;78:1121–1127.
30. de Feyter PJ, DeScheerder I, van den Brand M, et al. Emergency stenting for refractory acute coronary artery occlusion during coronary angioplasty. Am J Cardiol 1990;66:1147–1150.
31. Haude M, Erbel R, Straub U, et al. Results of intracoronary stents for management of coronary dissection after balloon angioplasty. Am J Cardiol 1991;67: 691–696.
32. Fischman DL, Savage MP, Leon MB, et al. Effect on intracoronary stenting on intimal dissection after balloon angioplasty: Results of quantitative and qualitative coronary analysis. J Am Coll Cardiol 1991;18:1445–1451.
33. Roubin GS, Cannon AD, Agrawal SK, et al. Intracoronary stenting for acute and threatened closure complicating percutaneous transluminal coronary angioplasty. Circulation 1992;85:916–927.
34. Herrmann HC, Buchbinder M, Clemen MW, et al. Emergent use of balloonexpandable coronary artery stenting for failed percutaneous transluminal coronary angioplasty. Circulation 1992;86:812–819.

35. Lincoff AM, Topol EJ, Chapekis AT, et al. Intracoronary stenting compared with conventional therapy for abrupt vessel closure complicating coronary angioplasty: A matched case-control study. J Am Coll Cardiol 1993;21:866–875.
36. Maiello L, Colombo A, Gianrossi R, et al. Coronary stenting for treatment of acute or threatened closure following dissection after coronary balloon angioplasty. Am Heart J 1993;125:1570–1575.
37. George BS, Voorhees WD III, Roubin GS, et al. Multicenter investigation of coronary stenting to treat acute or threatened closure after percutaneous transluminal coronary angioplasty: Clinical and angiographic outcomes. J Am Coll Cardiol 1993;22:135–143.
38. Warren SG, Barnett JC. Guiding catheter exchange during coronary angioplasty. Cathet Cardiovasc Diagn 1990;3:23–26.
39. Hinohara T, Selmon MR, Robertson GC, et al. Directional atherectomy: new approaches for treatment of obstructive coronary and peripheral vascular disease. Circulation 1990;81(suppl IV):IV-79-91.
40. Hinohara T, Rowe MH, Robertson GC, et al. Effect of lesion characteristics on outcome of directional coronary atherectomy. J Am Coll Cardiol 1991;17:1112–1120.
41. Safian RD, Erny RE, Gelbfish JS, et al. Coronary atherectomy: clinical, angiographic and histological findings and observations regarding potential mechanisms. Circulation 1990;82:69–79.
42. Topol EJ, Leya F, Pinkerton CA, et al. A comparison of directional atherectomy with coronary angioplasty in patients with coronary artery disease. N Engl J Med 1993;329:221–227.
43. Adelman AG, Cohen EA, Kimball BP, et al. A comparison of directional atherectomy with balloon angioplasty for lesions of the left anterior descending coronary artery. N Engl J Med 1993;329:228–233.
44. Bell MR, Kaufman UP, Vlietstra RE, Holmes DR Jr. Combined percutaneous coronary atherectomy and coronary angioplasty in 19 consecutive patients. J Am Coll Cardiol 1990;15:1146–1150.
45. Lee TC, Hartzler GO, Rutherford BD, McConahay DR. Removal of an occlusive coronary dissection flap by using an atherectomy catheter. Cathet Cardiovasc Diagn 1990;20:185–188.
46. Smucker ML, Sarnat WS, Kil D, et al. Salvage from cardiogenic shock by atherectomy after failed emergency coronary artery angioplasty. Cathet Cardiovasc Diagn 1990;21:23–25.
47. Warner M, Chami Y, Johnson D, Cowley MJ. Directional coronary atherectomy for failed angioplasty due to occlusive coronary dissection. Cathet Cardiovasc Diagn 1991;24:28–31.
48. Vetter J, Simpson J, Robertson G, et al. Rescue directional coronary atherectomy for failed balloon angioplasty (abstr). J Am Coll Cardiol 1991;17:384A.
49. Whitlow PL, Robertson GC, Rowe MH, et al. Directional coronary atherectomy for failed percutaneous transluminal coronary angioplasty (abstr). Circulation 1990;82(suppl III):III-1.
50. Hofling B, Gonschior P, Simpson L, et al. Efficacy of directional coronary atherectomy in cases unsuitable for percutaneous transluminal angioplasty (PTCA) and after unsuccessful PTCA. Am Heart J 1992;124:341–348.

51. McKeever LS, Marek J, Kerwin PM, et al. Bail-out directional atherectomy for abrupt coronary artery occlusion following conventional angioplasty. Cathet Cardiovasc Diagn 1993;1:31–36.
52. Whitlow PL. Guiding catheters for directional coronary atherectomy. Cathet Cardiovasc Diagn 1993;1:72–75.
53. van Suylen RJ, Serruys PW, Simpson JB, et al. Delayed rupture of right coronary artery after directional atherectomy for bail-out. Am Heart J 1991;121: 914–916.
54. Mabin TA, Holmes DR, Smith HC, Vlietstra RE, Bove AA, Reeder GS, Chesebro JH, Bresnahan JF, Orszulak TA. Intracoronary thrombus: role in coronary occlusion complicating percutaneous transluminal coronary angioplasty. J Am Coll Cardiol 1985;5:198–202.
55. Arora RR, Platko WP, Bhadwar K, Simpfendorfer C. Role of intracoronary thrombus in acute complications during percutaneous transluminal coronary angioplasty. Cathet Cardiovasc Diagn 1989;16:226–229.
56. Sugrue DD, Holmes DR, Smith HC, et al. Coronary artery thrombus as a risk factor for acute vessel occlusion during percutaneous transluminal coronary angioplasty: improving results. Br Heart J 1986;56:62–66.
57. Deligonul U, Gabliani GI, Caralis DG, Kern MJ, Vandormael MG. Percutaneous transluminal coronary angioplasty in patients with intracoronary thrombus. Am J Cardiol 1988;62:474–476.
58. Gulba DC, Daniel WG, Simon R, Jost S, Barthels M, Amende I, Rafflenbeul W, Lichtlen PR. Role of thrombolysis and thrombin in patients with acute coronary occlusion during percutaneous transluminal coronary angioplasty. J Am Coll Cardiol 1990;16:563–568.
59. Pavlides GS, Schreiber TL, Gangadharan V, Puchrowicz S, O'Neill WW. Safety and efficacy of urokinase during elective coronary angioplasty. Am Heart J 1991;121:731–737.
60. Schieman G, Cohen BM, Kozina J, Erickson JS, Podolin RA, Peterson KL, Ross J, Buchbinder M. Intracoronary urokinase for intracoronary thrombus accumulation complicating percutaneous transluminal coronary angioplasty in acute ischemic syndromes. Circulation 1990;82:2052–2060.
61. Suryapranata H, de Feyter PJ, Serruys PW. Coronary angioplasty in patients with unstable angina pectoris: is there a role for thrombolysis? J Am Coll Cardiol 1988;12:69A–77A.
62. Samaha JK, Quigley P, Kereiakes DJ, et al. Intracoronary thrombolytic therapy in patients with refractory thrombus after intravenous treatment. J Am Coll Cardiol 1989;13:92A.
63. Topol EJ. Tissue-type plasminogen activator in acute MI. Cardio 1988;(April): 57–60.
64. Currier JW, Ruocco NA, Jacobs AK, et al. Does low dose intracoronary rt-PA lyse chronic thrombotic occlusions prior to PTCA? J Am Coll Cardiol 1990;15:1200.
65. Tiefenbrunn AJ. Tissue-type plasminogen activator: intracoronary applications. Cathet Cardiovasc Diagn 1990;19:108–115.
66. Verna E, Repetto S, Boscarini M, Onofri M, Qing LG, Binaghi G. Management of complicated coronary angioplasty by intracoronary urokinase and immediate re-angioplasty. Cathet Cardiovasc Diagn 1990;19:116–122.

67. Erbel R, Pop T, Henrichs KJ, et al. Percutaneous transluminal coronary angioplasty after thrombolytic therapy: a prospective controlled randomized trial. J Am Coll Cardiol 1986;8:485–495.

68. Simonton CA, Mark DB, Hinohara T, et al. Late restenosis after emergent coronary angioplasty for acute myocardial infarction: comparison with elective coronary angioplasty. J Am Coll Cardiol 1988;11:698–705.

69. Ferguson JJ, Dear WE, Leatherman LL, et al. A multicenter trial of laser balloon angioplasty for abrupt closure following PTCA (abstr). J Am Coll Cardiol 1990;15(suppl):25A.

70. Reis GJ, Pomerantz RM, Jenkins RD, et al. Laser balloon angioplasty: clinical, angiographic and histologic results. J Am Coll Cardiol 1991;18:193–202.

71. Smith DL, Walinsky P, Martinez-Hernandez A, et al. Microwave thermal balloon angioplasty in the normal rabbit. Am Heart J 1992;123:1516–1521.

72. Lee BI, Becker GJ, Waller BF, et al. Thermal compression and molding of atherosclerotic vascular tissue with use of radiofrequency energy: implications for radiofrequency balloon angioplasty. J Am Coll Cardiol 1989;13:1167–1175.

73. Deutsch E, Martin JL, Budjak R, et al. Low stress angioplasty at 60 degrees C: attenuated arterial barotrauma (abstr). Circulation 1990;82(suppl III):III-72.

74. Resar JR, Wolff ME, Hruban RH, Brinker JA. Endoluminal sealing of vascular wall disruptions with radiofrequency-heated balloon angioplasty. Cathet Cardiovasc Diagn 1993;29:161–167.

75. Heuser RR, Mehta S, Strumpf RK. ACS RX flow support catheter as a temporary stent for dissection or occlusion during balloon angioplasty: initial experience. Cathet Cardiovasc Diagn 1992;27:66–74.

76. Ishihara M, Sato H, Tateishi H, et al. Intraaortic balloon pumping as the postangioplasty strategy in acute myocardial infarction. Am Heart J 1991;122:385–389.

77. Ohman EM, Califf RM, George BS, et al. The use of intraaortic balloon pumping as an adjunct to reperfusion therapy in acute myocardial infarction. Am Heart J 1991;121:895–901.

78. Suneja R, Hodgson JM. Use of intraaortic balloon counterpulsation for treatment of recurrent acute closure after coronary angioplasty. Am Heart J 1993;125:530–532.

79. Ishihara M, Sato H, Tateishi H, et al. Effects of intraaortic balloon pumping on coronary hemodynamics after coronary angioplasty in patients with acute myocardial infarction. Am Heart J 1992;124:1133–1138.

80. Bates ER, McGillem MJ, Mickelson JK, et al. A monoclonal antibody against the platelet glycoprotein IIb/IIIa receptor complex prevents platelet aggregation and thrombosis in a canine model of coronary angioplasty. Circulation 1991;84:2463–2469.

81. Heras M, Chesebro JH, Webster MWI. Hirudin, heparin, and placebo during deep arterial injury in the pig: the in vivo role of thrombin in platelet-mediated thrombosis. Circulation 1990;82:1476–1484.

Index

About the Editors

CHRISTOPHER J. WHITE is Director of Invasive Cardiology at Health Care International Medical Center, Glasgow, Scotland. The author or coauthor of more than 175 professional publications, Dr. White is a Fellow of the European College of Cardiology, the American College of Cardiology, the American College of Angiology, the American Society of Cardiovascular Interventionists, and the American Heart Association, among others. He received the B.A. degree (1974) in biology from Oberlin College, Ohio, and the M.D. degree (1978) from Case Western Reserve University, Cleveland, Ohio.

STEPHEN R. RAMEE is Director of Interventional Cardiology, Cardiac Catheterization Laboratory, Ochsner Medical Institutions, New Orleans, Louisiana. The author or coauthor of over 130 professional publications, Dr. Ramee is a Fellow of the American Heart Association and the American College of Cardiology, and a member of the Society for Cardiac Angiography and Intervention and the American Society of Cardiovascular Interventionists. He received the B.A. degree (1974) from Vanderbilt University, Nashville, Tennessee, the M.S. degree (1976) from Georgetown University, Washington, D.C., and the M.D. degree (1980) from George Washington University, Washington, D.C.